Prognostic and Predictive Factors in Gynecologic Cancers

Prognostic and Predictive Factors in Gynecologic Cancers

Edited by

Charles F Levenback MD, Anil K Sood MD,
Karen H Lu MD, and Robert L Coleman MD

The University of Texas
MD Anderson Cancer Center
Houston, Texas
USA

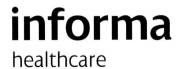

informa
healthcare

First published in 2007 by Informa Healthcare, Telephone House, 69-77 Paul Street, London EC2A 4LQ, UK.

Simultaneously published in the USA by Informa Healthcare, 52 Vanderbilt Avenue, 7th Floor, New York, NY 10017, USA.

Informa Healthcare is a trading division of Informa UK Ltd. Registered Office: 37–41 Mortimer Street, London W1T 3JH, UK. Registered in England and Wales number 1072954.

A CIP record for this book is available from the British Library.

Library of Congress Cataloging-in-Publication Data available on application

ISBN-13: 9780415391726

Orders may be sent to: Informa Healthcare, Sheepen Place, Colchester, Essex CO3 3LP, UK
Telephone: +44 (0)20 7017 5540
Email: CSDhealthcarebooks@informa.com
Website: http://informahealthcarebooks.com/

For corporate sales please contact: CorporateBooksIHC@informa.com
For foreign rights please contact: RightsIHC@informa.com
For reprint permissions please contact: PermissionsIHC@informa.com

Printed and bound by CPI Group (UK) Ltd, Croydon, CR0 4YY

Transferred to Digital Print 2012

Dedications

All my love and gratitude to my precious wife Ginny, my wonderful sons Sam and Ben, my father Bob, and my sister Liz, my in-laws Mary, Harold, Aby, Julie, Charlie and Kelly, and my many friends especially Max, Robert, Marc, Brad, Chip, Ron, Carol Ann, Joni, and Bill.

C.F.L

I dedicate this book to my wife, Kelly, and our kids, Nathan and Meghan, for their patience and support.

A.K.S

To my husband Charlie and my children Ned, David, and Kate, for thier constant love, joy and support. And to my patients, who inspire the work that I do.

K.H.L

To my folks, Gary and Marlene Beatty whose laughter, encouragement and love, inspire me. To my father Bob and stepmother Sharon Coleman for their unending love, support and humor I adore. To my wife, Fay, whose insight, continous love and daily self-sacrifice enable all that I accomplish and make my life whole. To my children, Jay, Christina, Kay, Joe, Mary, and Teresa, who bring true color, happiness and hope. And, to my assistant Liz, who so expertly "manufactured" the time and space to accomplish this project.

R.L.C

Contents

Contents

Contributors

Sarah Adams MD

Center for Research on Reproduction and
  Women's Health
University of Pennsylvania
Philadelphia, PA
USA

Ioannis Alagkiozidis MD

Center for Research on Reproduction and
  Women's Health
University of Pennsylvania
Philadelphia, PA
USA

Michael A Bidus MD

Department of Obstetrics and Gynecology
Walter Reed Army Medical Center and the
  United States Military Cancer Institute
Washington, DC
USA

Michael J Birrer MD PhD

National Cancer Institutes
Key West Research Center
Rockville, MD
USA

Robert E Bristow MD

Department of Gynecology and Obstetrics
The Johns Hopkins Medical Institutions
Baltimore, MD
USA

Russell R Broaddus MD PhD

Department of Pathology
The University of Texas
MD Anderson Cancer Center
Houston, TX
USA

Jubilee Brown MD

Department of Gynecologic Oncology
The University of Texas
MD Anderson Cancer Center
Houston, TX
USA

Mark Cadungog MD

Center for Research on Reproduction and
  Women's Health
University of Pennsylvania
Philadelphia, PA
USA

John K Chan MD

Division of Gynecologic Oncology
Department of Obstetrics and Gynecology
University of California
and
School of Medicine
San Francisco, CA
USA

Christina S Chu MD

Department of Obstetrics and Gynecology
University of Pennsylvania Medical Center
Hospital of the University of Pennsylvania,
Philadelphia, PA
USA

Robert L Coleman MD

Department of Gynecologic Oncology
The University of Texas
MD Anderson Cancer Center
Houston, TX
USA

José Ramon Conejo-Garcia MD

Department of Microbiology and
  Immunology and of Medicine
Dartmouth Medical School
Lebanon, NH
USA

George Coukos MD PhD

Abramson Cancer Research Institute
University of Pennsylvania
Philadelphia, PA
USA

Tyler Curiel MD

San Antonio Cancer Institute
San Antonio, TX
USA

Ben Davidson MD PhD

Department of Pathology
Rikshospitalet–Radiumhospitalet
  Medical Center
Montebello
Oslo
Norway

Teresa P Díaz-Montes MD

Department of Gynecology and
  Obstetrics
The Johns Hopkins Medical Institutions
Baltimore, MD
USA

Sean C Dowdy MD

Department of Obstetrics and Gynecology
Mayo Clinic
Rochester, MN
USA

Elizabeth D Euscher MD

Department of Pathology
The University of Texas
MD Anderson Cancer Center
Houston, TX
USA

John H Farley MD

Department of Obstetrics and Gynecology
Uniformed Services University of the Health
  Sciences
Bethesda, MD
USA

Michael Frumovitz MD MPH

Department of Gynecologic Oncology
The University of Texas
MD Anderson Cancer Center
Houston, TX
USA

Ginger J Gardner MD

Department of Gynecology and
  Obstetrics
The Johns Hopkins Medical Institutions
Baltimore, MD
USA

Phyllis Gimotty MD

Department of Biostatistics and
  Epidemiology
University of Pennsylvania
Philadelphia, PA
USA

Perry W Grigsby MD

Department of Radiation Oncology
Washington University School
  of Medicine
St Louis, MO
USA

Warner K Huh MD

Department of Obstetrics and Gynecology
University of Alabama–Birmingham
Birmingham, AL
USA

Robert B Jaffe MD

University of California
San Francisco Center for Reproductive
  Sciences
San Francisco, CA
USA

Anuja Jhingran MD

Department of Radiologic Oncology
The University of Texas
MD Anderson Cancer Center
Houston, TX
USA

Daniel S Kapp MD PhD

Department of Radiation Oncology
Stanford Cancer Center
Stanford University School of Medicine
Stanford, CA
USA

Dionysios Katsaros

Department of Obstetrics and
  Gynecology
University of Turin
Italy

Sarah Kim MD

Department of Obstetrics and Gynecology
University of Pennsylvania
Philadelphia, PA
USA

Robin A Lacour MD

Department of Gynecologic Oncology
The University of Texas
MD Anderson Cancer Center
Houston, TX
USA

Grainger S Lanneau MD

Department of Obstetrics and Gynecology
University of Oklahoma Health Sciences
  Center
Oklahoma City, OK
USA

Jayanthi S Lea MD

Division of Gynecologic Oncology
UT Southwestern Medical Center
Dallas, TX
USA

Charles F Levenback MD

Department of Gynecologic Oncology
The University of Texas
MD Anderson Cancer Center
Houston, TX
USA

Yvonne G Lin MD

Department of Gynecologic Oncology
The University of Texas
MD Anderson Cancer Center
Houston
TX, USA

Karen H Lu MD

Department of Gynecologic Oncology
The University of Texas
MD Anderson Cancer Center
Houston, TX
USA

D Scott McMeekin MD

Department of Obstetrics and
  Gynecology
University of Oklahoma Health Sciences
  Center
Oklahoma City, OK
USA

Andrea Mariani MD

Department of Obstetrics and Gynecology
Mayo Clinic
Rochester, MN
USA

G Larry Maxwell MD

Gynecologic Oncology Disease Center
Walter Reed Army Medical Center
  and the US Military Cancer Institute
Washington, DC
USA

Bradley J Monk MD

Division of Gynecologic Oncology
University of California Irvine Medical Center
Orange, CA
USA

Carolyn Y Muller MD

Division of Gynecologic Oncology
University of New Mexico
Albuquerque, NM
USA

Karl C Podratz MD PhD

Department of Obstetrics and
  Gynecology
Mayo Clinic
Rochester, MN
USA

Matthew A Powell MD

Department of Obstetrics and Gynecology
Washington University School of Medicine
St Louis, MO
USA

Lois M Ramondetta MD

Department of Gynecologic Oncology
The University of Texas
MD Anderson Cancer Center
Houston, TX
USA

Reuven Reich PhD

Department of Pharmacology and
  Experimental Therapeutics
School of Pharmacy
The Hebrew University of Jerusalem
Jerusalem
Israel

John I Risinger PhD

Laboratory of Biosystems and Cancer
National Institutes of Health/National
  Cancer Institute
Bethesda, MD
USA

Stephen L Rose MD

Division of Gynecologic Oncology
The University of Wisconsin
Madison, WI
USA

Stephen C Rubin MD

Department of Obstetrics and Gynecology
University of Pennsylvania Medical Center
Hospital of the University of Pennsylvania
Philadelphia, PA
USA

Brian M Slomovitz MD

Department of Obstetrics and Gynecology
Weill Medical College of Cornell University
New York Presbyterian Hospital
New York, NY
USA

Anil K Sood MD

Departments of Gynecologic Oncology and
    Cancer Biology
The University of Texas
MD Anderson Cancer Center
Houston, TX
USA

Davansu Tewari MD

Division of Gynecologic Oncology
University of California Irvine Medical
    Center
Orange, CA
USA

Claes G Trope MD PhD

Department of Gynecologic Oncology
University of Oslo
Rikshospitalet–Radiumhospitalet Medical
    Center
Montebello
Oslo
Norway

Jason D Wright MD

Department of Obstetrics and
    Gynecology
Columbia University
New York, NY
USA

Lin Zhang MD

Department of Biostatistics and Epidemiology
University of Pennsylvania
Philadelphia, PA
USA

Kristen K Zorn MD

Department of Obstetrics, Gynecology and
    Reproductive Sciences
Division of Gynecologic Oncology
Pittsburgh, PA
USA

Weiping Zou MD

Department of Surgery
University of Michigan
Ann Arbor, MI
USA

Preface

Experienced clinicians have long recognized limitations with regard to predicting the course of disease in individual patients. We rely heavily on the traditional prognostic and predictive factors such as tumor stage, histologic subtype and grade to provide broad guidelines for treatment recommendations. At the extremes of the prognostic spectrum, for example stage I and IV cervix cancer, traditional prognostic factors are fairly reliable. Nevertheless, we also know that occasionally patients with a favorable prognosis will suffer from recurrent cancer and conversely, patients with a terrible prognosis survive. In more ambiguous categories (for example stage II and III epithelial ovarian cancer), prognostication for individual patients can be particularly difficult. This high degree of uncertainty contributes to the patient's (and provider's) anxiety and leads to over-treatment of large numbers of patients.

There is a growing number of new prognostic and predictive factors that have been derived from molecular discoveries. These newly described molecular pathways and genetic markers are starting to become the basis of therapeutic intervention. We anticipate that in the coming years, treatment planning will be based on molecular profiling to a greater extent. Eventually, the traditional prognostic factors that we rely on so heavily now may be either complemented or superceded by molecular factors.

Our purpose in writing this book is to provide a single up-to-date resource of prognostic and predictive factors from both traditional and molecular categories for gynecologic malignancies. We hope that this book will be an easy to use resource for oncologists, translational and basic researchers, as well as fellows, residents and students who have an interest in gynecologic cancers. In order to provide a concise resource, we elected to focus on specific aspects of the major gynecologic cancers including ovarian, endometrial, and cervical cancer. Our hope is that this book will not only help clinicians at the bedside make informed treatment recommendations, but also stimulate scientists to continue to search for better prognostic and predictive markers for our patients.

CFL, AKS, KHL, RLC

Section I
Ovary

Section Editor: Anil K Sood

Clinical predictors of outcome in epithelial ovarian carcinoma   1

Teresa P Díaz-Montes and Robert E Bristow

INTRODUCTION

In the USA, ovarian cancer is the fourth most common cause of cancer-related death among women, and the most common cause of death among women with gynecologic malignancies.[1] The American Cancer Society (ACS) estimates that there will be 22 430 new cases of ovarian cancer and 15 280 deaths during 2007.[1] Seventy percent of women with ovarian cancer are diagnosed with advanced-stage disease, and approximately 60% of them will die within 5 years.[2] Also, at least 60% of advanced-stage ovarian cancer patients who are without any evidence of disease after completing primary therapy will ultimately develop recurrent disease.[3]

The prediction of clinical outcome and the use of prognostic factors in the selection of the most appropriate treatment have become important parts of the management of patients diagnosed with ovarian cancer. Prognostic factors are defined as phenotypes that correlate with overall survival. In general, they reflect the intrinsic biology of the tumor, and include histologic subtype, tumor grade, disease extent, and the capacity of the patient to cope with the morbidity associated with the tumor and its treatment. As clinical tools, prognostic factors can help facilitate individualized treatment planning for patients. As research tools, prognostic factors can help in identifying subgroups

Table 1.1 Prognostic factors in ovarian cancer

- Age
- Performance Status
- FIGO* Stage
- Extent of Disease
- Histologic Subtype
- Tumor Grade
- Presence of Ascites
- Tumor DNA Ploidy
- Initial Serum CA-125 Levels
- Residual Disease following Cytoreductive Surgery
- Platinum Sensitivity/Resistance

*FIGO = The International Federation of Gynecology and Obstetrics

of patients with an especially poor prognosis who may benefit from alternative treatment strategies. In clinical trials, prognostic factors are used to balance patients between treatment arms in order to minimize the risk of confounding. In this chapter, we describe factors currently thought to have prognostic significance for patients with ovarian cancer (Table 1.1).

PROGNOSTIC FACTORS

Tumor stage

Proper clinical management of patients with suspected ovarian cancer begins with surgery, which is necessary to confirm the diagnosis, accurately assess disease extent and assign stage, and achieve minimal residual disease through cytoreduction in patients with large-volume metastatic disease.[4] Surgical reduction of bulky ovarian tumors may enhance the potential efficacy of adjuvant chemotherapeutic strategies by alleviating the decrease in tumor growth fraction and the poor blood supply that are characteristic of large tumors.[5] On debulking a tumor, the growth fraction should increase[6] and the number of poorly perfused anoxic cells should decrease. By reducing the number of cancer cells, the chance of these cells undergoing spontaneous mutations resulting in drug resistance should decrease.[7] All of these effects are believed to enhance sensitivity to chemotherapy. Cytoreductive surgery may also improve patients' comfort, reduce the adverse metabolic consequences of the tumor, and enhance the patients' ability to maintain their nutritional status.[8] Currently, primary cytoreductive surgery with the goal of resecting as much macroscopic tumor as possible followed by combination chemotherapy with paclitaxel and a platinum compound is the accepted management for advanced ovarian cancer.[9]

The extent of tumor growth and spread at the time of diagnosis is the most important variable influencing the prognosis of patients with ovarian cancer. The extent of disease is conventionally expressed as the International Federation of Gynecology and Obstetrics (FIGO) stage. The distribution of ovarian cancer patients according to stage at diagnosis is as follows: stage I (23–33%), stage II (9–13%), stage III (46–47%), and stage IV (12–16%).[10,11] In earlier series in which women did not undergo careful surgical staging, the overall 5-year survival rate for those with apparent stage I disease was reported to be only 60%.[12,13] However, with proper surgical staging, the 5-year survival rate for stage I disease is actually

about 90%.[14,15] The 5-year survival rates for stages IIIA, IIIB, and IIIC were 49.2%, 40.8%, and 28.9% (Table 1.2).[16] Stage IV patients have a 5-year survival rate of 13.4%.[16]

A gynecologic oncologist should be asked to participate in the surgical procedure if an ovarian malignancy is suspected preoperatively or found intraoperatively.[17] Occult metastases are not uncommon in women with apparent clinical stage I or II disease.[13,18-20] The frequency with which this occurs was illustrated in a study by Young et al,[13] who reported on 100 patients with apparent stage I or II disease who were referred for additional staging surgery. More advanced disease was discovered in 29% of patients initially thought to have stage I disease and 43% thought to have stage II disease. Overall, one-quarter of patients were upstaged to stage III disease.

Patterns-of-care studies have consistently shown that gynecologic oncologists are more likely than other surgical specialists to perform a complete staging operation.[21] Earle et al[21] studied the associations between physician

Table 1.2 Five-year survivals by FIGO* stage for patients with ovarian cancer 1996-1998 FIGO statistics[†].

FIGO Stage	5-year survival (Percent)
IA	89.3
IB	64.8
IC	78.2
IIA	79.2
IIB	64.3
IIC	68.2
IIIA	49.2
IIIB	40.8
IIIC	28.9
IV	13.4

*FIGO = The International Federation of Gynecology and Obstetrics
[†]From Heintz AP, Odicino F, Maisonneuve P, et al. Carcinoma of the ovary: FIGO annual report. Int J Gynaecol Obstet 2003; 83:135-166.

specialty and outcomes in a population-based cohort of elderly ovarian cancer surgery patients. Among 3067 ovarian cancer patients who underwent surgery, 1017 (33%) were treated by gynecologic oncologists, 1377 (45%) by general gynecologists, and 673 (22%) by general surgeons. Among patients with stage I or II disease, those treated by a gynecologic oncologist (60%) were more likely to undergo lymph node dissection than those treated by a general gynecologist (36%) or a general surgeon (16%). Patients with stage III or IV disease were more likely to undergo a cytoreductive procedure if the initial surgery was performed by a gynecologic oncologist (58%) than by a general gynecologist (51%) or a general surgeon (40%; $p<0.00$), and were more likely to receive postoperative chemotherapy when operated on by a gynecologic oncologist (79%) or a general gynecologist (76%) than by a general surgeon (62%; $p<0.00$). Survival among patients operated on by gynecologic oncologists (hazard ratio (HR) 0.85, 95% confidence interval (CI) 0.76–0.95) or general gynecologists (HR 0.86, 95% CI 0.78–0.96) was better compared with patients operated on by general surgeons. Mayer et al[22] reported a series of 47 patients with stage I–II ovarian cancer treated with chemotherapy after surgical staging, and observed that the specialty of the operating surgeon was identified as a poor prognostic indicator. The 5-year actuarial survival and disease- free survival rates for stage I–II patients surgically staged by a gynecologic oncologist were 83% ± 7% and 76% ± 8%, respectively, compared with 59% ± 11% ($p<0.05$) and 39% ± 11% ($p<0.03$) for those operated upon by a nongynecologic oncologist.

Volume of residual disease

The concept of primary cytoreductive surgery for epithelial ovarian cancer has evolved since 1935, when Meigs[23] first suggested that as much tumor as possible should be removed to enhance the effect of postoperative radiotherapy. In 1975, Griffiths[24] was the first to conclusively demonstrate an inverse relationship between residual tumor size after primary debulking surgery and survival. In that study, patients left with no residual tumor had a median survival of 39 months, whereas patients with residual tumor >1.45 cm in greatest dimension survived a median of 12.7 months. An equally important observation from this landmark study was that even extensive tumor resection that failed to remove all tumors >1.5 cm had little influence on survival. In 1983, Hacker et al[25] reported a series of 47 patients undergoing surgery for advanced ovarian cancer and observed that primary cytoreduction to residual disease <0.5 cm was associated with a median survival time of 40 months, but decreased to 18 months when the largest residual tumor measured 0.5–1.5 cm. Both of these groups enjoyed superior survival when compared with patients left with bulky residual tumor >1.5 cm (median survival 6 months; $p<0.001$). Since then, virtually every study evaluating the prognostic impact of residual disease volume has confirmed that primary surgical cytoreduction resulting in minimal residual tumor is associated with an increased likelihood of complete clinical response to chemotherapy and superior overall survival compared with bulky (>1–2 cm) residual disease.[26]

Two studies by Hoskins et al,[27,28] reporting for the Gynecologic Oncology Group (GOG), illustrate both the potential benefits and shortcomings of primary cytoreductive surgery. In evaluating patients according to the volume of residual disease, these investigators identified three distinct groups: microscopic residual disease, residual disease ≤2 cm, and residual disease >2 cm. Patients left with microscopic disease had a 4-year survival rate of approximately 60%, whereas patients with gross disease <2 cm in greatest dimension had a 4-year survival rate of approximately 35%. Conversely, patients who could not be cytoreduced to disease <2 cm had a 4-year survival rate of <20% (Figure 1.1). Importantly, primary cytoreductive surgery failed to have any effect on survival if the largest residual tumor dimension exceeded 2 cm, regardless of the extent of resection (Figure 1.2).[27,28]

Eisenkop et al,[29] while evaluating prospectively a cohort of ovarian cancer patients with stage IIIC and IV disease, reported on the feasibility of complete cytoreduction and its impact on survival. Between 1990 and 1996, 163 consecutive patients underwent primary cytoreduction with the goal of excision or ablation of all visible disease prior to initiation of systemic platinum-based combination chemotherapy. A total of 139 patients (85.3%) underwent removal of all visible tumor, 22 (13.5%) had cytoreduction to ≤1 cm residual disease, and 2 (1.2%) had unresected bulky disease. The median survival and estimated 5-year survival rate for the entire cohort were 54 months and 48%. The probability of achieving complete cytoreduction was influenced independently by the preoperative GOG performance status (0–1 vs 2–3; $p=0.04$), the number of mesenteric and intestinal serosal implants (≤75 vs >75 implants; $p=0.00$), and stage (IIIC vs IV; $p=0.01$). The probability of survival was independently influenced by age (≤61 vs >61 years; $p=0.00$), volume of ascites (≤1 vs >1 liter; $p=0.01$), stage (IIIC vs IV; $p=0.04$), histology (clear cell and mucinous vs all other;

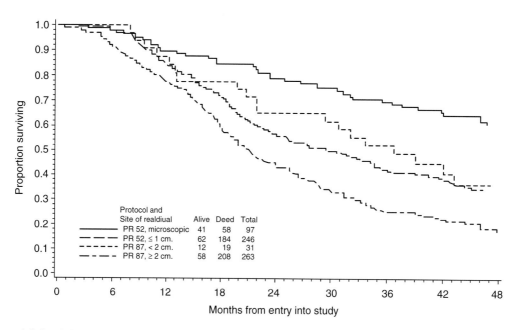

Figure 1.1 Survival time by residual disease.
*Copyright permission requested and in process from Elsevier to use Figure 2 from Hoskins WJ, McGuire WP, Brady MR, et al. The effect of diameter of largest residual disease on survival after primary cytoreductive surgery in patients with suboptimal residual epithelial ovarian carcinoma. Am J Obstet Gynecol 1994;170:974–979.

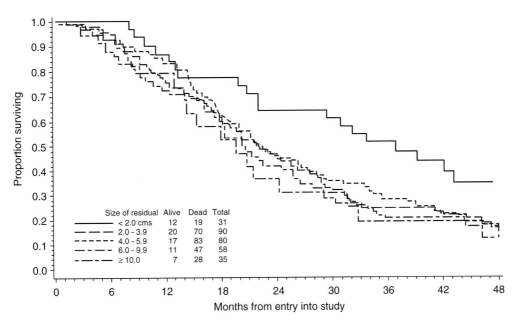

Figure 1.2 Survival time by maximum diameter of residual disease.
*Copyright permission requested and in process from Elsevier to use Figure 1 from Hoskins WJ, McGuire WP, Brady MR, et al. The effect of diameter of largest residual disease on survival after primary cytoreductive surgery in patients with suboptimal residual epithelial ovarian carcinoma. Am J Obstet Gynecol 1994;170:974–979.

$p=0.03$), and completeness of cytoreductive operation (complete vs incomplete cytoreduction; $p=0.02$).

Complete cytoreduction of all macroscopic disease is feasible and is associated with improved survival outcomes, as illustrated in the previous studies. Recently, Armstrong et al[30] reported an improved survival outcome in optimally cytoreduced stage III ovarian cancer patients treated with intravenous paclitaxel plus intraperitoneal cisplatin and paclitaxel. A randomized phase III trial conducted by the GOG compared intravenous paclitaxel plus cisplatin with intravenous paclitaxel plus intraperitoneal cisplatin and paclitaxel in patients with stage III ovarian cancer. Patients with stage III ovarian or primary peritoneal cancer with no residual mass greater than 1.0 cm were randomized to receive 135 mg

of intravenous paclitaxel/m² body surface area over a 24-hour period followed by either 75 mg of intravenous cisplatin per/m² on day 2 (intravenous therapy group) or 100 mg of intraperitoneal cisplatin/m² on day 2 and 60 mg of intraperitoneal paclitaxel/m² on day 8 (intraperitoneal therapy group). Treatment was given every 3 weeks for six cycles. Of 429 patients who underwent randomization, 415 were eligible for the study. Grade 3 and 4 pain, fatigue, and hematologic, gastrointestinal, metabolic, and neurologic toxic effects were more common in the intraperitoneal therapy group than in the intravenous therapy group ($p\leq0.00$). Only 42% of the patients in the intraperitoneal therapy group completed six cycles of the assigned therapy, but the median durations of progression-free survival in the intravenous and intraperitoneal therapy groups were 18.3 and 23.8 months, respectively ($p=0.05$). The median durations of overall survival in the intravenous and intraperitoneal therapy groups were 49.7 and 65.6 months, respectively ($p=0.03$).

Histologic grade

Histopathology is the evaluation of cancerous cells at a microscopic level, and is the basis for assigning tumor grading depending on the degree of differentiation, or maturity, of the cells. Tumors are graded on a scale of 1–3. Grade 1 (well-differentiated) tumors look most like normal tissue, grade 2 (moderately well-differentiated) tumors look somewhat like normal tissue, and grade 3 (poorly differentiated) tumors appear very abnormal. Grade 1 tumors have the best prognosis, and grade 3 tumors the worst. At present, grading of ovarian carcinoma is an important prognostic factor for stage I patients. Young et al[31] have demonstrated that stage I patients with grade 1 or grade 2 tumors have a 5-year survival rate of >90% when treated with surgery alone. In contrast, patients with stage I and grade 3 histology have a significantly worse survival, and prospective therapy is indicated.[32–34]

A variety of histologic grading systems for ovarian carcinoma have been used, but there is no widely accepted system. Binary grading systems are inherently superior to the more common three-grade systems, because they are more reproducible and they correspond to the number of options in the binary treatment decision for which grade is considered important: the use of or withholding of chemotherapy. During the last two decades, researchers at the MD Anderson Cancer Center have designed and refined a two-tier grading system (low-grade and high-grade) for invasive serous carcinoma of the ovary. Malpica et al[35] based the system primarily on the assessment of nuclear atypia, with the mitotic rate being used as a secondary feature. Cases assigned to the low-grade category were characterized by the presence of mild to moderate nuclear atypia. As a secondary feature, they tended to show ≤12 mitoses per 10 high-power fields (HPFs), whereas those in the high-grade category had marked nuclear atypia and as a secondary feature >12 mitoses per 10 HPFs. For comparison, the tumors were also graded using the Shimizu/Silverberg and FIGO grading systems. All of the serous carcinomas considered low-grade in the two-tier system were either grade 1 or grade 2 in the Shimizu/Silverberg and FIGO grading systems and, with one exception, all of those considered high-grade were either grade 2 or grade 3 in the latter systems. Malpica et al[35] concluded that there is usually a good correlation between the two-tier grading system and the Shimizu/Silverberg and FIGO grading systems. Because this system is based on defined criteria that are easy to follow and because it involves only two diagnostic categories, it should provide better reproducibility in the grading of ovarian serous carcinoma.

Histologic subtype

In general, the histologic type has less prognostic significance than other clinical factors such as stage, volume of residual disease, and histologic tumor grade. Clear cell ovarian cancer accounts for approximately 3% of ovarian epithelial cancer.[36] Approximately 50% of patients with clear cell cancer of the ovary present with FIGO stage I disease, while 15% will have stage II disease.[14] There is conflicting data on the behavior of these tumors, with some studies reporting a prognosis similar to that of other ovarian cancers[37,38] and others suggesting that patients with clear cell ovarian cancer have worse survival outcomes.[14,39–41]

Mucinous ovarian cancer is uncommon, representing approximately 4% of all ovarian epithelial cancer.[36] Approximately 63% of patients have stage I disease.[14] The overall prognosis for mucinous cancer of the ovary is better than that for serous carcinoma, largely due to a more favorable stage distribution. However, when stratified by stage, the clinical outcome of mucinous cancer is similar to that of serous ovarian cancer.[14,42–44] Advanced-stage mucinous carcinoma is uniformly fatal.

Endometrioid ovarian cancer accounts for 6% of ovarian epithelial cancer.[36] A high proportion of endometrioid carcinomas of the ovary are diagnosed at an early stage, with 52% of cases presenting with stage I or II disease.[14] The reported association of endometrioid ovarian cancer with endometriosis is around 40%.[45] It has been stated that endometrioid ovarian cancer has a better prognosis than serous ovarian cancer, but this is most likely related to the fact that a great majority of the patients present with early-stage disease.

Malignant mixed mesodermal tumors (MMMTs) of the ovary comprise less than 1% of ovarian epithelial cancers.[36] Approximately 74% of patients present with advanced-stage disease.[46] MMMTs are aggressive and rapidly fatal tumors, with a median survival of approximately 1 year.[47–49]

Tumor DNA ploidy

During the last decade, there has been increased interest in the prognostic significance of DNA content measured by flow cytometry in ovarian cancer. Most studies indicate that DNA ploidy or DNA index (the ratio between the aneuploid peak and the diploid peak on histograms from flow cytometry) provides useful prognostic information in early[34] and advanced[50] ovarian cancer, independent of other clinical and pathologic variables. Nevertheless, the precise role of DNA ploidy analysis in predicting the clinical behavior of epithelial ovarian tumors remains controversial. Zanetta et al[51] showed that DNA content of tumors in advanced-stage ovarian cancer, expressed in terms of either DNA ploidy or DNA index, was a significant independent prognostic factor, in addition to the stage of disease and the amount of residual tumor. Among patients with no residual disease after primary cytoreductive surgery, those with a DNA index of <1.3 had a more favorable outcome than those with a higher index. Gajewski et al[52] reported from a series of 87 patients that the survival for patients with DNA diploid tumors (68%) was significantly longer than for DNA aneuploid tumors (49%; $p=0.003$). When patients were separated into early-stage and advanced-stage disease, DNA content was a significant prognostic variable for survival in stage I and II patients ($p=0.05$). In stage III and IV patients, however, DNA content had no independent prognostic significance. There were 33 patients who underwent second-look surgery. Of 15 patients with negative second-look surgery 7 (47%) were DNA-aneuploid, whereas of 18 patients with positive second-look surgery, 17 (94%) were DNA-aneuploid. Stated another way, there was a much higher likelihood of positive second-look surgery in the DNA-aneuploid group (17/24) compared with the DNA-diploid group (1/9) ($p = 0.003$). In addition, for those patients with negative second-look surgery, none (0/8) of the DNA-diploid tumors recurred; however, 3 of 7 (43%) of the DNA-aneuploid tumors recurred and died. Cox proportional hazards analysis showed that DNA content was an independent prognostic factor for survival in epithelial ovarian cancer. Gajewski et al[52] concluded that aneuploid DNA content in ovarian cancer is also correlated with more aggressive biologic behavior, and therefore a worse clinical course.

CA-125 level

CA-125 was first identified in 1981, and since then has been one of the most studied molecular markers in the management of ovarian cancer patients. Overall, approximately 83% of patients with epithelial ovarian cancer have CA-125 levels of >35 U/ml.[53] Meyer and Rustin[54] have reported that levels at presentation correlate with the risk of malignancy, stage of disease, and histology. In addition, changes in CA-125 levels can be used to predict response to chemotherapy, while changes during follow-up can predict relapse with a lead time of approximately 60 days. A number of CA-125 indices have also been extensively evaluated to predict their prognostic significance.

Makar et al[55] evaluated the prognostic significance of serum CA-125 levels in 687 patients with invasive epithelial ovarian malignancies. The samples were collected preoperatively in 200 patients and postoperatively in 487. The serum CA-125 levels were elevated preoperatively in 90% of cases, with a median value of 429 U/ml. In patients with evidence of disease at the time of sampling, the serum CA-125 levels correlated directly with tumor stage, tumor load, and histologic grade. By multivariate analysis, the preoperative serum CA-125 levels had no independent prognostic significance. In patients without residual disease after primary surgery, histologic type ($p<0.00$), postoperative CA-125 levels >35 U/ml ($p = 0.00$), and tumor grade ($p = 0.03$) were independent prognostic factors for survival. For those with residual tumor after primary surgery, histologic type ($p<0.00$), postoperative treatment ($p = 0.00$), size of residual disease ($p = 0.00$), and postoperative serum CA-125 levels >65 U/ml ($p = 0.00$) were independent prognostic factors.

Mogensen[56] studied the prognostic value of CA-125 levels in patients with advanced ovarian cancer. In this report, serum CA-125 was measured during early chemotherapy in 121 patients with FIGO stage III or IV ovarian cancer. CA-125 was determined before the start of chemotherapy and 1 month after the first, second, and third courses. The antigen level before the start of chemotherapy held no prognostic information. However, CA-125 was a significant prognostic parameter in all three courses, but its correlation with survival improved with the number of courses. Patients with high marker levels (>100 U/ml) 1 month after the third course had a median survival of 7 months. Patients with CA-125 levels between 10 and 100 U/ml had a median survival of 22 months. Cox regression analysis of the covariation between survival, CA-125, and five variables (age, FIGO stage, histopathology, tumor grade, and residual tumor bulk) showed that the CA-125 value was the most significant prognostic parameter.

Additional prognostic factors

Other factors that influence the survival outcome of patients with ovarian cancer include: age, performance status, and presence of ascites. An analysis of a GOG database including over 2000 ovarian cancer patients reported that major prognostic factors associated with improved outcome were young age, low volume of residual disease, and high performance status. With regard to the effect of age, patients older than 69 years exhibited significantly shorter survival than those younger, even after correcting for stage, residual disease, and performance status. The adverse impact of older age was unaffected by variations in drugs, doses, and schedules; but there was no evidence that older patients tolerated intensive schedules less well than younger patients.[57] Omura et al[58] reported the experience of the long-term follow-up of 76 patients with advanced ovarian cancer managed according to the GOG protocols. A multivariate analysis demonstrated that cell type other than clear cell or mucinous, cisplatin-based treatment, good performance status, younger age, lower stage, clinically nonmeasurable disease, smaller residual tumor volume, and absence of ascites were favorable characteristics for overall survival ($p<0.05$). Loizzi et al[59] reported on survival outcomes in patients with recurrent ovarian cancer who were treated with chemoresistance assay-guided chemotherapy. Fifty patients who were treated with chemotherapy based on extreme drug resistance assay guidance were compared with 50 well-balanced control subjects who were treated empirically. In the platinum-sensitive group, patients with extreme drug resistance-directed therapy had an overall response rate of 65%, compared with 35% of the patients who were treated empirically ($p = 0.02$). The overall and progression-free median survivals were 38 and 15 months, respectively, in the extreme drug resistance assay group, compared with 21 and 7 months in the control group ($p = 0.00$, overall; $p = 0.00$, progression free). In the platinum-resistant group, there was no improved outcome in the patients who underwent assay-guided therapy. Multivariate analysis showed that platinum-sensitive disease, extreme drug resistance-guided therapy, and early stage of disease were independent predictors for improved survival.

In conclusion, favorable/low risk prognostic factors include early stage, well-differentiated tumor, nonclear cell or nonmucinous histology, absence of ascites, none to minimal residual disease (<1 cm) following cytoreductive surgery, younger age, and good performance status.

REFERENCES

1. American Cancer Society. Cancer Facts and Figures 2007. http://www.cancer.org/docroot/stt/stt_0.asp.

2. Ries LAG, Eisner MP, Kosary BK, et al, eds SEER Cancer Statistics Review, 1975–2001. Bethesda, MD: National Cancer Institute (http://www.seer.cancer.gov/csr/1975_2001).

3. Burke TW, Morris M. Secondary cytoreductive surgery for ovarian cancer. Obstet Gynecol Clin North Am 1994;21:167–78.

4. NIH Consensus Conference: Ovarian cancer: screening, treatment, and follow-up. JAMA 1995;273:491.

5. Boente MP, Chi DS, Hoskins WJ. The role of surgery in the management of ovarian cancer: primary and interval cytoreductive surgery. Semin Oncol 1998;25:326–34.

6. Norton L, Simon R. Tumor size, sensitivity to therapy, and design of treatment schedules. Cancer Treat Rep 1977;61:1307–17.

7. Goldie JH, Coldman AJ. A mathematic model for relating the drug sensitivity of tumors to their spontaneous mutation rate. Cancer Treat Rep 1979;63:1727–33.

8. Blythe JG, Wahl TP. Debulking surgery: does it increase the quality of survival? Gynecol Oncol 1982;14:396–408.

9. McGuire WP, Hoskins WJ, Brady MF, et al. Cyclophosphamide and cisplatin compared with paclitaxel and cisplatin in patients with stage III and stage IV ovarian cancer. N Engl J Med 1996;334:1–6.

10. International Federation of Gynecology and Obstetrics Report, 1991: 248.

11. Heintz AP, Odicino F, Maisonneuve P, et al. Carcinoma of the ovary. J Epidemiol Biostat 2001;6:107–38.

12. Berek JS, Hacker NF. Staging and second-look operations in ovarian cancer. In: Alberts DS, Surwit EA, eds. Ovarian Cancer. Boston: Martinus Nijhoff, 1985:109–27.

13. Young RC, Decker DG, Wharton JT, et al. Staging laparotomy in early ovarian cancer. JAMA 1983;250:3072–6.

14. Pecorelli S. FIGO annual report on the results of treatment in gynaecological cancer. J Epidemiol Biostat 1998;23:1–168.

15. Munoz KA, Harlan LC, Trimble EL. Patterns of care for women with ovarian cancer in the United States. J Clin Oncol 1997;15:3408–15.

16. Heinz AP, Odicino F, Maisonneuve P, et al. Carcinoma of the ovary: FIGO Annual Report. Int J Gynaecol Obstet 2003;83:135–66.

17. Guidelines for referral to a gynecologic oncologist: rationale and benefits. The Society of Gynecologic Oncologists. Gynecol Oncol 2000;78:S1–13.

18. Buchsbaum HJ, Lifshitz S. Staging and surgical evaluation of ovarian cancer. Semin Oncol 1984;11:227–37.

19. Knapp RC, Friedman EA. Aortic lymph node metastases in early ovarian cancer. Am J Obstet Gynecol 1974;119:1013–17.

20. Guthrie D, Davy ML, Philips PR. A study of 656 patients with 'early' ovarian cancer. Gynecol Oncol 1984;17:363–9.

21. Earle CC, Schrag D, Neville BA, et al. Effect of surgeon specialty on processes of care and outcomes for ovarian cancer patients. J Natl Cancer Inst 2006;98:172–80.

22. Mayer AR, Chambers SK, Graves E, et al. Ovarian cancer staging: does it require a gynecologic oncologist? Gynecol Oncol 1992;47:223–7.

23. Meigs JV. Tumors of the Female Pelvic Organs. New York: McMillan, 1935.

24. Griffiths CT. Surgical resection of tumor bulk in the primary treatment of ovarian carcinoma. Monogr Natl Cancer Inst 1975;42:101–4.

25. Hacker NF, Berek JS, LaGasse LD, et al. Primary cytoreductive surgery for epithelial ovarian cancer. Obstet Gynecol 1983;61:413–20.

26. Hoskins WJ, Rubin SC. Surgery in the treatment of patients with advanced ovarian cancer. Semin Oncol 1991;18:213–21.

27. Hoskins WJ, Bundy BN, Thigpen JT, Omura GA. The influence of cytoreductive surgery on recurrence-free interval and survival in small-volume stage III epithelial ovarian cancer: a Gynecologic Oncology Group study. Gynecol Oncol 1992;47:159–66.

28. Hoskins WJ, McGuire WP, Brady MF, et al. The effect of diameter of largest residual disease on survival after primary cytoreductive surgery in patients with suboptimal residual epithelial ovarian carcinoma. Am J Obstet Gynecol 1994;170:974–80.

29. Eisenkop SM, Friedman RL, Wang HJ. Complete cytoreductive surgery is feasible and maximizes survival in patients with advanced epithelial ovarian cancer: a prospective study. Gynecol Oncol 1998;69:103–8.

30. Armstrong DK, Bundy B, Wenzel L, et al. Intraperitoneal cisplatin and paclitaxel in ovarian cancer. N Engl J Med 2006;354:34–43.

31. Young RC, Walton LA, Ellenberg SS, et al. Adjuvant therapy in stage I and stage II epithelial ovarian cancer. Results of two prospective randomized trials. N Engl J Med 1990;322:1021–7.

32. Ahmed FY, Wiltshaw E, A'Hern RP, et al. Natural history and prognosis of untreated stage I epithelial ovarian carcinoma. J Clin Oncol 1996;14:2968–75.

33. Dembo AJ, Davy M, Steinwig AE, et al. Prognostic factors in patients with stage I epithelial ovarian cancer. Obstet Gynecol 1990;75:263–73.

34. Vergote IB, Kaern J, Abeler VM, et al. Analysis of prognostic factors in stage I epithelial ovarian carcinoma: importance of degree of differentiation and deoxyribonucleic acid ploidy in predicting relapse. Am J Obstet Gynecol 1993;169:40–52.

35. Malpica A, Deavers MT, Lu K, et al. Grading ovarian serous carcinoma using a two-tier system. Am J Surg Pathol 2004;28:496–504.

36. Seidman JD, Russell P, Kurman RJ. Surface epithelial tumors of the ovary. In: Kurman RJ, ed. Blaunstein's Pathology of the Female Genital Tract. New York: Springer-Verlag, 2002:810–904.

37. Crozier MA, Copeland LJ, Silva EG, et al. Clear cell carcinoma of the ovary: a study of 59 cases. Gynecol Oncol 1989;35:199–203.

38. Jenison EL, Montag AG, Griffiths CT, et al. Clear cell adenocarcinoma of the ovary: a clinical analysis and comparison with serous carcinoma. Gynecol Oncol 1989;32:65–71.

39. O'Brien ME, Schofield JB, Tan S, et al. Clear cell epithelial ovarian cancer (mesonephroid): bad prognosis only in early stages. Gynecol Oncol 1993;49:250–4.

40. Kennedy AW, Markman M, Biscotti CV, et al. Survival probability in ovarian clear cell adenocarcinoma. Gynecol Oncol 1999;74:108–14.

41. Tammela J, Geisler JP, Eskew PN Jr, et al. Clear cell carcinoma of the ovary: poor prognosis compared to serous carcinoma. Eur J Gynaecol Oncol 1998;19:438–40.

42. Chaitin BA, Gershenson DM, Evans HL. Mucinous tumors of the ovary: a clinicopathologic study of 70 cases. Cancer 1985;55:1958–62.

43. Hoerl HD, Hart WR. Primary ovarian mucinous cystadenocarcinomas: a clinicopathologic study of 49 cases with long-term follow-up. Am J Surg Pathol 1998;22:1449–62.

44. Kikkawa F, Kawai M, Tamakoshi K, et al. Mucinous carcinoma of the ovary: clinicopathologic analysis. Oncology 1996;53:303–7.

45. Sainz de la Cuesta R, Eichhorn JH, Rice LW, et al. Histologic transformation of benign endometriosis to early epithelial ovarian cancer. Gynecol Oncol 1996;60:238–44.

46. Le T, Krepart GV, Lotocki RJ, et al. Malignant mixed mesodermal ovarian tumor treatment and prognosis: a 20-year experience. Gynecol Oncol 1997;65:237–40.

47. Andersen WA, Young DE, Peters WA, et al. Platinum-based combination chemotherapy for malignant mixed mesodermal tumors of the ovary. Gynecol Oncol 1989;32:319–22.

48. Boucher D, Tetu B. Morphologic prognostic factors of malignant mixed mullerian tumors of the ovary: a clinicopathologic study of 15 cases. Int J Gynecol Pathol 1994;13:22–8.

49. Dehner LP, Norris HJ, Taylor HB. Carcinosarcomas and mixed mesodermal tumors of the ovary. Cancer 1971;27:207–16.

50. Kaern J, Trope CG, Kristensen GB, et al. Evaluation of deoxyribonucleic acid ploidy and S-phase fraction as prognostic parameters in advanced epithelial ovarian carcinoma: a prospective study. Am J Obstet Gynecol 1994;170:479–87.

51. Zanetta G, Keeney GL, Cha SS, et al. Flow cytometric analysis of DNA content in advanced ovarian carcinoma: its significance to long-term survival. Am J Obstet Gynecol 1996;175:1217–25.

52. Gajewski WH, Fuller AF Jr, Pastel-Ley C, et al. Prognostic significance of DNA content in epithelial ovarian cancer. Gynecol Oncol 1994;53:5–12.

53. Canney PA, Moore M, Wilkinson PM, James RD. Ovarian cancer antigen CA125: a prospective clinical assessment of its role as a tumour marker. Br J Cancer 1984;50:765–9.

54. Meyer T, Rustin GJ. Role of tumour markers in monitoring epithelial ovarian cancer. Br J Cancer 2000;82:1535–8.

55. Makar AP, Kristensen GB, Kaern J, et al. Prognostic value of pre- and postoperative

serum CA 125 levels in ovarian cancer: new aspects and multivariate analysis. Obstet Gynecol 1992;79:1002–10.

56. Mogensen O. Prognostic value of CA 125 in advanced ovarian cancer. Gynecol Oncol 1992;44:207–12.

57. Thigpen T, Brady MF, Omura GA, et al. Age as a prognostic factor in ovarian carcinoma. The Gynecologic Oncology Group experience. Cancer 1993;71:606–14.

58. Omura GA, Brady MF, Homesley HD, et al. Long-term follow-up and prognostic factor analysis in advanced ovarian carcinoma: the Gynecologic Oncology Group experience. J Clin Oncol 1991;9:1138–50.

59. Loizzi V, Chan JK, Osann K, et al. Survival outcomes in patients with recurrent ovarian cancer who were treated with chemoresistance assay-guided chemotherapy. Am J Obstet Gynecol 2003;189:1301–7.

Influence of *BRCA1* and *BRCA2* on ovarian cancer survival

2

Christina S Chu and Stephen C Rubin

INTRODUCTION

Epithelial ovarian cancer (EOC) accounts for one-quarter of all gynecologic cancers, but is responsible for the majority of deaths.[1,2] A woman's lifetime risk of ovarian cancer is about 1 in 55, and the American Cancer Society (ACS) estimates that in 2007 in the USA, 22 430 women will be diagnosed with ovarian cancer and that 15 280 will die of their disease.[3]

Many risk factors associated with EOC have been identified (Table 2.1), the most significant of which is family history of the disease. In 1966, Lynch et al[4] were the first to suggest that a woman's hereditary factors contributed to the risk of developing ovarian cancer. Since that initial report, a family history of ovarian cancer as well as a personal history of breast cancer has been noted in several case–control studies[5–7] to increase the risk of EOC. Schildkraut and Thompson[7] noted a familial clustering of ovarian cancer cases. They examined 493 women with newly diagnosed EOC in comparison with 2465 controls. The odds ratios for ovarian cancer in first- and second-degree relatives were 3.6 (95% confidence interval (CI) 1.8–7.1) and 2.9 (95% CI 1.6–5.3), respectively, compared with women with no family history of ovarian cancer. A decade later, Stratton et al[8] performed a large meta-analysis, incorporating data from nearly 18 000 women, and showed that the relative risk of ovarian cancer for women with a first-degree relative with ovarian cancer was 3.1 (95% CI 2.6–3.7). Although the lifetime risk of developing ovarian cancer in the general population is 1–2%, with even one affected family member, women see their risk increased to 4–5%. With two affected family members, the risk increases to 7%.[9,10]

The majority of cases of EOC are sporadic, with only approximately 10% being due to an inherited predisposition.[11–15] The majority of these cases are due to mutations in the *BRCA1* and *BRCA2* genes, with a small percentage being due to mutations in the DNA mismatch repair genes related to the hereditary nonpolyposis colorectal carcinoma syndrome.

Table 2.1 Risk factors associated with epithelial ovarian cancer

- Age >50 years
- Family history of breast and/or ovarian cancer: *BRCA1*, *BRCA2* mutation; DNA mismatch repair gene mutation
- Reproductive factors: early menarche, late menopause, infertility, nulliparity. Breastfeeding and oral contraceptive use are protective
- Demographics: Ashkenazi Jewish or White race; residence in industrialized nations (except Japan)
- Diet: high intake of fat, coffee; low intake of fiber, vitamin A
- Environmental exposure: use of talc on the perineum; viral infection with mumps or rubella; asbestos; radiation

Table 2.2 Major mutations associated with hereditary breast and ovarian cancer in the Ashkenazi Jewish population

Gene	Chromosome location	Contribution to overall ovarian cancer cases (%)
BRCA1: 185delAG 5382insC	17q21	4.1
BRCA2: 6174delT	13p12	3.3

Significant specific mutations for these genes are described in Table 2.2. For carriers of mutations in the *BRCA* genes, the lifetime risk of ovarian cancer is estimated to be 15–60%. Unlike sporadic cancers, over 90% of *BRCA*-associated ovarian cancers are of serous histologic subtype (Figures 2.1 and 2.2).

BRCA1 AND *BRCA2*

The *BRCA1* gene was initially cloned in 1994 at chromosome 17q21,[16] and a year later, the *BRCA2* gene was isolated at chromosome 13q12.[17]

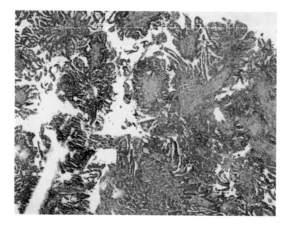

Figure 2.1 Papillary serous adenocarcinoma, 5x. Serous carcinomas are characterized by nuclear atypia, cellular budding, and areas of confluence.

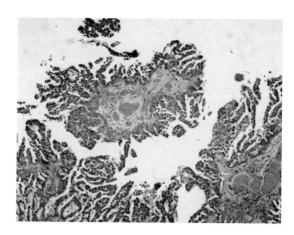

Figure 2.2 Papillary serous adenocarcinoma, 10x. The extent of papillation may vary, but the structures generally display prominent vasculature in the stromal cores.

Both genes appear to function as tumor suppressor genes, playing a role in DNA damage repair, replication fidelity, and regulation of gene expression. Approximately 80% of mutations are frameshift or loss-of-function mutations,[18] which are transmitted in an autosomal dominant fashion. Germline mutations in *BRCA1* are responsible for approximately 90% of hereditary ovarian cancers, with mutations in *BRCA2* accounting for the majority of the remainder. In addition to breast cancer, mutations in both *BRCA1* and *BRCA2* appear to confer a predilection for fallopian tube and primary peritoneal carcinomas as well.[19]

BRCA1 and *BRCA2* mutations are important factors in hereditary ovarian cancer, but do not appear to play a significant role in the development of sporadic tumors, although *BRCA* 'silencing' by other mechanisms, including promoter hypermethylation, has been reported in sporadic ovarian cancers. Mutations in *BRCA1* occur in only 1 of 800 people in the general population, and in only 3–6% of all patients with epithelial ovarian carcinoma,[7,20] but prevalence varies considerably with ethnicity and personal and family history. Among individuals of Ashkenazi Jewish heritage, the prevalence of mutations may be as high as 2.5%.[21,22] Among these individuals, three founder mutations (the 185delAG and 5382insC mutations in *BRCA1*, and the 6174delT mutation in *BRCA2*) account for 90% of the cases of breast and ovarian cancer.[21,22] Among Ashkenazi women with a personal history of breast cancer, the prevalence rises to 10%;[23,24] for those with a personal history of ovarian cancer, the rate is as high as 40%.[25,26] Even in the general population, a diagnosis of breast cancer may confer a 3% risk of mutation, but that rate rises to 22.8% for those who also have a family history of ovarian cancer.[27] In high-risk families with multiple cases of breast and/or ovarian cancer, individual women may have a risk as high as 40% of carrying a mutation in either *BRCA1* or *BRCA2*.[27]

PENETRANCE

Not all mutation carriers develop cancer: overall, mutations may carry a lifetime risk of 15–60%.[28–31] The particular risk of developing a tumor may be affected by the specific mutation involved, patient age, and population studied. When examining high-risk families carrying mutations in *BRCA1*, the Breast Cancer Linkage Consortium reported the risk of developing ovarian cancer by age 70 years to be 44–63%,[31] and similar studies showed the rate to be 27% for those carrying *BRCA2* mutations.[28] Ashkenazi women who carry mutations, even those unselected for family history, have been found to suffer a risk of ovarian cancer of 16–37%.[29,30] This contrasts sharply with the risk in the general population of about 1.4%, where penetrance of *BRCA* mutations tends to be lower.[31]

CLINICAL COURSE

Several studies have examined the effect of *BRCA* mutations on survival in patients with ovarian cancer (Table 2.3). While the majority of studies have demonstrated a more favorable outcome for mutation carriers in comparison with sporadic ovarian cancers,[25,32–37] some have not confirmed this finding.[38,39] Even before *BRCA1* was cloned, Buller et al[40] in 1993 first provided indirect evidence of a survival advantage. Their study examined 11 members of four families who had two or more first-degree relatives diagnosed with ovarian cancer. Of these patients, 1 was stage II, 6 were stage III, 3 were stage IV, and 1 was unstaged. For a comparison group, the authors selected 34 consecutively treated patients of similar age with stage III disease. They noted that patients with familial ovarian cancer exhibited a 67% 5-year survival rate, compared with only 17% in patients with nonfamilial cases (*p* <0.04). More recently, in 2000, a large population-based US Surveillance, Epidemiology, and End Results (SEER) database study identified 25 637 white women with epithelial ovarian cancer.[41] Of these patients, 824 women had a prior diagnosis of breast cancer. These women had an overall estimated 5-year survival rate of 49%, compared with 45% among women without a history of prior breast cancer. However, the survival advantage was significantly higher in women with advanced disease, and those diagnosed over the age of 55. Although these women did not undergo genetic testing, it has been estimated that 88% of women with both breast and ovarian cancer are carriers of *BRCA1* mutations,[42] providing further indirect evidence that *BRCA* mutation confers a survival advantage. Although this study is limited by lack of data on well-established clinical prognostic factors (such as residual disease and chemotherapy), as well as the potential

Table 2.3 Survival in patients with mutations in BRCA1 and BRCA2

Study	Year	Mutation	Population	n	Stage	5-year survival rate (%)		p-value
						Cases	Controls	
Rubin et al[32]	1996	BRCA1	Unselected for family history	43	III, IV	(77 months median survival)	(43 months median survival)	<0.001
Aida et al[34]	1998	BRCA1	Breast–ovarian cancer families	25	I, III, IV	78.6	30.0	<0.05
Johannsson et al[38]	1998	BRCA1	Breast–ovarian cancer families	38	I–IV	32	37	Not significant
Pharoah et al[39]	1999	BRCA1, BRCA2	Breast–ovarian cancer families	151	I–IV	21 (BRCA1) 25 (BRCA2)	30	0.005
Boyd et al[25]	2000	BRCA1, BRCA2	Consecutive cases diagnosed at single institution, patients of Jewish origin	81	III, IV	45	25	0.004
Ben David et al[35]	2002	BRCA1, BRCA2	Unselected for family history, Jewish women	234	III, IV	60.3 (3-year)	44.5 (3-year)	Not stated
Cass et al[36]	2003	BRCA1, BRCA2	Tumor registry, Jewish women	29	III, IV	65	48	0.046
Majdak et al[37]	2005	BRCA1, BRCA2	Consecutive cases from single institution	36	I–IV	40 (3-year)	31 (3-year)	0.019

for incomplete data regarding breast cancer history, the study's main strength is its ability to minimize selection bias given the large number of patients identified through a population-based system.

Of the studies directly examining survival in populations of ovarian cancer patients with documented mutations in the BRCA genes, the first was performed by Rubin et al[32] in 1996. The investigators examined 53 advanced-stage patients with germline mutations in BRCA1 in comparison with sporadic age- and stage-matched controls. BRCA1 mutation carriers had a median survival of 77 months, compared with only 29 months for patients with sporadic cancers ($p < 0.001$). The study was criticized for not reporting information on

clinical prognostic factors, potential differences in treatment, and for possible selection biases in formulating the control group, but it was the first to report a significant survival advantage for mutation carriers. Two years later, Aida et al[34] analyzed 25 patients with germline mutations of BRCA1 from several high-risk families in Japan. They selected age- and treatment-matched controls for comparison, and noted 5-year survival rates of 78.6% and 30.3%, respectively ($p < 0.05$). Similarly, a significant advantage in median disease-free interval was also noted, of 91.4 months versus 40.9 months, respectively ($p < 0.05$).

These reports were followed by two showing no survival advantage for mutation carriers. Johannsson et al[38] conducted a population-based study of 38 patients with *BRCA1* mutations diagnosed with ovarian cancer (7 also had breast cancer) identified from genetic analysis of breast cancer families from southern Sweden. Although survival in the first years after diagnosis appeared better for the mutation carriers than for age- and stage-matched patients from the general population, long-term survival was not significantly different. In fact, multivariate analysis showed a statistically worse survival for *BRCA1* patients than controls, although the nonparallel survival curves made direct comparison difficult. Pharoah et al[39] did note a significantly worse prognosis for patients with *BRCA1* and *BRCA2* mutations compared with sporadic cases. These authors examined patients with ovarian cancer from breast–ovarian cancer families. They identified 151 patients from 57 documented *BRCA1* and *BRCA2* families and 199 patients from 62 families in which a *BRCA1* or *BRCA2* mutation was not found after genetic testing. Utilizing an age-matched set of 552 population control cases, the investigators noted that overall survival in familial ovarian cancer cases as a whole was significantly worse than for population controls: the 5-year survival rates were 21% in patients from *BRCA1* families, 25% in those from *BRCA2* families, and 19% in those from families with no identified mutation, versus 30% in population controls (p <0.005). Unfortunately, the results must be interpreted with caution, given that the familial cases had a significantly higher proportion of stage III and IV tumors (83%) than the population controls (56%; p <0.001), and thus would be expected, based on stage alone, to have a worse prognosis. In addition, the authors made a fundamental assumption that all patients diagnosed with ovarian cancer in families with documented mutations were mutation carriers, without performing actual confirmational genetic analysis.

In 2000, more evidence for a survival advantage was reported by Boyd et al.[25] They performed a retrospective cohort study to examine a consecutive series of 933 ovarian cancer patients diagnosed and treated at Memorial Sloan-Kettering Cancer Center. Of these patients, they identified 189 women who identified themselves as Jewish, and, among these, 88 found to have *BRCA1* or *BRCA2* mutations were utilized for study. Mutation carriers were noted to have longer median time to recurrence (7 months vs 14 months; p <0.001) as well as increased survival ($p = 0.004$). The presence of a *BRCA* mutation was associated with a 25% reduction in the relative risk of death when compared with sporadic cancers, and was noted to be an independent prognostic factor among patients with stage III tumors. In the study by Boyd et al,[25] selection bias was avoided by utilizing all cases from a large consecutive series of ovarian cancer patients using archival material, thereby eliminating preferential inclusion of living patients in the mutation-carrier group. In addition, treatment-related differences were also minimized, given the use of patients and controls treated at the same institution over the same period of time.

Several other studies support a more favorable prognosis for patients with mutations in *BRCA1* and *BRCA2* as well. Ben David et al[35] performed a nationwide study collecting blood and tissue samples at the time of primary surgery from women with ovarian cancer in Israel in order to perform testing for the three major founder mutations in *BRCA1* and *BRCA2* (185delAG, 5382insC, and 6174delT). Of 896 specimens analyzed, 234 women were found to carry a mutation. Mutation carriers had a significantly better survival than noncarriers, with 3-year survival rates of 65.8% and 51.9%, respectively ($p = 0.001$). Even among those with advanced-stage disease, 3-year survival rates were 60.3% and 44.5%, respectively (*p* not stated). Women with mutations were significantly younger (56.5 years vs 59 years; *p* = 0.001), although the authors found that the survival benefit persisted even after controlling for age. Cass et al[36] examined 34 Jewish ovarian cancer patients with the three founder mutations in *BRCA1* and *BRCA2* in comparison with 35 women with sporadic cancers. *BRCA1* carriers were noted to be younger than *BRCA2* carriers (48 years vs 57 years; *p* = 0.01). Among advanced-stage patients, the rate of surgical cytoreduction was found to be equal. Although recurrence rates were statistically similar, mutation carriers displayed a more favorable 5-year survival rate (65% vs 48%), disease-free survival (49 months vs 19 months; *p* = 0.16), and improved response rate to therapy (72% vs 36%; *p* = 0.01). Finally, most recently, Majdak et al[37] screened a series of 205 consecutive patients with ovarian cancer at the Medical University of Gdansk in Poland by conformational sensitive gel electrophoresis and direct sequencing. They only discovered 16 unclassified variant mutations in *BRCA1* or *BRCA2* and 18 pathogenic mutations in *BRCA1*. On multivariate analysis, a pathogenic mutation in *BRCA1*, but not unclassified variant mutation, was an independent factor in predicting a decreased risk of recurrence and improved survival.

MECHANISMS FOR *BRCA*-ASSOCIATED SURVIVAL ADVANTAGE

The mechanism for the apparent survival advantage conferred by *BRCA* mutation is unknown. One theory proposes that *BRCA*-associated cancers display a more indolent rate of tumor growth, while another posits greater susceptibility to chemotherapy. In support of the latter,

mutation carriers have been noted to have a longer disease-free interval after surgery and chemotherapy,[25,36] and Levine et al[43] have noted a significantly higher growth fraction in *BRCA*-associated tumors compared with sporadic tumors, speculating that increased rates of proliferation might contribute to improved chemosensitivity. Evidence suggests the *BRCA* genes may be involved in DNA repair, the maintenance of genomic integrity, and cell cycle checkpoint control.[44–50] Although *BRCA1* has been linked to a number of cellular functions, the only known function of *BRCA2* is to interact with RAD51 to facilitate homologous recombination DNA repair. Cells with mutated BRCA proteins may be less able to repair DNA damage induced by chemotherapy, thereby leading to an improved tumor response to treatment. In fact, Husain et al[51] studied cisplatin-resistant breast and ovarian cancer cell lines and noted increased levels of BRCA1 protein. In the ovarian cancer cell line SKOV-3 CDDP/R, DNA damage repair was correspondingly improved. Antisense inhibition of *BRCA1* induced a decreased efficiency of DNA repair, enhanced apoptosis, and restoration of cisplatin sensitivity. Intriguing data by Cass et al[36] have demonstrated in a small subset of patients that in vitro chemosensitivity testing is predictive of response to treatment with platinum and paclitaxel in patients with hereditary cancers, but not in patients with sporadic tumors. Although *p53* (*TP53*) mutations have been documented in a high percentage of patients with *BRCA*-associated ovarian cancers, Cass et al[36] could not demonstrate a link between *p53* mutation status and survival among *BRCA* mutation carriers.

RISK MODIFICATION

Women with documented disease-associated mutations in *BRCA1* and *BRCA2* have three options for ovarian cancer risk modification: surveillance, chemoprophylaxis, and prophylactic surgery. Although many efforts have been made to define effective screening regimens, no method exists that can reliably identify patients with early ovarian cancer.[52] The National Institutes of Health Consensus Conference on Ovarian Cancer[53] recommended a combination of pelvic bimanual examination, transvaginal ultrasound, and serum CA-125 determination performed on an annual or semiannual basis. The Cancer Genetics Studies Consortium has recommended the use of transvaginal ultrasound and CA-125, starting between the ages of 25 and 35.[54] Clinical trials underway in the USA and the UK are evaluating the Risk of Ovarian Cancer Algorithm (ROCA), which utilizes a computerized Bayesian algorithm to calculate risk based on longitudinal yearly CA-125 measurements.[55] Despite these recommendations, no methods have been shown to impact survival, and both CA-125 determination and transvaginal ultrasound are troubled by a significant number of false positives. In addition, studies have consistently shown that despite a well-documented increased risk of cancer, women often do not comply with recommendations for screening. Although breast cancer screening seems to be more accepted, less than one-third of mutation carriers complied with recommendations for a transvaginal ultrasound in the first year after genetic testing, and the rate dropped even lower to 11% by the second year after testing.[56] Even a more convenient, less invasive test such as CA-125 testing was only utilized by 32% of women in the first year after mutation testing.[56] Efforts directed towards developing proteomic methods of early detection appear promising.[57]

Although several chemopreventatives, such as retinoids, COX-2 inhibitors, and vitamin D, are under evaluation, the chief agent in use is the oral contraceptive pill (OCP). Since 1979, OCPs have been noted to reduce the risk of ovarian cancer by up to 40% in the general population,[9] and in 1998, Narod et al[58] found a similar pattern of risk reduction among patients with mutations in *BRCA1* and *BRCA2*. In a study comparing 207 mutation carriers suffering from ovarian cancer compared with 161 of their cancer-free sisters, any past use of OCPs reduced the risk by 50% without a significant increase in the rate of breast cancer. Findings by Modan et al[59] disputed these conclusions. The authors compared 840 Jewish women with ovarian cancer with 751 controls and noted that OCP use only appeared to affect the risk of women who were mutation-free. Among mutation carriers, the reduction in risk was only 0.2% per year of use. Although the protective mechanisms of OCPs have not been fully elucidated, evidence suggests that ovulation suppression is not solely responsible. Work in primates indicates that progesterone may mediate apoptosis of ovarian epithelial cells, as well as changes in transforming growth factor β (TGF-β) production.[60,61] Clinically, progestin-only contraceptives, which do not reliably prevent ovulation, have also been noted to be as effective as combination OCPs in lowering risk of ovarian cancer,[62] and pills with higher levels of progesterone seem to confer greater benefit than those with lower doses.[63]

Without question, prophylactic surgery to remove the fallopian tubes and ovaries provides the greatest reduction in ovarian cancer risk for women carrying mutations in *BRCA1* and *BRCA2*. Generally, the procedure may be safely performed laparoscopically, as an outpatient procedure. Rebbeck et al[64] examined 259 mutation carriers undergoing prophylactic surgery in comparison with 292 matched controls. Among the mutation carriers, 6 women (2.3%) were diagnosed with occult ovarian carcinoma at the time of surgery and 2 (0.8%) went on to develop primary peritoneal cancer. In comparison, 58 control patients (19.9%) who did not undergo surgical prophylaxis developed subsequent ovarian cancer. Kauff et al[65] noted that prophylactic surgery decreased the risk of both ovarian cancer and breast cancer in mutation carriers. In a computer model of outcomes in a simulated cohort of 30-year-old mutation carriers, Grann et al[66] found that prophylactic oophorectomy was associated with a 2.6-year gain in life expectancy compared with surveillance alone. Another decision analysis by Schrag et al[67] noted a gain in life expectancy of 0.2–1.8 years for prophylactic oophorectomy.

As expected, this gain was most marked in women with high-penetrance mutations.

CONCLUSIONS

Patients with mutations at *BRCA1* and *BRCA2* are at high risk of developing ovarian cancer, although present evidence suggests that cancers in mutation carriers may present at earlier ages and have a more indolent course. Increased surveillance is an option for management, but risk-reducing options such as OCP use appear to be somewhat effective. Prophylactic removal of the fallopian tubes and ovaries appears to have the greatest potential to attenuate risk.

REFERENCES

1. Baker TR, Piver MS. Etiology, biology, and epidemiology of ovarian cancer. Semin Surg Oncol 1994;10:242–8.

2. Tortolero-Luna G, Mitchell MF, Rhodes-Morris HE. Epidemiology and screening of ovarian cancer. Obstet Gynecol Clin North Am 1994;21:1–23.

3. American Cancer Society. Cancer Facts and Figures 2007. http://www. cancer. org/docroot/ stt/stt _0.asp.

4. Lynch HT, Shaw MW, Magnuson CW, et al. Hereditary factors in cancer. Study of two large midwestern kindreds. Arch Intern Med 1966; 117:206–12.

5. Koch M, Gaedke H, Jenkins H. Family history of ovarian cancer patients: a case–control study. Int J Epidemiol 1989;18:782–5.

6. Hartge P, Schiffman MH, Hoover R, et al. A case–control study of epithelial ovarian cancer. Am J Obstet Gynecol 1989;161:10–16.

7. Schildkraut JM, Thompson WD. Familial ovarian cancer: a population-based case–control study. Am J Epidemiol 1988; 128:456–66.

8. Stratton JF, Pharoah P, Smith SK, et al. A systematic review and meta-analysis of family history and risk of ovarian cancer. Br J Obstet Gynaecol 1998;105:493–9.

9. Casagrande JT, Louie EW, Pike MC, et al. 'Incessant ovulation' and ovarian cancer. Lancet 1979;ii:170–3.

10. Kerlikowske K, Brown JS, Grady DG. Should women with familial ovarian cancer undergo prophylactic oophorectomy? Obstet Gynecol 1992;80:700–7.

11. Schildkraut JM, Risch N, Thompson WD. Evaluating genetic association among ovarian, breast, and endometrial cancer: evidence for a breast/ovarian cancer relationship. Am J Hum Genet 1989;45: 521–9.

12. Houlston RS, Collins A, Slack J, et al. Genetic epidemiology of ovarian cancer: segregation analysis. Ann Hum Genet 1991;55:291–9.

13. Bewtra C, Watson P, Conway T, et al. Hereditary ovarian cancer: a clinicopathological study. Int J Gynecol Pathol 1992;11: 180–7.

14. Narod SA, Madlensky L, Bradley L, et al. Hereditary and familial ovarian cancer in southern Ontario. Cancer 1994;74:2341–6.

15. Lynch HT, Lynch JF, Conway TA. Hereditary ovarian cancer. In: Rubin SC, Sutton GP, eds. Ovarian Cancer. New York: McGraw-Hill, 1993:189–217.

16. Miki Y, Swensen J, Shattuck-Eidens D, et al. A strong candidate for the breast and ovarian cancer susceptibility gene *BRCA1*. Science 1994;266:66–71.

17. Wooster R, Bignell G, Lancaster J, et al. Identification of the breast cancer suscepti-bility gene *BRCA2*. Nature 1995;378: 789–92.

18. Boyd J, Rubin SC. Hereditary ovarian cancer: molecular genetics and clinical implications. Gynecol Oncol 1997;64:196–206.

19. Bandera CA, Muto MG, Welch WR, et al. Genetic imbalance on chromosome 17 in papillary serous carcinoma of the peritoneum. Oncogene 1998;16:3455–9.

20. Takahashi H, Behbakht K, McGovern PE, et al. Mutation analysis of the *BRCA1* gene in ovar-ian cancers. Cancer Res 1995;55:2998–3002.

21. Malone KE, Daling JR, Thompson JD, et al. *BRCA1* mutations and breast cancer in the general population: analyses in women before age 35 years and in women before age 45 years with first-degree family history. JAMA 1998; 279:922–9.

22. Couch FJ, Hartmann LC. *BRCA1* testing – advances and retreats. JAMA 1998;279:955–7.

23. Robson M, Levin D, Federici M, et al. Breast conservation therapy for invasive breast cancer in Ashkenazi women with *BRCA* gene founder mutations. J Natl Cancer Inst 1999; 91:2112–17.

24. Ford D, Easton DF, Bishop DT, et al. Risks of can-cer in *BRCA1*-mutation carriers. Breast Cancer Linkage Consortium. Lancet 1994;343:692–5.

25. Boyd J, Sonoda Y, Federici MG, et al. Clinicopathologic features of *BRCA*-linked and sporadic ovarian cancer. JAMA 2000;283: 2260–5.

26. Moslehi R, Chu W, Karlan B, et al. *BRCA1* and *BRCA2* mutation analysis of 208 Ashkenazi Jewish women with ovarian cancer. Am J Hum Genet 2000;66:1259–72.

27. Newman B, Mu H, Butler LM, et al. Frequency of breast cancer attributable to *BRCA1* in a population-based series of American women. JAMA 1998;279:915–21.

28. Ford D, Easton DF, Stratton M, et al. Genetic heterogeneity and penetrance analysis of the *BRCA1* and *BRCA2* genes in breast cancer families. The Breast Cancer Linkage Consortium. Am J Hum Genet 1998;62:676–89.

29. Struewing JP, Hartge P, Wacholder S, et al. The risk of cancer associated with specific mutations of *BRCA1* and *BRCA2* among Ashkenazi Jews. N Engl J Med 1997;336:1401–8.

30. Risch HA, McLaughlin JR, Cole DE, et al. Prevalence and penetrance of germline *BRCA1* and *BRCA2* mutations in a popula-tion series of 649 women with ovarian cancer. Am J Hum Genet 2001;68:700–10.

31. Easton DF, Bishop DT, Ford D, et al. Genetic linkage analysis in familial breast and ovarian cancer: results from 214 families. The Breast Cancer Linkage Consortium. Am J Hum Genet 1993;52:678–701.

32. Rubin SC, Benjamin I, Behbakht K, et al. Clinical and pathological features of ovarian cancer in women with germ-line mutations of *BRCA1*. N Engl J Med 1996;335:1413–16.

33. Boyd J. Molecular genetics of hereditary ovarian cancer. In: Rubin SC, Sutton GP, eds. Ovarian Cancer, 2nd edn. Philadelphia: Lippincott Williams & Wilkins, 2001:3–22.

34. Aida H, Takakuwa K, Nagata H, et al. Clinical features of ovarian cancer in Japanese women with germ-line mutations of *BRCA1*. Clin Cancer Res 1998;4:235–40.

35. Ben David Y, Chetrit A, Hirsh-Yechezkel G, et al. Effect of *BRCA* mutations on the length

of survival in epithelial ovarian tumors. J Clin Oncol 2002;20:463–6.

36. Cass I, Baldwin RL, Varkey T, et al. Improved survival in women with *BRCA*-associated ovarian carcinoma. Cancer 2003; 97:2187–95.

37. Majdak EJ, Debniak J, Milczek T, et al. Prognostic impact of *BRCA1* pathogenic and *BRCA1/BRCA2* unclassified variant mutations in patients with ovarian carcinoma. Cancer 2005;104:1004–12.

38. Johannsson OT, Ranstam J, Borg A, et al. Survival of *BRCA1* breast and ovarian cancer patients: a population-based study from southern Sweden. J Clin Oncol 1998;16: 397–404.

39. Pharoah PD, Easton DF, Stockton DL, et al. Survival in familial, *BRCA1*-associated, and *BRCA2*-associated epithelial ovarian cancer. United Kingdom Coordinating Committee for Cancer Research (UKCCCR) Familial Ovarian Cancer Study Group. Cancer Res 1999;59:868–71.

40. Buller RE, Anderson B, Connor JP, et al. Familial ovarian cancer. Gynecol Oncol 1993;51:160–6.

41. McGuire V, Whittemore AS, Norris R, et al. Survival in epithelial ovarian cancer patients with prior breast cancer. Am J Epidemiol 2000;152:528–32.

42. Frank TS, Manley SA, Olopade OI, et al. Sequence analysis of *BRCA1* and *BRCA2*: correlation of mutations with family history and ovarian cancer risk. J Clin Oncol 1998; 16:2417–25.

43. Levine DA, Federici MG, Reuter VE, et al. Cell proliferation and apoptosis in *BRCA*-associated hereditary ovarian cancer. Gynecol Oncol 2002;85:431–4.

44. Xu X, Weaver Z, Linke SP, et al. Centrosome amplification and a defective G2-M cell cycle checkpoint induce genetic instability in *BRCA1* exon 11 isoform-deficient cells. Mol Cell 1999;3:389–95.

45. Yang H, Jeffrey PD, Miller J, et al. *BRCA2* function in DNA binding and recombination from a *BRCA2*-DSS1-ssDNA structure. Science 2002;297:1837–48.

46. Patel KJ, Yu VP, Lee H, et al. Involvement of *BRCA2* in DNA repair. Mol Cell 1998; 1:347–57.

47. Tirkkonen M, Johannsson O, Agnarsson BA, et al. Distinct somatic genetic changes associated with tumor progression in carriers of *BRCA1* and *BRCA2* germ-line mutations. Cancer Res 1997;57:1222–7.

48. Gretarsdottir S, Thorlacius S, Valgardsdottir R, et al. *BRCA2* and *p53* mutations in primary breast cancer in relation to genetic instability. Cancer Res 1998;58:859–62.

49. Xu X, Wagner KU, Larson D, et al. Conditional mutation of *BRCA1* in mammary epithelial cells results in blunted ductal morphogenesis and tumour formation. Nat Genet 1999;22:37–43.

50. Scully R, Anderson SF, Chao DM, et al. *BRCA1* is a component of the RNA polymerase II holoenzyme. Proc Natl Acad Sci USA 1997;94:5605–10.

51. Husain A, He G, Venkatraman ES, et al. *BRCA1* up-regulation is associated with repair-mediated resistance to *cis*-diamminedichloroplatinum(II). Cancer Res 1998;58:1120–3.

52. Mackey SE, Creasman WT. Ovarian cancer screening. J Clin Oncol 1995;13:783–93.

53. NIH consensus conference. Ovarian cancer. Screening, treatment, and follow-up. NIH Consensus Development Panel on Ovarian Cancer. JAMA 1995;273:491–7.

54. Burke W, Daly M, Garber J, et al. Recommendations for follow-up care of individuals with an inherited predisposition to cancer. II. *BRCA1* and *BRCA2*. Cancer Genetics Studies Consortium. JAMA 1997; 277:997–1003.

55. Skates SJ, Pauler DK, Jacobs IJ. Screening based on the risk of cancer calculation from

bayesian hierarchical changepoint and mixture models of longitudinal markers. J Am Stat Assoc 2001;96:429.

56. Botkin JR, Smith KR, Croyle RT, et al. Genetic testing for a *BRCA1* mutation: Prophylactic surgery and screening behavior in women 2 years post testing. Am J Med Genet 2003;118A:201–9.

57. Petricoin EF, Ardekani AM, Hitt BA, et al. Use of proteomic patterns in serum to identify ovarian cancer. Lancet 2002;359:572–7.

58. Narod SA, Risch H, Moslehi R, et al. Oral contraceptives and the risk of hereditary ovarian cancer. Hereditary Ovarian Cancer Clinical Study Group. N Engl J Med 1998;339:424–8.

59. Modan B, Hartge P, Hirsh-Yechezkel G, et al. Parity, oral contraceptives, and the risk of ovarian cancer among carriers and noncarriers of a *BRCA1* or *BRCA2* mutation. N Engl J Med 2001;345:235–40.

60. Rodriguez GC, Nagarsheth NP, Lee KL, et al. Progestin-induced apoptosis in the Macaque ovarian epithelium: differential regulation of transforming growth factor-beta. J Natl Cancer Inst 2002;94:50–60.

61. Rodriguez GC, Walmer DK, Cline M, et al. Effect of progestin on the ovarian epithelium of macaques: cancer prevention through apoptosis? J Soc Gynecol Invest 1998;5:271–6.

62. Rosenberg L, Palmer JR, Zauber AG, et al. A case–control study of oral contraceptive use and invasive epithelial ovarian cancer. Am J Epidemiol 1994;139:654–61.

63. Schildkraut JM, Calingaert B, Marchbanks PA, et al. Impact of progestin and estrogen potency in oral contraceptives on ovarian cancer risk. J Natl Cancer Inst 2002;94:32–8.

64. Rebbeck TR, Lynch HT, Neuhausen SL, et al. Prophylactic oophorectomy in carriers of *BRCA1* or *BRCA2* mutations. N Engl J Med 2002;346:1616–22.

65. Kauff ND, Satagopan JM, Robson ME, et al. Risk-reducing salpingo-oophorectomy in women with a *BRCA1* or *BRCA2* mutation. N Engl J Med 2002;346:1609–15.

66. Grann VR, Jacobson JS, Thomason D, et al. Effect of prevention strategies on survival and quality-adjusted survival of women with *BRCA1/2* mutations: an updated decision analysis. J Clin Oncol 2002;20:2520–9.

67. Schrag D, Kuntz KM, Garber JE, et al. Life expectancy gains from cancer prevention strategies for women with breast cancer and *BRCA1* or *BRCA2* mutations. JAMA 2000; 283:617–24.

Cell cycle and apoptotic markers

3

*John H Farley**

INTRODUCTION

The struggle between life and death in a cell is constant. This is the relentless battle being waged both at the molecular genomic level and at the cellular level. When there is an imbalance in these finely tuned processes, uncontrolled growth of the cellular population, or cancer, can be the outcome. Ovarian cancer is the most lethal gynecologic malignancy.[1] Despite the advent of multiple screening technologies, the majority of ovarian cancer patients still present at an advanced stage, and the survival for patients with advanced-stage disease is poor.[2] The recent genomic revolution has provided enormous information concerning the molecular characteristics of cancer. Identification and characterization of the genes and their protein products that contribute to the malignant phenotype can provide researchers with novel molecular targets that can be exploited in an attempt to improve ovarian cancer survival. In gynecologic oncology, we are now just beginning to investigate these new biologic therapies in the treatment of ovarian cancer.[3] There are a variety of cell surface receptors, signaling pathways, and nuclear proteins that stimulate cellular proliferation or inhibit cell death.

*The views expressed herein are those of the author and do not reflect the official policy or opinion of the Department of Defense or the United States Army or Navy.

An understanding of the cellular proteins that affect growth deregulation in ovarian cancers can provide a framework for the rational application and testing of these novel therapies.[4] This chapter will summarize our knowledge of these proteins and any association that they might have with prognosis and survival.

CELL CYCLE

Tumor suppressor genes

TP53

TP53 (encoding the p53 protein) is a tumor suppressor gene that inhibits cell cycle progression and responds to DNA damage, and its mutation is the most frequent genetic event described in ovarian cancer.[5,6] According to immunohistochemical evaluation, overexpression of p53 occurs in 45–55% of epithelial ovarian cancers.[6–9] In a univariate analysis p53 overexpression was a significant poor prognostic factor; however, after adjustment for stage, p53 overexpression did not retain statistical significance.[6]

The Gynecologic Oncology Group (GOG) sought to explain the apparent disparities in the literature regarding p53 overexpression and prognostic significance in epithelial ovarian cancer.[10] Overexpression (>30%) of p53 occurred in 56% of tumors, including 100% of patients with only missense mutation(s), 32% with truncation mutations, and 40% lacking a mutation in exons 2–11. Overexpression of p53 was associated with tumor grade but not with patient outcome. The median survival of patients with low p53 expression was 45 months, while overexpression was associated with a median survival of only 39 months (Figure 3.1).[10] These results intimate that it is the mutation in the *TP53* gene, not overexpression of p53, that is the significant molecular genetic event, and can be associated with a short-term survival benefit.[10] The prognostic implications of *TP53*/p53 are discussed in detail in Chapter 4.

nm23

Nucleoside diphosphate kinase (*nm23-H1*) is a candidate metastasis suppressor gene first characterized in breast cancer.[11] Along with absence of axillary lymph node metastases and hormonal therapy, nm23 protein expression was found to positively affect survival in breast cancer patients. In epithelial ovarian cancers,

expression of the nm23 kinase protein by immunohistochemistry is strongly upregulated, with 88% of ovarian cancers staining positively.[11] There is a trend towards decreased survival with focal staining of nm23 kinase. Although no statistical significance was found with nm23 protein expression in ovarian cancers, the pattern and intensity of protein staining may identify patients at high risk of tumor progression.[11]

BRCA1

While only responsible for approximately 5–10% of all new ovarian cancer cases, mutation of the breast and ovarian cancer susceptibility gene *BRCA1* has been associated with a 40–63% risk of developing ovarian cancer over a lifetime.[12] *BRCA1* is a putative tumor suppressor gene responsible for a hereditary ovarian cancer syndrome. BRCA1 protein expression has been analyzed by immunohistochemistry in normal ovarian surface epithelium and 119 epithelial ovarian tumors (19 benign, 24 borderline, and 76 malignant tumors).[13]

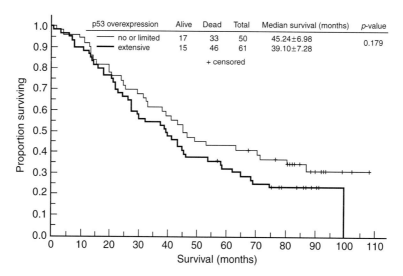

Figure 3.1 Kaplan–Meier survival analysis for p53 overexpression. Reproduced from Havrilesky et al. J Clin Oncol 2003;21:3814–25[10] with permission from the American Society of Clinical Oncology.

Ovarian surface epithelial cells were found to express BRCA1 protein. Decreased expression of BRCA1 was found in 16% of benign tumors, 38% of borderline tumors, and 72% of carcinomas. Methylation of *BRCA1* was not detected in benign or borderline tumors, but was present in 31% of carcinomas. Reduced expression of BRCA1 protein correlated with the presence of gene methylation. Unfortunately, the prognosis of ovarian carcinoma patients did not correlate with BRCA1 protein expression or genetic status.[13]

Loss of heterozygosity (LOH) at 17q21, the *BRCA1* locus, however, is seen in 40–70% of invasive ovarian cancers.[14] The frequency of *BRCA1* promoter hypermethylation as an epigenetic means of *BRCA1* inactivation has been evaluated for a large population-based cohort of ovarian cancer patients.[14] *BRCA1* hypermethylation was seen in 15% of the sporadic cancers analyzed in this study. Additionally, *BRCA1* methylation was only seen in ovarian cancer patients without a family history suggestive of a breast/ovarian cancer syndrome. Interestingly, none of the 12 tumors with *BRCA1* promoter hypermethylation demonstrated BRCA1 protein expression by immunohistochemistry. These findings suggested that reduced expression of BRCA1 protein along with genetic and epigenetic changes in the *BRCA1* gene play an important role in the development of sporadic ovarian carcinomas. As a result, promoter hypermethylation may be an alternative to mutation in causing the inactivation of the *BRCA1* tumor suppressor gene in sporadic ovarian cancer.[14]

RB2/p130

Members of the retinoblastoma protein (pRb) function as cell cycle regulators and modulate the sensitivity of cancer cells to chemotherapy.[15–17] pRb reactivity is found in approximately 47% of epithelial ovarian cancers.[16] Immunohistochemical analysis of 69 ovarian carcinomas for pRb expression revealed no association between pRb levels and certain clinicopathologic factors such as International Federation of Gynecologic Oncology (FIGO) stage, grade, and histologic type.[16] However, *RB2/p130* a member of the retinoblastoma gene family, maps to human chromosome 16q12.2, a region in which deletions have been found in ovarian carcinoma.[15] An examination of 45 ovarian cancer specimens by immunohistochemical and western blot analysis found pRb2/p130 expression to be localized to the nucleus. In contrast to benign non-neoplastic epithelium, where pRb2/p130 was localized to the nuclei, ovarian adenocarcinomas showed cytoplasmic staining as well. Primary ovarian adenocarcinomas showed loss or decrease of pRb2/p130 expression in 40% of tumors analyzed. pRb2/p130 expression was inversely related to tumor grade, with 73% of grade 1 and 2 cancers showing positive expression of pRb2/p130, while 61% of grade 3 tumors were negative for protein expression.[15] This suggests that *RB2/p130* may play a role as a tumor suppressor gene in ovarian cancer.

Protein kinases

Protein kinases are enzymes that covalently attach phosphates to the side-chains of serine, threonine, or tyrosine residues of specific proteins inside cells. Such phosphorylation of proteins can control their enzymatic activity, interactions with other proteins and molecules, and propensity for degradation by proteases. Perturbation of protein kinase signaling by mutations and other genetic alterations can result in deregulated kinase activity and malignant transformation.

Receptor tyrosine kinases

All receptor tyrosine kinases (RTKs) share several structural features. They are glycoproteins possessing an extracellular ligand-binding domain, which conveys ligand specificity, and a single hydrophobic transmembrane domain, which anchors the receptor to the membrane. Intracellular sequences typically contain regulatory regions in addition to the catalytic domain. Ligand binding induces activation of the intracellular tyrosine kinase domain, leading to the initiation of signaling events specific for the receptor. RTKs are organized into families based on sequence homology, structural characteristics, and distinct motifs in the extracellular domain. There are currently 19 known families in vertebrates. The various subfamilies include receptors for epidermal growth factor (EGF), platelet-derived growth factor (PDGF), vascular endothelial growth factor (VEGF), fibroblast growth factor (FGF), and hepatocyte growth factor (HGF). In malignant tumors, a number of receptors are overexpressed or mutated, leading to abnormal cell proliferation.

The epidermal growth factor receptor family (Erb family)

One of the best characterized pathways initiating malignant change in cell is the EFG receptor (EGFR) family of membrane proteins.[18] The EGFR family consists of four structurally similar RTK proteins: ErbB-1 (EGFR), ErbB-2 (HER2/neu), ErbB-3, and ErbB-4.[18] These receptors are activated by binding of ligands, including EGF, transforming growth factor α (TGF-α), amphiregulin, and the neuregulins. Dimerization of the EGFR complex then induces activation of Ras, Raf, mitogen-activated protein kinase (MAPK), and ultimately gene activation.[19] The biologic effects mediated by the EGFR family are quite broad, and include mediation of cell proliferation, development, differentiation, and oncogenesis.[18]

EGFR

In 96 cases of ovarian cancer, EGFR protein expression by immunohistochemistry was present in 39.8% of cancers analyzed.[20] The clinical significance of EGFR protein expression in the development and progression of human ovarian carcinoma was studied in 7 ovarian cystadenomas, 6 mucinous tumors of low malignant potential (LMP), and 25 invasive adenocarcinomas by immunohistochemistry. EGF and EGFR expression was found to be significantly higher in mucinous cystadenocarcinomas than in mucinous cystadenomas or mucinous tumors of LMP.[21] In a series of 226 patients with early-stage epithelial ovarian carcinomas, FIGO stages IA–IIC, a number of clinicopathological factors were studied in relation to p53 and EGFR protein expression.[22] In a Cox multivariate analysis, tumor grade, p53 status, and EGFR status were all independent and significant prognostic factors with regard to disease-free survival (DFS). A prognostic model proposed using these factors (grade 3, p53-positivity, and EGFR-positivity) found the poorest prognosis (39% DFS) for patients possessing all of these clinical factors.[22]

HER2

Studies have shown that the HER2 (ERBB2) oncogene is overexpressed in approximately 25–30% of ovarian carcinoma cases, but to date no consensus regarding overexpression and prognosis has been possible.[23,24] HER2 immunohistochemical staining of ovarian tissue is primarily a cytoplasmic stain; however, there is varying intensity of staining, requiring interpretation (Figure 3.2).[23] An immunohistochemical

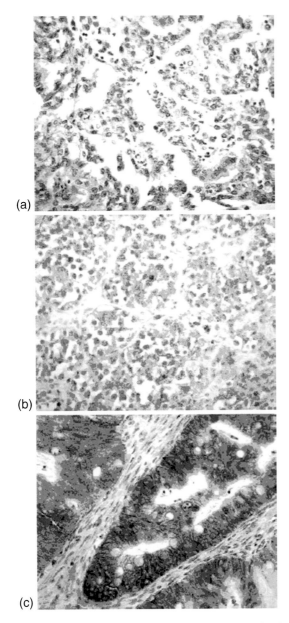

(a)

(b)

(c)

Figure 3.2 Examples of ovarian carcinoma tissue stained positively for HER2. Reproduced from Hogdall et al. Cancer 2003;98:66–73[23] with permission from John Wiley and Sons, Inc.

evaluation of HER2 protein expression performed on the first 181 patients included in the Danish MALOVA study diagnosed with epithelial ovarian carcinoma provided contrasting results.[23] HER2 overexpression was found in 52.5%

of these cases, in which 74.7% were weakly positive (1+) and 25.3% were moderately (2+) to intensely positive (3+). In this study, increased HER2 expression was found to be correlated with reduced survival.[23] Significant differences in survival between patients with positive HER2 expression and those without HER2 overexpression were found for the subgroups of FIGO stage I, stage III, and stage IV. For stage I, the 5-year survival rate for HER2-negative patients approached 100% compared with 71% for HER2-positive patients. For stage III and IV, the

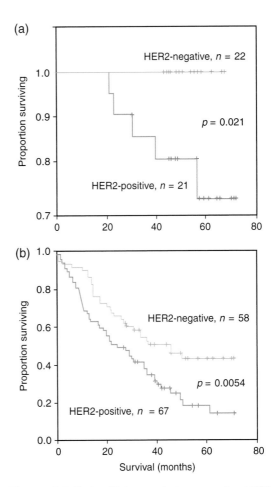

Figure 3.3 Kaplan–Meier survival curves for HER2 expression for FIGO stage I (a) and stage III/IV (b). Reproduced from Hogdall et al. Cancer 2003;98:66–73[23] with permission from John Wiley and Sons, Inc.

5-year survival rate for HER2-negative patients was approximately 45%, while for HER2-positive patients it was only 18% (Figure 3.3).[23] Multivariate survival analyses demonstrated HER2 overexpression to be a prognostic marker.

In another study that could explain the conflicting results in the literature regarding HER2 protein expression and survival, HER2 protein expression, and the frequency of HER2 amplification were examined in a series of 103 high-grade, advanced-stage (FIGO stage III or IV) ovarian surface epithelial carcinomas.[24] Only 5 of 102 (4.9%) tumors were positive for HER2 protein expression by immunohistochemistry. Over one-third (33.3%) of tumors, however, showed *HER2* amplification. Only 25% of cancers that showed *HER2* amplification by fluorescence in situ hybridization (FISH) were positive for HER2 protein overexpression by immunohistochemistry. There was no correlation between HER2 expression and survival.[24] Thus, the strong correlation between HER2 immunostaining and amplification characteristic of breast carcinoma might not be observed in ovarian carcinoma.

Endothelial growth factors; vascular endothelial growth factor

Angiogenesis is the formation of new blood vessels, a process required by many biologic processes, including the development of cancer.[25] New vessel formation can be stimulated by a variety of factors, including VEGF.[26,27] The VEGF family of glycoproteins consists of seven related growth factors: VEGF-A (known simply as VEGF) through VEGF-E and placental growth factor-1 and -2.[28] VEGF mediates angiogenic signals to the vascular endothelium through high-affinity RTKs that are thought to activate the MAPK pathway. Although many stimulators and inhibitors of angiogenesis have been identified, the trigger that causes a dormant tumor to transform into a proangiogenic tumor remains elusive.[29] Expression of VEGF in ovarian carcinomas by immunohistochemistry revealed focal or diffuse strong immunostaining in 48–51%.[30,31] In early-stage ovarian cancer, increased VEGF expression by immunohistochemistry was associated with a decreased disease-free survival of 18 months versus >120 months for VEGF nonexpressors.[32] In a multivariate analysis, only VEGF expression was associated with poorer survival in these early-stage ovarian cancer patients. Significant associations between VEGF expression and FIGO stage, histologic grade, and patient outcome have been observed.[31] The survival of patients with high VEGF expression was significantly worse than that of patients with low and absent VEGF expression. Multivariate analysis revealed that disease stage and VEGF expression were significant and independent prognostic indicators of overall survival time.

Inhibitors of cell cycle regulators

Phosphorylation of pRb by serine/threonine kinases known as cyclin-dependent kinases (cdks) inactivates pRb. The cdks form complexes with proteins called cyclins. There are at least nine cdks (cdk1,...,cdk9) and 15 cyclins (cyclin A,..., cyclin T).[33] cdk4 and cdk6 along with their D-type cyclins are responsible for the cell's progression through G_1 phase. cdk2 and cyclin E are responsible for the progression from G_1 to S phase. cdk2 and cyclin A are responsible for the progression through S phase, and cdk1 and cyclin B are required for mitosis. These complexes are in turn inhibited by a combination of small proteins called cdk inhibitors (CKIs). The INK4 (inhibitor of cdk4) family consists of p16^{INK4A}, p15^{INK4B}, p18^{INK4C}, and p19^{INK4D}, and specifically inhibit cyclin D-associated kinases. The protein kinase inhibitor protein family of p21$^{Waf1/Cip1}$, p27^{Kip1}, and p57^{Kip2} inhibit the cyclin E/cdk2 and cyclin A/cdk2 complexes. Loss of expression of CKIs confers a poor prognosis in a variety of cancers.[33]

Cyclin D

Cyclin D1 was evaluated in a panel of 79 epithelial ovarian carcinomas by immunohistochemical staining.[34] Expression of cyclin D1 was detected in 32.4% of epithelial cancers, 69.6% of borderline tumors, and 72.7% of benign tumors. Cyclin D1 expression correlated inversely with tumor grade.[34] Cyclin D1 overexpression was more frequently detected in borderline and grade 1 tumors than in grade 2 and grade 3 tumors. The expression of cyclin D1 was also examined in a consecutive series of 134 serous epithelial ovarian carcinomas using immunohistochemistry, and the results correlated with disease outcome. Nineteen percent of epithelial ovarian carcinomas were found to overexpress cyclin D1.[35] On multivariate analysis, overexpression of cyclin D1 combined with other molecular markers to include combined loss of p21$^{Waf1/Cip1}$ in the presence of p53 overexpression were independent predictors of reduced overall survival.[35] In another study of 70 patients with epithelial ovarian carcinomas followed for 8 years, the cyclin D1 content was analyzed by western blotting.[36] Patients with highly positive cyclin D1 tumors had shorter overall survival than patients with positive cyclin D1 (median survival 31 months vs 49 months). For patients with high cyclin D1 expression and residual disease >2 cm, the relative risks of death were 2.48 and 3.7, respectively.[36]

Cyclin E

Immunohistochemical expression of cyclin E was evaluated in 139 suboptimally debulked advanced epithelial ovarian cancer specimens from patients treated on GOG Protocol 111.[37] High cyclin E expression (≥40% cyclin E-positive tumor cells) was seen in 62 (45%) of the suboptimally debulked advanced ovarian cancer patients. Expression of cyclin E was not associated with age, race, stage, grade, cell type, or amount of residual disease. High versus low cyclin E expression was associated with a shorter median survival (29 months vs 35 months) and worse overall survival ($p < 0.05$) (Figure 3.4).[37] High cyclin E expression was also associated with a decreased survival when patients were stratified by FIGO stage III (Figure 3.5a), serous histology (Figure 3.5b), and platinum-based chemotherapy (Figure 3.6). High cyclin E expression was an independent poor prognostic factor for patients with advanced ovarian cancer, and it was associated with amplification of the cyclin E gene (*CCNE*) (Figure 3.7).[37] Clear cell carcinoma exhibits significantly increased expression of cyclin E.[38] The incidence of cyclin E staining was significantly higher in clear cell carcinoma (100%) than in either endometrioid carcinoma (50%) or poorly differentiated carcinoma (20%).

CKIs

p16^{INK4A}

Approximately 40–43% of epithelial ovarian cancers will overexpress p16^{INK4A} protein, while most benign tumors will show no p16^{INK4A} expression in the tumor cells.[39–41] The prognostic significance of the G$_1$ pathway was evaluated by immunohistochemical technique in 59 epithelial ovarian cancer patients undergoing surgery and platinum-based chemotherapy.[40] Abnormal expression of p16^{INK4A} was observed in 33.9% of studied cases. Abnormal G$_1$ pathway, alteration in p16^{INK4A}, pRb, or

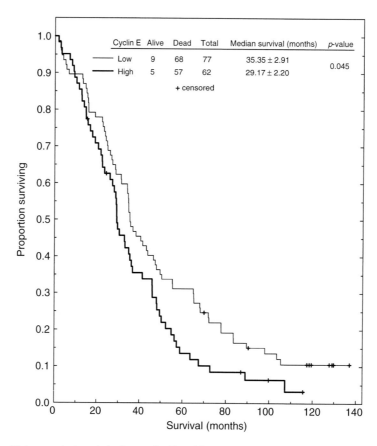

Cyclin E	Alive	Dead	Total	Median survival (months)	p-value
Low	9	68	77	35.35 ± 2.91	
High	5	57	62	29.17 ± 2.20	0.045

+ censored

Figure 3.4 Kaplan–Meier survival analysis for cyclin E-positive tumor cells in women with suboptimally debulked advanced ovarian cancer. Reproduced from Farley et al, Cancer Res 2003;63:1235–41[37] with permission from the American Association for Cancer Research.

cyclinD1/cdk4 were detected in 49.2% of cases. Although individually p16[INK4A] overexpression was not of prognostic significance, univariate analyses identified abnormal G_1 pathway (HR 2.935; $p = 0.03$) as prognostic factors for overall survival.[40] When the combined phenotypes of cdk4/p16[INK4A] expression are examined, patients with cdk4-positive/p16[INK4A]-negative expression have a reduced overall survival.

p21[Waf1/Cip1] and p27[Kip1]

The CKI family of protein inhibitors p21[Waf1/Cip1], p27[Kip1], and p57[Kip2] inhibit cdk2–cyclin complexes. Using immunohistochemistry, the frequency of expression and the possible prognostic significance have been examined in a series of 185 uniformly treated patients with stage III ovarian cancer.[42] p21[Waf1/Cip1] has been found to be overexpressed in 48% of cases.[42,43] Neither p21[Waf1/Cip1] nor p27[Kip1] expression was of prognostic significance for the whole group of patients. Western blot analysis of p21[Waf1/Cip1], however, appeared to confirm the significance of this CKI in ovarian cancer prognosis. p21[Waf1/Cip1] levels were examined in a series of 102 ovarian tissue samples, including normal ovary, primary ovarian tumors, omental metastasis, recurrent disease, and residual tumor after chemotherapy.[44] p21[Waf1/Cip1] was detectable in

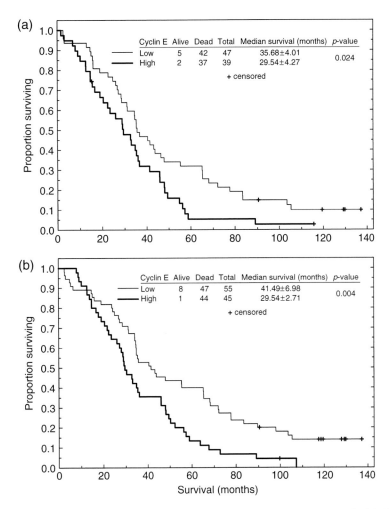

Figure 3.5 Kaplan–Meier survival analysis for cyclin E expression in women with suboptimally debulked ovarian cancer by tumor stage (FIGO stage III) (a) and cell type (serous adenocarcinoma) (b). Reproduced from Farley et al, Cancer Res 2003;63:1235–41[37] with permission from the American Association for Cancer Research.

74% of ovarian tissue samples. In the subgroup of stage III–IV ovarian cancer patients, p21[Wafl/Cip1]-positive cases showed a more favorable prognosis, with a 3-year time to progression (TTP) rate of 58% for p21[Wafl/Cip1]-positive patients, compared with 33% for p21[Wafl/Cip1]-negative patients.

CDKN1B, encoding p27[Kip1], is a potential tumor suppressor gene. p27[Kip1] expression has been evaluated by immunohistochemistry and western blot analysis in a series of 82 epithelial ovarian tumors, 16 of which were classified as LMP and 66 as primary ovarian adenocarcinomas.[45] Analysis revealed frequent loss of p27[Kip1] expression in 33% of primary ovarian adenocarcinomas, compared with only 6% of LMP tumors. In addition to nuclear staining, cytoplasmic localization of p27[Kip1] was noted in 55%. There was a significant correlation between presence of p27[Kip1] staining and a longer time to progression.[45] p27[Kip1] status was then assessed by immunohistochemical analysis of tissue sections from primary tumors of 99 patients with stages III–IV ovarian carcinoma.

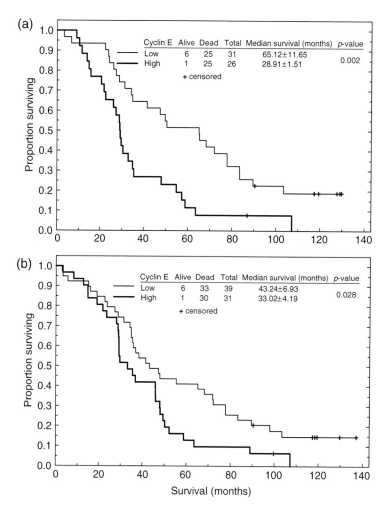

Figure 3.6 Kaplan–Meier survival analysis for cyclin E expression in women with suboptimally debulked ovarian cancer by residual disease (nonmeasurable tumor) (a) and treatment (cisplatin plus paclitaxel) (b). Reproduced from Farley et al, Cancer Res 2003;63:1235–41[37] with permission from the American Association for Cancer Research.

p27[Kip1] expression was detected in 47% patients.[46] Although p27[Kip1] expression did not correlate with any of the classical clinicopathologic parameters, the 5-year TTP rate in p27[Kip1]-positive patients was 50% compared with 11% in p27[Kip1]-negative patients. p27[Kip1]-positive cases showed a 5-year overall survival rate of 53%, compared with 43% for p27[Kip1]-negative cases. In multivariate analysis, p27[Kip1] expression was an independent predictor of progression of disease and survival.[46]

The location of p27[Kip1] staining in the cell appears to be of clinical importance when interpreting p27[Kip1] immunohistochemical staining (Figure 3.8).[47,48] Analysis by the present author of p27[Kip1] nuclear staining in advanced ovarian cancer revealed no difference in survival for p27[Kip1] expressors versus nonexpressors. Decreased nuclear staining has been associated with shorter survival, as has cytoplasmic localization of p27[Kip1].[47,48] Subcellular localization of p27[Kip1] was evaluated

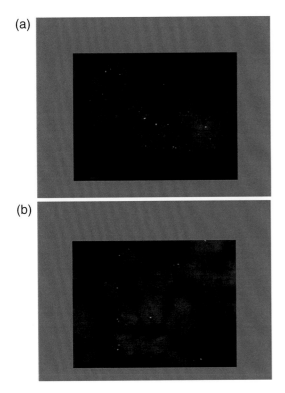

(a)

(b)

Figure 3.7 Representative fluorescence in situ hybridization (FISH) analysis of low cyclin E expressor by immunohistochemistry (a) and high cyclin E protein expressor by immunohistochemistry and corresponding amplification of chromosome 19q (b). Reproduced from Farley et al, Cancer Res 2003;63:1235–41[37] with permission from the American Association for Cancer Research.

using tissue microarrays containing 421 cases of ovarian carcinoma.[48] Nuclear-only staining was associated with a 58% 5-year survival rate, while negative (<5%) and cytoplasmic staining was associated with only a 30–32% 5-year survival rate (Figure 3.9a). The presence of p27[Kip1] in the cytoplasm regardless of the nuclear stain correlated strongly with late-stage disease, extent of cytoreduction, and shorter disease-specific survival (Figure 3.9b).

MAPK pathway; Ras proteins

The *RAS* superfamily of genes encodes small guanosine triphosphate (GTP)-binding proteins that are responsible for regulation of many cellular processes, including differentiation, cytoskeletal organization, and protein trafficking. Each Ras protein consists of approximately 190 amino acid residues.[49] Activated Ras activates Raf, which is a serine/threonine kinase. Raf activates MEK (MAPK/ERK kinase, also known as MAPKK), which in turn activates mitogen-activated protein kinase (MAPK, also know as extracellular regulated kinase, ERK). The central kinase in this pathway, MEK, is a critical signaling protein for multiple oncogenic pathways, including the EGFR family, VEGF, PDGF, and activated Ras. MAPK activation also results in phosphorylation and activation of ribosomal S6 kinase and transcription factors such as Jun, Myc, and Fos, resulting in the switching on of a number of genes associated with proliferation. Mutant oncogenic forms of Ras (H-Ras, N-Ras, K-Ras A, and K-Ras B) have been found in up to 30% of all human cancers and 4% of epithelial ovarian cancers. The presence of *RAS* mutations in gynecologic malignancies appears to be a rare event. In one extensive study, only one cystadenoma (5%), six LMP tumors (30%), and one ovarian carcinoma (4%) demonstrated an activated *KRAS* gene.[50]

ARHI

No more than 20% of invasive cancers exhibit *RAS* mutations. Functional activation of the Ras pathway in the absence of genetic mutations has, however, been reported in a majority of ovarian cancer cell lines.[51,52] As a result, certain members of the *RAS* superfamily may act as tumor suppressor genes rather than as protooncogenes. Ras homolog gene family, member I (*ARHI*) is a maternally imprinted putative human tumor suppressor gene that maps to chromosome 1p31 and that encodes a 26 kDa small G-protein with 60% homology

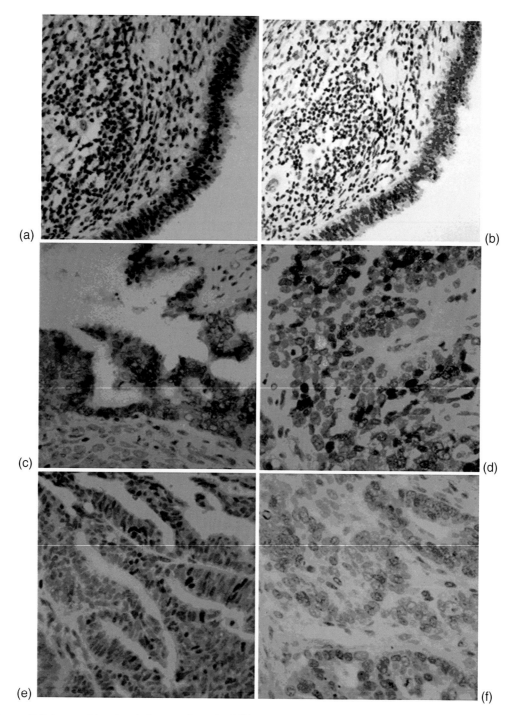

Figure 3.8 Immunohistochemical expression of p27^{Kip1} in benign and invasive ovarian cancers. Photomicrographs of representative p27^{Kip1} staining in a benign ovarian epithelial tumor (a: 600×), a corresponding benign negative control (b: 600×), an epithelial low-malignant-potential tumor (c: 700×), a stage I epithelial ovarian tumor (d: 1000×), a stage II epithelial ovarian tumor (e: 700×), and a stage III epithelial adenocarcinoma (f: 700×). Reproduced from Hurteau et al. Gynecol Oncol 2001;83:292–8[47] with permission from Academic Press.

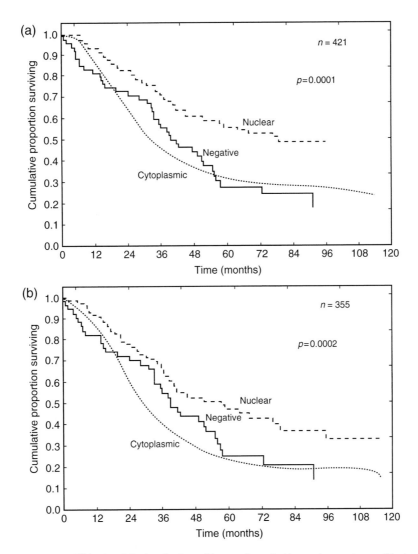

Figure 3.9 Association of p27^{Kip1} subcellular localization with overall survival in ovarian carcinoma (Kaplan–Meier analysis): (a) all ovarian cancer cases; (b) late-stage disease. Reproduced from Rosen et al. Clin Cancer Res 2005;11:632-7[48] with permission from the American Association for Cancer Research.

to Rap and Ras.[52] *ARHI* is expressed in normal ovarian epithelial cells but downregulated in most ovarian cancer cell lines.[52] Analysis by immuno-histochemistry demonstrates strong ARHI protein expression in the surface epithelial cells of benign ovarian cysts and follicles. This protein expression is reduced in LMP tumors of the ovary, and in frankly malignant invasive ovarian cancers ARHI protein was downregulated in

63% and expression of the gene was lost altogether in 47%.[52] A 5-year survival rate of 39% was observed in patients whose tumors had strong expression of ARHI, 43% in those with weak expression, compared with 33% in those with negative expression. ARHI expression correlated with p21$^{Waf1/Cip1}$ protein expression and was associated with a prolonged disease-free survival but not overall survival.

MAPK

MAPK plays a pivotal role in signal transduction. Evaluation of the expression of active MAPK in ovarian serous carcinomas was assessed by immunohistochemistry in 207 cases.[53] Forty-five percent of ovarian serous carcinomas were positive for MAPK expression. There was a lower frequency of expression of active MAPK in high-grade ovarian serous carcinomas (41%) compared with low-grade serous tumors (81%). Active MAPK was present in all of the 19% low-grade tumors with either *KRAS* or *BRAF* mutations, as well as in 41% of tumors with wild-type *KRAS* and *BRAF*.[53] In advanced FIGO stage serous ovarian carcinomas, expression of active MAPK alone served as a good survival indicator in the 2-year follow-up but not in the 5-year follow-up. Active MAPK appears to be more frequently expressed in low-grade than in high-grade ovarian serous carcinomas, and as a result may provide a therapeutic target in these tumors. Active MAPK could also serve as a good prognostic marker in patients with high-grade serous carcinomas.

APOPTOSIS

Bcl-2 family

The Bcl-2 and p53 gene products have both been linked to cell death by apoptosis. The expression of Bcl-2 was studied in normal ovaries and in ovarian tumors by immunohistochemical analysis.[54] Normal epithelium was strongly stained positive for Bcl-2 in all ovaries examined. Forty-eight percent of malignant tumors showed strong Bcl-2 staining. The expression of Bcl-2 in malignant tumor cells appeared to be inversely correlated with the expression of p53, and this has been confirmed in

other studies.[55] Bcl-2 expression correlated with survival and with significantly reduced survival in weakly and unstained groups compared with those patients having strongly stained malignant tumor cells. Using molecular and immunohistochemical analyses, p53 and the products of its downstream genes $p21^{Waf1/Cip1}$, Bax, and Bcl-2 were evaluated in ovarian tumor tissues.[56] Bcl-2 expression was not associated with increased rates of progression and death. Bax expression was found to be associated with both progression-free and overall survival. Those patients who simultaneously expressed Bax and Bcl-2 had longer progression-free and overall survivals compared with patients whose tumors did not express Bcl-2.[56]

Survivin

Survivin is a newly discovered member of the IAP (inhibitors of apoptosis proteins) family, selectively overexpressed in common human cancers but not in normal adult tissues, and associated with aggressiveness of the disease and unfavorable outcomes. Analysis of serial frozen sections for survivin protein expression in 26 patients with ovarian epithelial carcinoma and 10 patients with benign cystadenoma of the ovary by fluorescent immunohistochemistry revealed that survivin was weakly detected in some benign ovarian cystadenomas (0–12.1%).[57] There was, however, abundant survivin immunoreactivity in the nucleus and/or cytoplasm of the epithelial ovarian carcinoma cells. An immunohistochemical analysis of 103 cases of epithelial ovarian tumors showed survivin overexpression in 21.2% of benign tumors, 47.8% of borderline tumors, and 51.1% (24 of 47) of ovarian carcinomas.[58] Overexpression of survivin was significantly correlated with the size of residual disease.[58]

Patients with survivin overexpression were also found to have a short overall survival. Survivin was also investigated in 110 primary ovarian cancer patients by immunohistochemistry.[35] Cytoplasmic survivin immunoreaction was observed in 84.5% cases, while nuclear survivin immunostaining was observed in 29.1% of cases. There was no relationship between cytoplasmic survivin positivity rate and any of the clinical parameters examined. Serous tumors showed a lower percentage of nuclear survivin positivity with respect to other histotypes (20.5% vs 48.6%, respectively). Bcl-2 and p53 expression was not correlated with survivin status. There was no difference in time to progression and overall survival according to survivin status in ovarian cancer patients.[35]

Cellular apoptosis susceptibility protein

The cellular apoptosis susceptibility (*CAS*) gene is the human homolog of the yeast chromosome segregation gene *CSE* and is located on 20q13.[59] CAS protein is a cytoplasmic antigen that is highly expressed in proliferating cells, but only at low levels in cells that do not proliferate. In normal cells, CAS is considered to function as a 'switch', determining whether a cell will proliferate or undergo apoptosis.[59] Investigation of CAS in serous ovarian carcinoma by immunohistochemistry revealed CAS expression to be negative in serous cystadenomas and LMP tumors. In contrast, moderate or strong immunostaining was observed in

34 of 41 cases (83%) of serous carcinomas.[59] Another study analyzed CAS protein expression immunohistochemically and compared it with prognosis and the expression of the cell cycle-associated proteins pRb, cyclin D1, and p53 on paraffin-embedded tissue from 69 ovarian carcinomas. CAS reactivity was present in 100% of these cancers analyzed, pRb in 54%, cyclin D1 in 47%, and p53 in 49%.[16] Significant reciprocal correlation was observed between high levels of CAS and histologic type, FIGO stage III, and grade 3. In univariate analysis, CAS levels predicted outcome.[16]

CONCLUSIONS

With the discovery and mapping of the human genome, molecular approaches to the treatment of cancer are becoming even more pervasive. Logical, systematic, targeted approaches to the treatment of all malignancies in general and gynecologic malignancies specifically are becoming the standard of care. The shotgun approach of chemotherapy or radiotherapy is rapidly becoming a modality of the past. Recently, bevacizumab, (rhuMAb VEGF), a recombinant humanized version of a murine anti-human VEGF monoclonal antibody has displayed activity in refractory ovarian cancer.[60] A minimal understanding of the basic concepts of life and death in the cell is essential for the gynecologic oncologist as we approach this new molecular era. Hopefully, this review will provide some of these building blocks.

REFERENCES

1. American Cancer Society. Cancer Facts and Figures 2007. http://www.cancer.org/docroot/stt/stt_0.asp.

2. McGuire WP, Hoskins WJ, Brady MF, et al. Comparison of combination therapy with paclitaxel and cisplatin versus cyclophosphamide and cisplatin in patients with suboptimal stage III and stage IV ovarian cancer: a Gynecologic Oncology Group study. Semin Oncol 1997;24:S2-13–16.

3. Bookman MA. Biologic therapies for gynecologic cancer. Curr Opin Oncol 1995;7: 478–84.

4. Bookman MA. Biological therapy for gynecologic malignancies. Cancer Treat Res 1998;95:115–47.

5. Casey G, Lopez ME, Ramos JC, et al. DNA sequence analysis of exons 2 through 11 and immunohistochemical staining are required to detect all known *p53* alterations in human malignancies. Oncogene 1996;13:1971–81.

6. Eltabbakh GH, Belinson JL, Kennedy AW, et al. p53 overexpression is not an independent prognostic factor for patients with primary ovarian epithelial cancer. Cancer 1997;80: 892–8.

7. Geisler JP, Geisler HE, Miller GA, et al. p53 and bcl-2 in epithelial ovarian carcinoma: their value as prognostic indicators at a median follow-up of 60 months. Gynecol Oncol 2000;77:278–82.

8. Baekelandt M, Kristensen GB, Nesland JM, Trope CG, Holm R. Clinical significance of apoptosis-related factors p53, Mdm2, and Bcl-2 in advanced ovarian cancer. J Clin Oncol 1999;17:2061.

9. Hartmann LC, Podratz KC, Keeney GL, et al. Prognostic significance of p53 immunostaining in epithelial ovarian cancer. J Clin Oncol 1994;12:64–9.

10. Havrilesky L, Darcy M, Hamdan H, et al. Prognostic significance of *p53* mutation and p53 overexpression in advanced epithelial ovarian cancer: a Gynecologic Oncology Group Study. J Clin Oncol 2003;21:3814–25.

11. Srivatsa PJ, Cliby WA, Keeney GL, et al. Elevated nm23 protein expression is correlated with diminished progression-free survival in patients with epithelial ovarian carcinoma. Gynecol Oncol 1996;60:363–72.

12. Romagnolo D, Annab LA, Thompson TE, et al. Estrogen upregulation of *BRCA1* expression with no effect on localization. Mol Carcinog 1998;22:102–9.

13. Wang C, Horiuchi A, Imai T, et al. Expression of BRCA1 protein in benign, borderline, and malignant epithelial ovarian neoplasms and its relationship to methylation and allelic loss of the *BRCA1* gene. J Pathol 2004;202: 215–23.

14. Baldwin RL, Nemeth E, Tran H, et al. *BRCA1* promoter region hypermethylation in ovarian carcinoma: a population-based study. Cancer Res 2000;60:5329–33.

15. D'Andrilli G, Masciullo V, Bagella L, et al. Frequent loss of pRb2/p130 in human ovarian carcinoma. Clin Cancer Res 2004; 10:3098–103.

16. Peiro G, Diebold J, Lohrs U. *CAS* (cellular apoptosis susceptibility) gene expression in ovarian carcinoma: correlation with 20q13.2 copy number and cyclin D1, p53, and Rb protein expression. Am J Clin Pathol 2002; 118:922–9.

17. Tonini T, Gabellini C, Bagella L, et al. pRb2/p130 decreases sensitivity to apoptosis induced by camptothecin and doxorubicin but not by taxol. Clin Cancer Res 2004; 10:8085–93.

18. Arteaga CL, Khuri F, Krystal G, Sebti S. Overview of rationale and clinical trials with signal transduction inhibitors in lung cancer. Semin Oncol 2002;29:15–26.

19. Vogel CL, Cobleigh MA, Tripathy D, et al. Efficacy and safety of trastuzumab as a single agent in first-line treatment of HER2-overexpressing metastatic breast cancer. J Clin Oncol 2002;20:719–26.

20. Owens OJ, Stewart C, Leake RE, McNicol AM. A comparison of biochemical and immunohistochemical assessment of EGFR expression in ovarian cancer. Anticancer Res 1992;12:1455–8.

21. Niikura H, Sasano H, Sato S, Yajima A. Expression of epidermal growth factor-related proteins and epidermal growth factor receptor in common epithelial ovarian tumors. Int J Gynecol Pathol 1997;16:60–8.

22. Skirnisdottir I, Seidal T, Sorbe B. A new prognostic model comprising p53, EGFR, and tumor grade in early stage epithelial ovarian carcinoma and avoiding the problem of inaccurate surgical staging. Int J Gynecol Cancer 2004;14:259–70.

23. Hogdall EV, Christensen L, Kjaer SK, et al. Distribution of HER-2 overexpression in ovarian carcinoma tissue and its prognostic value in patients with ovarian carcinoma: from the Danish MALOVA Ovarian Cancer Study. Cancer 2003;98:66–73.

24. Lee CH, Huntsman DG, Cheang MC, et al. Assessment of Her-1, Her-2, And Her-3 expression and Her-2 amplification in advanced stage ovarian carcinoma. Int J Gynecol Pathol 2005;24:147–52.

25. Paley PJ. Angiogenesis in ovarian cancer: molecular pathology and therapeutic strategies. Curr Oncol Rep 2002;4:165–74.

26. Pegram M, Hsu S, Lewis G, et al. Inhibitory effects of combinations of HER-2/neu antibody and chemotherapeutic agents used for treatment of human breast cancers. Oncogene 1999;18:2241–51.

27. Aguilar Z, Akita RW, Finn RS, et al. Biologic effects of heregulin/neu differentiation factor on normal and malignant human breast and ovarian epithelial cells. Oncogene 1999;18:6050–62.

28. Starling N, Cunningham D. Monoclonal antibodies against vascular endothelial growth factor and epidermal growth factor receptor in advanced colorectal cancers: present and future directions. Curr Opin Oncol 2004;16:385–90.

29. D'Amato RJ, Loughnan MS, Flynn E, Folkman J. Thalidomide is an inhibitor of angiogenesis. Proc Natl Acad Sci USA 1994;91:4082–5.

30. Brustmann H. Vascular endothelial growth factor expression in serous ovarian carcinoma: relationship with topoisomerase II alpha and prognosis. Gynecol Oncol 2004;95:16–22.

31. Shen GH, Ghazizadeh M, Kawanami O, et al. Prognostic significance of vascular endothelial growth factor expression in human ovarian carcinoma. Br J Cancer 2000;83:196–203.

32. Paley PJ, Staskus KA, Gebhard K, et al. Vascular endothelial growth factor expression in early stage ovarian carcinoma. Cancer 1997;80:98–106.

33. Farley JH, Birrer MJ. Biologic directed therapies in gynecologic oncology. Curr Oncol Rep 2003;5:459–67.

34. Sui L, Tokuda M, Ohno M, Hatase O, Hando T. The concurrent expression of p27^{kip1} and cyclin D1 in epithelial ovarian tumors. Gynecol Oncol 1999;73:202–9.

35. Bali A, O'Brien P, Edwards L, et al. Cyclin D1, p53, and p21$^{Wafl\Cip1}$ expression is predictive of poor clinical outcome in serous epithelial ovarian cancer. Clin Cancer Res 2004;10:5168–77.

36. Barbieri F, Lorenzi P, Ragni N, et al. Overexpression of cyclin D1 is associated with poor survival in epithelial ovarian cancer. Oncology 2004;66:310–15.

37. Farley J, Smith LM, Darcy KM, et al. Cyclin E expression is a significant predictor of survival in advanced, suboptimally debulked ovarian epithelial cancers: a Gynecologic Oncology Group study. Cancer Res 2003;63:1235–41.

38. Shimizu M, Nikaido T, Toki T, Shiozawa T, Fujii S. Clear cell carcinoma has an expression pattern of cell cycle regulatory molecules that is unique among ovarian adenocarcinomas. Cancer 1999;85:669–77.

39. Dong Y, Walsh MD, McGuckin MA, et al. Increased expression of cyclin-dependent kinase inhibitor 2 (CDKN2A) gene product P16^{INK4A} in ovarian cancer is associated with progression and unfavourable prognosis. Int J Cancer 1997;74:57–63.

40. Kusume T, Tsuda H, Kawabata M, et al. The p16–cyclin D1/CDK4–pRb pathway and clinical outcome in epithelial ovarian cancer. Clin Cancer Res 1999;5:4152–7.

41. Sui L, Dong Y, Ohno M, et al. Inverse expression of Cdk4 and p16 in epithelial ovarian tumors. Gynecol Oncol 2000;79:230–7.

42. Baekelandt M, Holm R, Trope CG, Nesland JM, Kristensen GB. Lack of independent prognostic significance of p21 and p27 expression in advanced ovarian cancer: an immunohistochemical study. Clin Cancer Res 1999;5:2848–53.

43. Harlozinska A, Bar JK, Montenarh M, Kartarius S. Relations between immunologically different p53 forms, p21^{WAF1} and PCNA expression in ovarian carcinomas. Oncol Rep 2002;9:1173–9.

44. Ferrandina G, Stoler A, Fagotti A, et al. p21$^{WAF1/CIP1}$ protein expression in primary ovarian cancer. Int J Oncol 2000;17: 1231–5.

45. Masciullo V, Sgambato A, Pacilio C, et al. Frequent loss of expression of the cyclin-dependent kinase inhibitor p27 in epithelial ovarian cancer. Cancer Res 1999;59:3790–4.

46. Masciullo V, Ferrandina G, Pucci B, et al. p27^{Kip1} expression is associated with clinical outcome in advanced epithelial ovarian cancer: multivariate analysis. Clin Cancer Res 2000; 6:4816–22.

47. Hurteau JA, Allison BM, Brutkiewicz SA, et al. Expression and subcellular localization of the cyclin-dependent kinase inhibitor p27^{Kip1} in epithelial ovarian cancer. Gynecol Oncol 2001;83:292–8.

48. Rosen DG, Yang G, Cai KQ, et al. Subcellular localization of p27^{kip1} expression predicts poor prognosis in human ovarian cancer. Clin Cancer Res 2005;11:632–7.

49. Adjei AA, Hidalgo M. Intracellular signal transduction pathway proteins as targets for cancer therapy. J Clin Oncol 2005;23: 5386–403.

50. Teneriello MG, Ebina M, Linnoila RI, et al. p53 and Ki-ras gene mutations in epithelial ovarian neoplasms. Cancer Res 1993;53: 3103–8.

51. Mammas IN, Zafiropoulos A, Spandidos DA. Involvement of the ras genes in female genital tract cancer. Int J Oncol 2005;26:1241–55.

52. Rosen DG, Wang L, Jain AN, et al. Expression of the tumor suppressor gene ARHI in epithelial ovarian cancer is associated with increased expression of p21$^{WAF1/CIP1}$ and prolonged progression-free survival. Clin Cancer Res 2004;10:6559–66.

53. Hsu CY, Bristow R, Cha MS, et al. Characterization of active mitogen-activated protein kinase in ovarian serous carcinomas. Clin Cancer Res 2004;10:6432–6.

54. Athanassiadou P, Petrakakou E, Sakelariou V, et al. Expression of p53, bcl-2 and heat shock protein (hsp72) in malignant and benign ovarian tumours. Eur J Cancer Prev 1998;7:225–31.

55. Chan WY, Cheung KK, Schorge JO, et al. Bcl-2 and p53 protein expression, apoptosis, and p53 mutation in human epithelial ovarian cancers. Am J Pathol 2000;156:409–17.

56. Schuyer M, van der Burg ME, Henzen-Logmans SC, et al. Reduced expression of BAX is associated with poor prognosis in patients with epithelial ovarian cancer: a multifactorial analysis of TP53, p21, BAX and BCL-2. Br J Cancer 2001;85:1359–67.

57. Takai N, Miyazaki T, Nishida M, Nasu K, Miyakawa I. Expression of survivin is associated with malignant potential in epithelial ovarian carcinoma. Int J Mol Med 2002;10:211–16.

58. Sui L, Dong Y, Ohno M, et al. Survivin expression and its correlation with cell proliferation and prognosis in epithelial ovarian tumors. Int J Oncol 2002;21:315–20.

59. Brustmann H. Expression of cellular apoptosis susceptibility protein in serous ovarian carcinoma: a clinicopathologic and immunohistochemical study. Gynecol Oncol 2004;92:268–76.

60. Monk BJ, Choi DC, Pugmire G, Burger RA. Activity of bevacizumab (rhuMAB VEGF) in advanced refractory epithelial ovarian cancer. Gynecol Oncol 2005;96:902–5.

TP53/p53 as a prognostic factor

4

Stephen L Rose

REVIEW OF TUMOR SUPPRESSOR GENES

Tumor suppressor genes are responsible for the inhibition of unchecked cellular proliferation. These genes were first speculated to exist when combinations of tumor cells and normal cells produced hybrids that lacked the proliferative capacities of malignant cells, but showed characteristics of the normal cell line.[1] While studying pediatric retinoblastoma in 1971, Knudson proposed that two allelic events or 'hits' were necessary for conversion to a malignant cell. In heritable cancers, the first event was proposed to be a germline mutation leading to allelic heterogeneity.[2] The second event would then be a somatic mutation leading to a loss of heterozygosity (LOH) and the malignant phenotype. This became known as the 'two-hit hypothesis' (Figure 4.1). In sporadic cancers, one 'hit' is usually a point mutation, while the second 'hit' is usually deletion of all or a part of a chromosome. In fact, the second 'hit' in both sporadic and heritable cancers may come from any number of mechanisms, including nondisjunction, mitotic recombination, deletion, point mutation, or silencing due to methylation. Although the two-hit hypothesis is a widely recognized model for the development of hereditary cancers, it should not be extrapolated to tumors beyond heritable pediatric cancers, for which it was originally described.[3]

The mutant tumor suppressor gene alone may or may not be sufficient for the development of cancer, and many adult tumors have been shown to require multiple mutations for tumorigenesis to occur. In fact, tumor suppressor genes may exert their effects in multiple ways, leading Kinzler and Vogelstein[4] to suggest that tumor suppressor genes be further subdivided into 'gatekeepers' and 'caretakers'. Gatekeepers are genes that directly inhibit the growth or promote the death of tumor cells. Examples of gatekeepers would include the retinoblastoma (*RB1*), von Hippel–Lindau (*VHL*), neurofibromatosis type 1 (*NF1*), and adenomatous polyposis coli (*APC*) genes, as well as *TP53*. The two-hit hypothesis provides the classic model for inactivation of these genes. Caretaker genes, on the other hand, are genes that maintain the integrity of the genome. Their inactivation does not directly lead to tumor initiation, but leads to genetic instability which then increases the risk of mutation in all genes. Examples of caretaker genes include the nucleotide excision repair genes that are responsible for xeroderma pigmentosa, the mismatch repair genes that cause hereditary nonpolyposis colorectal cancer, the *ATM* gene, and the *BRCA1* and *BRCA2* genes.

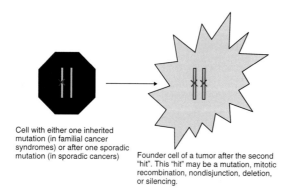

Cell with either one inherited mutation (in familial cancer syndromes) or after one sporadic mutation (in sporadic cancers)

Founder cell of a tumor after the second "hit". This "hit" may be a mutation, mitotic recombination, nondisjunction, deletion, or silencing.

Figure 4.1 The Knudson Two Hit Hypothesis. In hereditary cancers, the first allelic mutation is inherited, whereas in sporadic cancers the first hit may be a sporadic mutation or other mechanism of silencing. The second allelic "hit" which gives rise to the founder cell of a tumor may come from mutation, mitotic recombination, nondysjunction, deletion or silencing.

TP53 FUNCTION AND REGULATION

The *TP53* gene encompasses about 20 kb of DNA located on the short arm of chromosome 17 (17p13.1). Exons 2–11 encode a 53 kDa nuclear phosphoprotein that exists in virtually all normal cells at transiently low levels. The p53 protein contains five domains: an N-terminal transactivation domain, a sequence-specific DNA-binding domain, a C-terminal domain involved in DNA-binding regulation, a proline-rich regulatory domain, and an oligomerization domain (Figure 4.2). Figure 4.2(b) is a representation of the three-dimensional structure of the p53 DNA-binding domain, which is made up of β-sheets arranged in a scaffold that supports the flexible loops and helices that are in direct contact with DNA. Mutations that render the p53 protein dysfunctional in cancer either alter the DNA-binding sites or alter protein folding to interfere with DNA–p53 interaction. p53 is not necessary for human development, but lack of p53 confers a great risk of malignancy.[5] In fact, *TP53* mutation is associated with nearly 50% of all human cancers. In addition to mutation, p53 function may also be altered by post-translational modifications. p53 has been shown to be heavily post-translationally modified by a variety of mechanisms, including phosphorylation, acetylation, ubiquitination, sumoylation, glycosylation, methylation, and neddylation, which all serve to either increase or decrease the stability of p53.[6] In fact, p53 dysfunction may be more common than not when post-translational modifications are taken into account in addition to *TP53* mutation. *TP53* serves as a gatekeeper tumor suppressor gene, playing a crucial role in DNA surveillance and repair at the G_1 cell cycle checkpoint.[7] Wild-type p53 functions as a homotetrameric complex that binds DNA in a sequence-specific fashion to regulate gene transcription.[8] When DNA damage occurs, p53 mediates G_1 arrest by activating the expression of genes responsible for DNA damage response pathways such as *WAF1*, which encodes p21[Waf1/Cip1], a potent inhibitor of cyclin-dependent kinase (cdk)-dependent phosphorylation of retinoblastoma protein (pRb). Hypophosphorylated pRb binds the synthesis-promoting E2F-1 transcription factor, resulting in cell cycle arrest (Figure 4.3).[9] p53 may also inhibit G_1 by controlling the transcriptional activity of RNA polymerase II by inhibition of the cdk-activating kinase (CAK) complex cdk7/cyclin H1/Mat1.[10] In addition, G_1 arrest may be achieved by the ability of p53 to induce *PC3*, whose gene product reduces the cyclin D1 level, leading to inhibition of cdk4 and hypophosphorylation of pRb.[11] The G_1–S checkpoint is critical for DNA damage repair during cell cycle arrest.

p53 may also arrest the cell cycle at the G_2–M (gap 2–mitosis) transition (Figure 4.4).

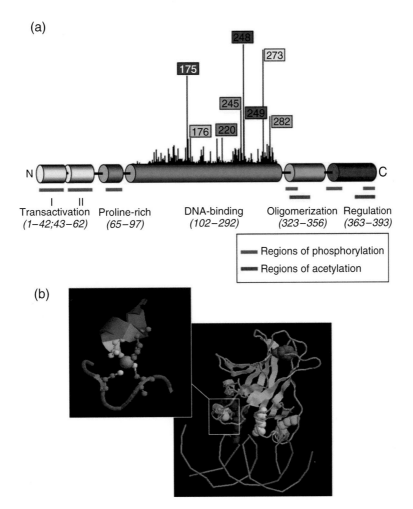

Figure 4.2 p53 Protein structure. A—Linear representation of p53. The protein can be divided into several functional domains, represented by colored cylinders on the figure: yellow, transactivation domains I and II; orange, proline-rich region; blue, DNA-binding domain; green, oligomerization domain; and red, regulation domain. p53 activity is modulated via post-translational modifications, such as phosphorylation (violet lines) and acetylation (pink lines), at the N- and C-terminal ends of the molecule. Vertical lines over the DNA-binding domain illustrate the distribution and the prevalence of point mutations found in TP53 gene in human tumors. The eight most frequently mutated codons ("hot spot" codons) are identified by color boxes. B—Three-dimensional representation of the p53 DNA-binding domain bound to DNA. The amino acids corresponding to "hot spot" codons are represented with the same color as in A, highlighting their role in protein conformation (R175, C176, Y220, G245, R249, and R282) or in DNA-binding (R248 and R273). Inset: Geometry of zinc coordination between protein loops 2 and 3. © 2004 From Critical Reviews in Clinical and Laboratory Sciences by Seeman S, et al. Reproduced by permission of Taylor & Francis Group.

p53 activation of target genes can effectively inhibit cyclin B1/cdc2 activity, which is essential for cells to enter mitosis. p21[Waf1/Cip1] also plays a role in G_2 arrest by direct inhibition of the cyclin B1/cdc2 complex.[12] In addition,

p53 induces GADD45, which can then bind cdc2, disrupting its ability to complex with cyclin B1.[13,14] In addition, p53 induces 14-3-3-σ, which not only binds and sequesters cdc2 in the cytoplasm, but also binds and inhibits

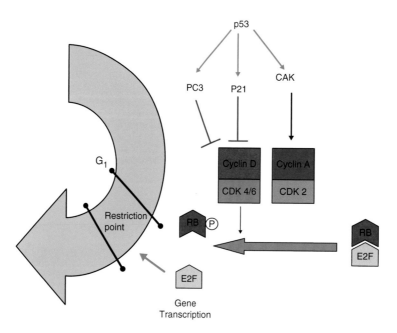

Figure 4.3 P53 mediated G1-S phase cell cycle arrest. This schematic depicts G1-S phase cell cycle arrest by p53 induction of p21, CAK and PC3. The green arrows represent activation of the target, and red blocking lines represent inhibition of the target.

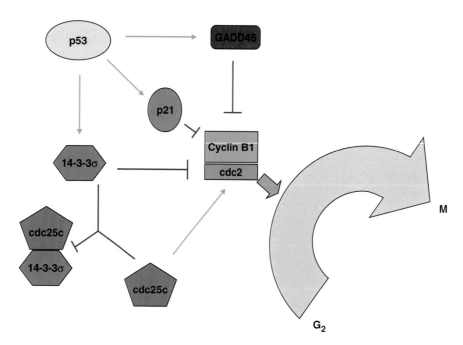

Figure 4.4 P53 mediated G2-M phase cell cycle arrest. This schematic depicts G2-M phase cell cycle arrest by p53 induction of p21, GADD45 and 14-3-3σ. The green arrows represent activation of the target, and red blocking lines represent inhibition of the target.

cdc25c, which is responsible for the dephosphorylation and activation of the cyclinB/cdc2 complex.[15–18] p53 has been deemed the 'guardian of the genome' because of its role in arresting the growth of cells with DNA damage.

p53 also controls cellular proliferation and genome integrity by the induction of apoptosis via the transcriptional activation of p53 target genes. It influences both the extrinsic and intrinsic apoptotic pathways by activation of downstream targets directly involved in the control of cell death. Figure 4.5 illustrates the interplay between the extrinsic and intrinsic pathways. The plasma membrane death receptors Fas, DR4, and DR5 have all been shown to be regulated by p53 in the extrinsic pathway.[19] p53 induces caspase-8, which in turn upregulates Bid. Bid inserts into the mitochondrial membrane, where it activates Bax and Bak. Bax and Bak initiate mitochondrial apoptosome formation. Bid also serves as the link between the extrinsic and intrinsic pathways. p53 regulates the intrinsic apoptotic pathway by direct induction of the Bcl-2 family members Bax, PUMA (p53-upregulated modulator of apoptosis), and Noxa, which are localized in the mitochondrial membrane and stimulate the release of cytochrome *c* and activation of the caspase pathway.[20,21] Apoptosome formation is dependent upon cytochrome *c*, Apaf-1, and caspase-9 association. Caspases 2, 8, 9, and 10 are initiator caspases that cleave the proenzyme caspases 3, 6, and 7, allowing for cellular digestion.[20,22] p53 does not work alone

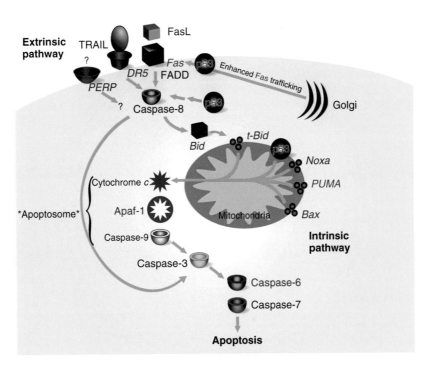

Figure 4.5 A model for p53-mediated apoptosis. This model depicts the involvement of p53 in the extrinsic and intrinsic apoptotic pathways. P53 target genes are shown in red. The convergence of the two pathways through Bid is shown. © 2003, From The Journal of Cell Science, by Haupt S, et al. Reproduced with permission of The Company of Biologists Ltd.

in transactivation, but rather appears to be governed by a wide array of co-activators and co-repressors that together effect gene transcription. For example, in colorectal cancer, the absence of acetyltransferase enzyme p300 has been shown to increase apoptosis in response to DNA damage.[23] This also correlated with an increased expression of PUMA and a decreased expression of p21[Wafl/Cip1]. In contrast, the same study found that the presence of p300 increased p21[Wafl/Cip1] expression, resulting in growth arrest. This example illustrates a situation in which p300 determines whether cells are programmed for apoptosis or cell cycle arrest, and raises the question of what is responsible for this decision: p53 or its co-activators?

p53 also plays an important role in angiogenesis. It has been shown to upregulate thrombospondin-1 (TSP1), brain-specific angiogenesis inhibitor 1 (BAI1), matrix metalloproteinase 2 (MMP2), and Eph receptor A2 (EphA2), all of which function to inhibit angiogenesis. In addition, p53 downregulates pro-angiogenic genes such as MMP1, cyclooxygenase-2 (COX-2), vascular endothelial growth factor A (VEGFA), and hypoxia-inducible factor 1α (HIF-1α).[24] Figure 4.6 illustrates these functions and the resultant impact on angiogenesis. Loss of wild-type p53 will therefore lead to a more angiogenic tumor phenotype. In fact, studies have revealed that wild-type p53, through alteration of TSP:VEGFA ratios, could induce dormancy and inhibit metastasis.[25,26]

p53 is degraded through ubiquitin-mediated proteolysis, which is regulated by Mdm2. Mdm2 is upregulated by an increase in p53 binding to its regulatory site. The increased amount of Mdm2 can then bind to p53, flagging the p53 protein for ubiquitination and degradation, creating a classic feedback loop. In addition, p53 may be stabilized by p14[ARF], which is an

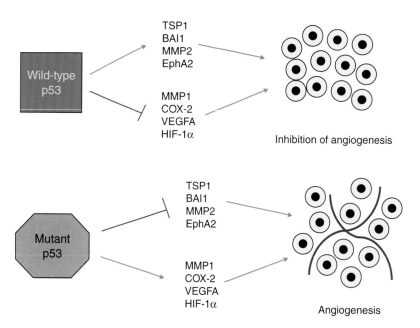

Figure 4.6 A model for p53 regulation of angiogenesis. Wild type p53 induction of genes that regulate angiogenesis is depicted. The green arrows represent activation and the red arrows represent inhibition.

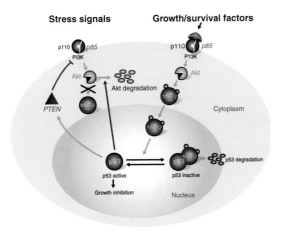

Stress signals   **Growth/survival factors**

Figure 4.7 A model for the regulation of p53 by the AKT pathway under growth/survival conditions and under stress signals. The negative regulation of p53 by AKT is induced in response to survival signals from Mdm2. The activation of this pathway leads to the inhibition and destruction of p53. Under stress conditions this pathway is blocked through the cleavage and degradation of AKT, and the inhibition of pl3K through PTEN. Both of these activities are induced by p53. In this model survival is achieved by inhibition of p53 by AKT, whereas apoptosis is achieved by counteracting AKT by p53. p53 target genes are shown in red. Green arrows represent activation, whereas red arrows represent inhibition. © 2003, From The Journal of Cell Science, by Haupt S, et al. Reproduced with permission of The Company of Biologists Ltd.

inhibitor of Mdm2.[27] These pathways were proposed in a model by Haupt et al,[20] as shown in Figure 4.7. In this model, p53 can be targeted for degradation in response to growth or survival signals. These signals induce Akt, which in turn phosphorylates Mdm2. Mdm2 phosphorylation leads to increased nuclear accumulation and decreased affinity for p14[ARF] all of which lead to degradation of p53. Stress signals, however, lead to the activation of PTEN by p53, which in turn inhibits Akt phosphorylation of Mdm2, allowing for growth inhibition and activation of the apoptotic pathways.

METHODS OF DETECTION

A review of the literature reveals a variety of methods that have been used to detect *TP53*/p53 dysfunction. These fall into three categories: prescreening technologies that look only at p53 inactivation, screening techniques designed to find known mutations, and scanning technologies aimed at known and unknown mutations.

The most widely used prescreening method is immunohistochemistry. This involves staining of the ovarian tumor with an enzyme-linked antibody to a specific p53 domain. The enzyme converts the substrate into a color that precipitates on the slide and can be observed microscopically (Figure 4.8). Wild-type p53 should not be detected with immuno-staining, because of its short half-life; however, mutant p53, which accumulates in the nucleus, should be detected. p53 immunostaining is rapid and inexpensive; however, the inability of immunohistochemistry to detect most null mutations, the inter- and intraobserver variation due to the subjective nature of scoring, and the differences in antibody specificity make this a somewhat unreliable method of detection.

Many screening techniques have been employed to detect *TP53* sequence abnormalities.

- Denaturing gradient gel electrophoresis (DGGE) identifies mutations based upon the fact that DNA molecules that differ by only one nucleotide have different melting temperatures. This will in turn affect the mobility of the molecule during gel electrophoresis. This method can be combined with the polymerase chain reaction (PCR) and is highly sensitive; however, it requires special primers and does not reveal the position of any changes.

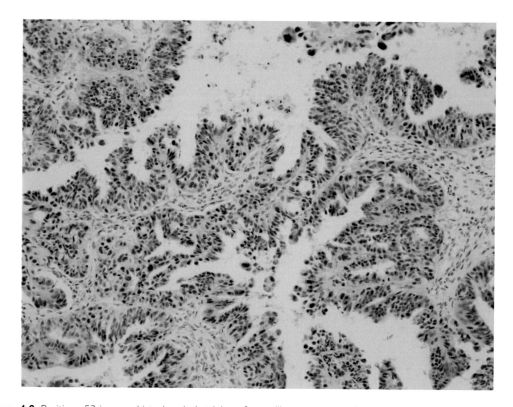

Figure 4.8 Positive p53 immunohistochemical staining of a papillary serous ovarian carcinoma with the D07 antibody.

- One of the most frequently used screening technologies is single-strand conformation polymorphism analysis (SSCP). Single-stranded DNA will take on a unique conformational structure that has a distinct electrophoretic mobility in a polyacrylamide gel. DNA is amplified with radiolabeled PCR primers and then denatured prior to gel electrophoresis next to control samples. Differing electrophoretic mobility will then arise if the DNA is mutated. SSCP is relatively quick and simple to perform; however, it does not pinpoint the position or the type of mutation detected.

- Heteroduplex analysis is based on the principle that if DNA from a heterozygous individual is denatured and allowed to re-anneal, some normal strands will anneal with mutant strands (a heteroduplex), and different conformations will arise. The heteroduplex will then have a different mobility in gel electrophoresis than a homoduplex.

The gold standard for mutation detection, however, is direct DNA sequencing. DNA sequencing can be achieved manually, but this requires time and is labor-intensive. Automated sequencing has now all but replaced manual sequencing. This has been shown to be reliable and efficient with multiple systems.

Most *TP53* gene mutations are missense, or single amino acid substitutions that do not result in a truncated protein. Proteins transcribed from the *TP53* gene with missense mutations have a much longer half-life than the respective products from wild-type *TP53*. Therefore, in the event of a missense mutation, the dysfunctional p53 products accumulate in the nucleus and are usually detectable by immunohistochemical staining. Null or truncating mutations, however, are missing the epitopes commonly targeted by commercial p53 antibodies, and are not identified when immunostaining is substituted for SSCP direct mutation analysis. Most (>80%) of the missense mutations occur in exons 5–8, the coding regions sensitive to p53 inactivation and responsible for the physical interaction between p53 and DNA.[28] Because of this, many investigators have limited their sequencing of the *TP53* gene to exons 5–8. However, an increase in null mutations is encountered when the complete open reading frame is included in analysis. Specifically, the addition of exons 4 and 9 have been shown to harbor many *TP53* null mutations.[29] While the most complete *TP53* mutational analysis would require direct sequencing of exons 2–11, we recommend SSCP screening of at least exons 4–9 with direct sequencing of abnormalities for an adequate analysis.

TP53 IN OVARIAN CANCER

TP53 mutations have been shown to occur in up to 50–80% of ovarian cancers.[30–33] They have been shown to be more common in late-stage disease, higher-grade tumors, older patients, and tumors of serous and endometrioid histology.[34,35] They are less likely to occur in tumors of clear cell histology.[35,36]

The early literature researching the role of *TP53* as a prognostic factor in ovarian cancer used immunohistochemistry as the means for *TP53* mutation detection. The evidence for p53 immunohistochemistry as a prognostic factor in ovarian cancer is conflicting, and different studies have employed different staining antibodies, which have resulted in an inability to adequately compare these studies.[34,37–53]

Table 4.1 lists details of studies of p53 as a prognostic factor. Many have found p53 immunohistochemistry to be an adverse prognostic factor in univariate analysis, but only a few have found it to be significant in a multivariate model. Baekelandt et al[47] and Tachibana et al[49] found that positive immunostaining with the D01 antibody was an independently poor prognostic variable, while Geisler et al[42] reached the same conclusion utilizing the PAb1801 antibody. In contrast, Shahin et al[34] found that tumors stained with the D07 antibody, known to have less intratumor heterogeneity, did not have prognostic significance. These findings are consistent with other reports in ovarian cancer employing the D07 antibody.[39,43–46,48–52] However, Shahin et al[34] also sequenced these tumors directly, finding a sequencing and immunohistochemistry mutation concordance of only 71%, and a 20.5% chance of positive D07 antibody staining without a sequenced mutation. Taking these results together, positive p53 immunostaining has been shown to confer a worse prognosis in many univariate analyses; however, most studies have not found it to be an independently poor prognostic factor.

Table 4.2 lists studies employing direct sequencing of *TP53* mutations to determine prognosis – again with conflicting results.[34,35,54–63] This table shows the 12 *TP53* sequencing and prognosis studies listed in the International Agency for Research on Cancer (IARC) *TP53* Mutational Database.[64] Only two studies show *TP53* mutation to be an adverse prognostic factor after multivariate analysis. Shahin et al[34] with direct sequencing, found only tumor *TP53* null mutants to be an independently poor prognostic factor, while Okuda et al[35] found tumor *TP53* mutations to confer a worse prognosis in 27 patients with endometrioid histology. In contrast, Havrilesky et al[59]

Table 4.1 Studies relating p53 immunostaining to survival

Ref	n	Antibody	Positive staining (%)	Univariate analysis	Multivariate analysis
37	107	PAb1801	50	NS	—
38	284	PAb1801	62	Worse prognosis	NS
39	93	D07	47	—	NS
40	89	CM1	45	Worse prognosis	NS
41	61	CM1, PAb240, PAb1801	52	NS	NS
42	83	PAb1801	Quantitative	Worse prognosis	Worse prognosis
43	54[a]	D07	72	NS	NS
44	187	D07	14	Worse prognosis	—
45	105	D07	44	NS	NS
46	162	D07	52	NS	—
47	185	D01	49	Worse prognosis	Worse prognosis
34	171	D07	48.5	NS	NS
48	90	D07	47	NS	NS
49	73	D01	Quantitative	Worse prognosis	Worse prognosis
		PAb1801		NS	—
		D07		Worse prognosis	NS
		RSP53		NS	—
		Bp53-12		Worse prognosis	NS
50	783	D07	53	Worse prognosis	NS
51	107	D07	48.6	NS	NS
52	134	D07	59	Worse prognosis	NS alone
53	82	D07/BP53-12	53.7	Worse prognosis	NS

[a]Stages III and IV only.
NS, not significant.

found that tumor *TP53* mutation conferred a short-term survival benefit. This benefit disappeared, however, with longer follow-up. We theorized that there may be wide variability in the prognosis of tumor missense mutations, depending on the severity of conformational deformity dictated by the specific mutation. To investigate this more closely, our group went on to analyze the effect of 82 *TP53* missense-mutant epithelial ovarian cancers utilizing the IARC *TP53* Mutational Database, which specifies the effects of *TP53* mutations on p53 core domain structure. We found no relationship between degree of p53 conformational deformity and outcome.[60] Leitao et al[62] and Wang et al[63]

sequenced only early-stage ovarian cancers for *TP53* mutation. Consistent with previous reports, they did find fewer *TP53* mutations in early-stage tumors. Wang et al[63] did not find any survival benefit for wild-type *TP53* tumors. In contrast, Leitao et al[62] did find *TP53* mutation to be a poor prognostic factor in a univariate analysis; however, no multivariate analysis was undertaken.

Taking these results together, while *TP53* mutation is more common in late-stage disease and high-grade tumors, there is no consistent evidence suggesting that *TP53* mutation alone is an independent adverse prognostic factor in ovarian cancer. However, it is important to note

Table 4.2 Studies relating *TP53* mutation by direct sequencing to survival

Ref	*n*	*Method*[a]	*Exons*	*Mutation rate (%)*	*Univariate analysis*	*Multivariate analysis*
54	178	SSCP/direct	2–11	55.6	Worse prognosis	NS
34	171	SSCP/direct	2–11	57.3	Null–worse prognosis	Null–worse prognosis
55	45	DGGE	2–11	64.4	NS	—
56	73	SSCP/direct	5–8	44	NS	—
57	82	SSCP/direct	5–8	39	NS	—
58	31	SSCP	4–8	41.9	NS	—
59	109	Direct	2–11	74	Improved prognosis in short term, lost in long term	—
60	267	SSCP/direct	4–10	47	NS[b]	—
35	27[c]	SSCP/direct	5–8	63	Worse prognosis	Worse prognosis
61	178[d]	TTGE/direct	2–11	28.9	NS	—
62	68[d]	Direct	2–11	32	Worse prognosis	—
63	109	TTGE/direct	2–11	73.4	NS	—

[a]SSCP, single-strand conformational polymorphism; DGGE, denaturing gradient gel electrophoresis; TTGE, temperature gradient gel electrophoresis.
[b]Missense mutations only analyzed for prognosis.
[c]Endometrioid histology only.
[d]Early-stage cancers only.
NS, not significant.

the types of sequenced mutations studied, as well as the completeness of analysis. Shahin et al[34] analyzed exons 2–11 and did find *TP53* null mutation to be an independently poor prognostic factor, while missense mutation alone was not found to impact survival. In contrast, Fallows et al[56] broke their analysis down into missense and nonmissense mutations and did not find a significant survival difference. However, only exons 5–8 were analyzed. Wang et al[63] did sequence exons 2–11, but did not find any survival difference even when mutational type was broken down into missense versus nonmissense. Results that do not break down *TP53* mutation by type may be confounded by the large number of missense mutations in ovarian cancers, and those that do

not include exons 4 and 9 may not have a significant number of null mutations to adequately study their effect on survival. Conversely, the lack of survival advantage seen in the studies may indicate that *TP53* mutation is a late event in ovarian carcinogenesis, or perhaps is one of many factors that play a role individually as well as cooperatively in this process.

STRATEGIES FOR RESTORING p53 FUNCTION

Due to the paucity of *TP53* mutations in early-stage, low-grade tumors, some reports of improved survival in wild-type *TP53* tumors, the dependence on wild-type p53 function of some anticancer drugs, and the promotion of an antiangiogenic phenotype by wild-type p53, restoration of wild-type p53 function has been investigated as a treatment strategy.

Gene therapy

One of the most widely heralded mechanisms for restoring p53 function is through the use of gene therapy. Gene therapy attempts to restore wild-type p53 function by replacing the mutant *TP53* gene with a functional wild-type copy, usually achieved through the intraperitoneal introduction of a viral vector. Different viral vectors have been investigated as candidates. Retroviral vectors integrate into the host genome and then require cell division for transduction; however, they may cause damage to the genome and have a relatively low transduction efficiency. Adenoviruses are more attractive candidates, as they have a relatively high transduction efficiency in a wide range of cells (Figure 4.9). Because they do not integrate into the host genome, concerns regarding mutagenesis are minimized. The double-stranded DNA adenovirus serotype 5 (Ad-p53)

has been the favored adenovirus for *TP53* gene replacement. Using replication-deficient rAd-p53, proliferation of the ovarian cancer cell lines SKOV3, OVCAR-3 and 2774 was significantly inhibited.[65] These preclinical findings led to a phase I/II trial in recurrent ovarian cancer.[66] This trial found that intraperitoneal rAd-p53 combined with platinum-based chemotherapy could lead to a significant reduction in serum CA-125 in heavily pretreated *TP53*-mutant ovarian cancer patients. These promising results, combined with an acceptable toxicity profile, led to the development of a large, international phase II/III trial of intraperitoneal rAd-p53 for first-line treatment in women with *TP53*-mutant ovarian cancer who had either no residual disease or residual disease ≤2 cm. Unfortunately, this trial was closed after the first interim analysis due to lack of an adequate therapeutic benefit.

Liposomal-bound p53

Another method of p53 restoration involves the injection of liposomes complexed with a

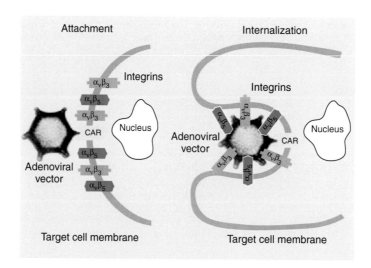

Figure 4.9 Entry of a serotype-5 adenovirus into a cell. Reprinted from The Lancet Oncology, Vol 4, Zeimet A, Marth C. Why did p53 gene therapy fail in ovarian cancer? 415-422, © 2003, with permission from Elsevier.

plasmid carrying wild-type *TP53*. The liposomes are then endocytosed into the target cells. This method is relatively nontoxic and nonimmunogenic. Kim et al[67] treated ovarian cancer cell lines with DDC, a cationic liposome composed of dioleoyltrimethylaminopropane, 1,2-dioleoyl-3-phosphophatidylethanolamine, and cholesterol, in complex with a wild-type *TP53* plasmid. They found increased *TP53* mRNA expression as well as growth inhibition in the transfected ovarian cancer cell lines. In addition, inoculation of tumors in nude mice with DDC/pp53-EGFP resulted in a greater than 60% reduction in tumor volume.

Modulation of aberrant p53

There are varying degrees of p53 dysfunction. While insertions or deletions in *TP53* cause stop codons and more severe dysfunction, missense mutations may affect p53 folding in varying degrees, depending upon how critical the area of mutation is and how severe the amino acid substitution is, as well as the resultant conformational change. Altered folding may then condense an important DNA-binding site, resulting in lack of DNA binding by mutant p53. Designing mechanisms to restore these conformational changes, thereby restoring wild-type function, is an attractive therapeutic target. Several small molecules have been developed to stabilize p53 structure. One of these,

CP31398, has been shown to stabilize p53 and induce apoptosis and cell cycle arrest in some human cancer cell lines.[68] In addition, small peptides such as CDB3 and ASPP may also be used to stabilize mutant p53 by the same mechanisms. The US National Cancer Institute (NCI) drug discovery program has contributed to the discovery of small chemicals that may play biologic roles in different cancer types. One of the most promising molecules to be discovered in this program is PRIMA-1, which has been shown to restore wild-type p53 function at many of the most common mutational sites. Although no direct interaction between PRIMA-1 and p53 has been established, PRIMA-1 has been shown to exhibit growth inhibition in *TP53*-mutant tumors without side-effects.[69,70]

In conclusion, while p53 dysfunction is the most common genetic alteration known in ovarian cancer, there is still much to learn about its role in the development and progression of this disease. p53 maintains the integrity of the genome through cell cycle arrest as well as induction of apoptotic pathways. While data for *TP53*/p53 as a prognostic factor are conflicting, there is some evidence to suggest that *TP53* null mutation may be an adverse prognostic factor. Finally, restoration of wild-type p53 function via gene replacement and modulation of aberrant p53 are viable targets for novel therapeutics.

REFERENCES

1. Anderson MJ, Stanbridge EJ. Tumor suppressor genes studied by cell hybridization and chromosome transfer. FASEB J 1993;7:826–33.

2. Knudson AG, Hethcote HW, Brown BW. Mutation and childhood cancer: a probabilistic model for the incidence of retinoblastoma. Proc Natl Acad Sci USA 1975;72:5116–20.

3. Knudson AG. Two genetic hits (more or less) to cancer. Nat Rev Cancer 2001;1:157–70.

4. Kinzler KW, Vogelstein B. Gatekeepers and caretakers. Nature 1997;386:761–3.

5. Harvey M, McArthur MJ, Montgomery CJ, et al. Spontaneous and carcinogen-induced

tumorigenesis in p53-deficient mice. Nat Genet 1993;5:225–9.

6. Lu X. p53: a heavily dictated dictator of life and death. Curr Opin Genet Dev 2005;15: 27–33.

7. Israels ED, Israels LG. The cell cycle. Oncologist 2000;5:510–13.

8. Kern SE, Kinzler KW, Bruskin A, et al. Identification of p53 as a sequence-specific DNA-binding protein. Science 1991;252: 1708.

9. Brehm A, Miska EA, McCance DJ, et al. Retinoblastoma protein recruits histone deacetylase to repress transcription. Nature 1998;391:597–601.

10. Schneider E, Montenarh M, Wagner P. Regulation of CAK kinase activity by p53. Oncogene 1998;17:2733–41.

11. Guardavaccaro D, Corrente G, Covone F. Arrest of G_1-S progression by the p53-inducible gene *PC3* is Rb dependent and relies on the inhibition of cyclin D1 transcription. Mol Cell Biol 2000;20:1797–815.

12. Flatt PM, Tang LJ, Scatena CD. p53 regulation of G2 checkpoint is retinoblastoma protein dependent. Mol Cell Biol 2000;20: 4210–23.

13. Jin S, Antinore MJ, Lung FD. The GADD45 inhibition of Cdc2 kinase correlates with GADD45-mediated growth suppression. J Biol Chem 2000; 275:16602–8.

14. Zhan Q, Antinore MJ, Wang XW. Association with Cdc2 and inhibition of Cdc2/Cyclin B1 kinase activity by the p53-regulated protein Gadd45. Oncogene 1999;18:2892–900.

15. Hermeking H, Lengauer C, Polyak K. 14-3-3-σ is a p53-regulated inhibitor of G2/M progression. Mol Cell 1997;1:3–11.

16. Peng CY, Graves PR, Thomas RS. Mitotic and G2 checkpoint control: regulation of 14-3-3 protein binding by phosphorylation of Cdc25C on serine-216. Science 1997;277: 1501–5.

17. Ferrell JE. How regulated protein translocation can produce switch-like responses. Trends Biochem Sci 1998;23:461–5.

18. Chan TA, Hermeking H, Lengauer C. 14-3-3-σ is required to prevent mitotic catastrophe after DNA damage. Nature 1999;401:616–20.

19. Yu J, Zhang L. The transcriptional targets of p53 in apoptosis control. Biochem Biophys Res Commun 2005;331:851–8.

20. Haupt S, Berger M, Goldberg Z, Haupt Y. Apoptosis – the p53 network. J Cell Sci 2003;116:4077–85.

21. Schuler M, Bossy-Wetzel E, Godstein JC, et al. p53 induces apoptosis by caspase activation through mitochondrial cytochrome *c* release. Biol Chem 2000;275:7337–42.

22. MacLachlan TK, El-Deiry WS. Apoptotic threshold is lowered by p53 transactivation of caspase-6. Proc Natl Acad Sci USA 2002; 99:9492–7.

23. Iyer NG, Chin S, Ozdag H, et al. p300 regulates p53 dependent apoptosis after DNA damage in colorectal cancer cells by modulation of PUMA/p21 levels. Proc Natl Acad Sci USA 2004;101:7386–91.

24. Bergers G, Benjamin LE. Tumorigenesis and the angiogenic switch. Nat Rev 2003;3:401–10.

25. Holmgren L, Jackson G, Arbiser J. p53 induces angiogenesis-restricted dormancy in a mouse fibrosarcoma. Oncogene 1998;17:819–24.

26. Gautam A, Densmore CL, Melton S, et al. Aerosol delivery of PEI–p53 complexes inhibits B16-F10 lung metastases through regulation of angiogenesis. Cancer Gene Ther 2002;9:28–36.

27. Zhang Y, Xiong Y, Yarbrough WG. ARF promotes MDM2 degradation and stabilizes p53: *ARF–INK4a* locus deletion impairs both the Rb and p53 tumor suppression pathways. Cell 1998;92:725.

28. Hollstein M, Sidransky D, Vogelstein B, Harris C. p53 mutations in human cancers. Science 1991;253:49.

29. Skilling JS, Sood AK, Niemann T, et al. An abundance of p53 null mutations in ovarian carcinoma. Oncogene 1996;13:117–23.

30. Okamoto A, Sameshima Y, Yokoyama S, et al. Frequent allelic losses and mutations of the p53 gene in human ovarian cancer. Cancer Res 1991;51:5171–6.

31. Kupryjanczyk J, Thor AD, Beauchamp R, et al. p53 gene mutations and protein accumulation in human ovarian cancer. Proc Natl Acad Sci USA 1993;90:4961–5.

32. Kohler MF, Marks JR, Wiseman RW, et al. Spectrum of mutation and frequency of allelic deletion of the p53 gene in ovarian cancer. J Natl Cancer Inst 1993;85:1513–19.

33. Wertheim I, Muto MG, Welsh WR, et al. p53 gene mutation in human borderline epithelial ovarian tumors. J Natl Cancer Inst 1994; 86:1549–51.

34. Shahin MS, Hughes JH, Sood AK, Buller RE. The prognostic significance of p53 tumor suppressor gene alterations in ovarian carcinoma. Cancer 2000;89:2006–17.

35. Okuda T, Otsuka J, Sekizawa A, et al. p53 mutations and overexpression affect prognosis of ovarian endometrioid cancer but not clear cell cancer. Gynecol Oncol 2003; 88:318–25.

36. Ho ES, Lai C, Hsich Y, Chen J. p53 mutation is infrequent in clear cell carcinoma of the ovary. Gynecol Oncol 2001;80:189–93.

37. Marks JR, Davidoff AM, Kerns BJ, et al. Overexpression and mutation of p53 in epithelial ovarian cancer. Cancer Res 1991; 51:2979–84.

38. Hartmann LC, Podratz KC, Keeney GL, et al. Prognostic significance of p53 immunostaining in epithelial ovarian cancer. J Clin Oncol 1994;12:64–9.

39. Sheridan E, Silcocks P, Smith J, et al. p53 mutation in a series of epithelial ovarian cancers from the UK, and its prognostic significance. Eur J Cancer 1994:1701–4.

40. Van der Zee AGJ, Hollema H, Suurmeijer AJH, et al. Value of P-glycoprotein, glutathione S-transferase pi, c-erbB-2, and p53 as prognostic factores in ovarian carcinomas. J Clin Oncol 1995;13:70–8.

41. Allan LA, Campbell MK, Milner BJ, et al. The significance of p53 mutation and over-expression in ovarian cancer prognosis. Int J Gynecol Cancer 1996;6:483–90.

42. Geisler JP, Geisler HE, Wiemann MC, et al. Quantification of p53 in epithelial ovarian cancer. Gynecol Oncol 1997;66:435–8.

43. Goff BA, Ries JA, Els LP, et al. Immunophenotype of ovarian cancer as predictor of clinical outcome: evaluation at primary surgery and second-look procedure. Gynecol Oncol 1998;70:378–85.

44. Marx D, Meden H, Ziemek T, et al. Expression of the p53 tumor suppressor gene as a prognostic marker in platinum-treated patients with ovarian cancer. Eur J Cancer 1998; 34:845–50.

45. Mano Y, Kikuchi Y, Yamamoto K, et al. Bcl-2 as a predictor of chemosensitivity and prognosis in primary epithelial ovarian cancer. Eur J Cancer 1999;35:1214–19.

46. Ferrandina G, Fagotti A, Salerno MG, et al. p53 overexpression is associated with cytoreduction and response to chemotherapy in ovarian cancer. Br J Cancer 1999;81:733–40.

47. Baekelandt M, Kristensen GB, Nesland JM, et al. Clinical significance of apoptosis-related factors p53, mdm2, and bcl-2 in advanced ovarian cancer. J Clin Oncol 1999;17: 2061–8.

48. Sagarra R, Andrade L, Martinez E, et al. p53 and Bcl-2 as prognostic predictors in epithelial ovarian cancer. Int J Gynecol Cancer 2002;12:720–7.

49. Tachibana M, Watanabe J, Matsushima Y, et al. Independence of the prognostic value of tumor suppressor protein expression in ovarian adenocarcinomas: a multivariate analysis of expression of p53, retinoblastoma, and

related proteins. Int J Gynecol Cancer 2003; 13:598–606.

50. Nielsen JS, Jakobsen E, Holund B, et al. Prognostic significance of p53, Her-2, and EGFR overexpression in borderline and epithelial ovarian cancer. Int J Gynecol Cancer 2004;14:1086–96.

51. Hashiguchi Y, Tsuda H, Inoue T, et al. Alteration of cell cycle regulators correlates with survival in epithelial ovarian cancer patients. Hum Pathol 2004;35:165–75.

52. Bali A, O'Brien PM, Edwards LS, et al. Cyclin D1, p53, and p21[Waf1/Cip1] expression is predictive of poor clinical outcome in serous epithelial ovarian cancer. Clin Cancer Res 2004;10:5168–77.

53. Dogan E, Saygili U, Tuna B, et al. p53 and mdm2 as prognostic indicators in patients with epithelial ovarian cancer: a multivariate analysis. Gynecol Oncol 2005;97:46–52.

54. Reles A, Wen WH, Schmider A, et al. Correlation of p53 mutations with resistance to platinum-based chemotherapy and shortened survival in ovarian cancer. Clin Cancer Res 2001;7:2984–97.

55. Smith-Sorensen B, Kaern J, Holm R, et al. Therapy effect of either paclitaxel or cyclophosphamide combination treatment in patients with epithelial ovarian cancer and relation to p53 gene status. Br J Cancer 1998;78:375–81.

56. Fallows S, Price J, Atkinson RJ, et al. p53 mutation does not affect prognosis in ovarian epithelial malignancies. J Pathol 2001;19: 68–75.

57. Schuyer M, van der Burg MEL, Henzen-Logmans SC, et al. Reduced expression of BAX is associated with poor prognosis in patients with epithelial ovarian cancer: a multifactorial analysis of TP53, p21, BAX and BCL-2. Br J Cancer 2001;85:1359–67.

58. Niwa K, Itoh M, Murase T, et al. Alteration of p53 gene in ovarian carcinoma: clinicopathological

correlation and prognostic significance. Br J Cancer 1994;70:1191–7.

59. Havrilesky L, Darcy KM, Hamdan H, et al. Prognostic significance of p53 mutation and p53 overexpression in advanced epithelial ovarian cancer: a Gynecologic Oncology Group study. J Clin Oncol 2003;21:3814–25.

60. Rose SL, Robertson AD, Goodheart MJ, et al. The impact of p53 protein core domain structural alteration in ovarian cancer survival. Clin Cancer Res 2003;9:4139–44.

61. Wang Y, Helland A, Holm R, et al. TP53 mutations in early-stage ovarian carcinoma, relation to long-term survival. Br J Cancer 2004;90: 678–85.

62. Leitao MM, Boyd J, Hummer A, et al. Clinicopathologic analysis of early-stage sporadic ovarian carcinoma. Am J Surg Pathol 2004;28:147–59.

63. Wang Y, Kringen P, Kristensen GB, et al. Effect of the codon 72 polymorphism (c.215G>C, p.Arg72Pro) in combination with somatic sequence variants in the TP53 gene on survival in patients with advanced ovarian carcinoma. Hum Mutat 2004;24:21–34.

64. Olivier M, Eeles R, Hollstein M, et al. The IARC TP53 Database: new online mutation analysis and recommendations to users. Hum Mutat 2002;19:607–14.

65. Mujoo K, Maneval DC, Anderson SC, Gutterman JU. Adenoviral-mediated p53 tumor suppressor gene therapy of human ovarian carcinoma. Oncogene 1996;18:1617.

66. Buller RE, Runnebaum IB, Karlan BY, et al. A phase I/II trial of rAd/p53 (SCH58500) gene replacement in recurrent ovarian cancer. Cancer Gene Ther 2002;9:553–66.

67. Kim CK, Choi EJ, Choi SH, et al. Enhanced p53 gene transfer to human ovarian cancer cells using the cationic nonviral vector, DDC. Gynecol Oncol 2003;90:265–72.

68. Takimoto R, Wang W, Dicker DT, et al. The mutant p53-conformation modifying drug,

CP-31398, can induce apoptosis of human cancer cells and can stabilize wild-type p53 protein. Cancer Biol Ther 2002;1:47–55.

69. Bykov VJ, Issaeva N, Shilov A, et al. Restoration of the tumor suppressor function to mutant p53 by a low-molecular-weight compound. Nat Med 2002;8:282–28.

70. Bykov VJ, Issaeva N, Selivanova G, et al. Mutant p53-dependent growth suppression distinguishes PRIMA-1 from known anti-cancer drugs: a statistical analysis of information in the National Cancer Institute Database. Carcinogenesis 2002;23:2011–18.

Molecular profiling in ovarian cancer   5

Michael J Birrer, Kristin K Zorn, and Ginger J Gardner

INTRODUCTION

The classic multihit hypothesis of tumorigenesis and the intricacies of molecular signaling pathways point to the complex biology involved in the development and growth of malignant epithelial cells. Until recently, molecular technologies only permitted the evaluation of a small group of genes or a particular signaling pathway at a given time. With the development of microarray technology, the opportunity to obtain a system-wide understanding of the machinery of a tumor cell is now possible.

Molecular profiling is defined as the characterization of tumors based on their patterns of gene and protein expression. Comprehensive molecular profiling includes the assessment of DNA (the genomic level), RNA (the transcriptional level), and proteins (the translational level), and provides an opportunity to utilize this data in the study of tumors of a particular clinical phenotype. The large body of data gathered by molecular profiling can serve as a watershed in the characterization of a tumor, as it sets the stage for detailed analysis on groups of genes or proteins that appear to have differential expression and activity.

This chapter will describe the currently available methods for molecular profiling, present the data from analysis of ovarian cancers, and discuss the important potential clinical implications of this data.

COMPARATIVE GENOMIC HYBRIDIZATION

Well-established cytogenetic techniques such as fluorescence in situ hybridization (FISH) have been the mainstay of assessing DNA copy number abnormalities. FISH allows the identification of specific locus of interest such as 3q26, which has an increased copy number in approximately 40% of ovarian cancers.[1] Comparative genomic hybridization (CGH) represents the first approach to scanning the entire genome for DNA copy number abnormalities. First described in 1992, the technique involves differentially labeling test and reference DNA with fluorescent dye followed by hybridization to metaphase chromosomes.[2] The ratio of the hybridization intensity of the test to the reference specimens gives an indication of relative copy number increases and decreases in DNA. Importantly, fresh or archival tissue generally can be used for CGH, allowing tissue banks of formalin-fixed, paraffin-embedded samples to be evaluated. CGH represents an advance in its ability to assess the whole genome, allowing, for example, multiple studies to reveal consistent aberrations in both ovarian and fallopian tube carcinomas. Consistent gains in 3q26–qter, 7q32–qter, 8q24–qter, 17q32–qter, and 20q13.2–qter, as well as losses in 4, 13q, 16qter, 18qter, and Xq12 have been documented (Figure 5.1).[3–6]

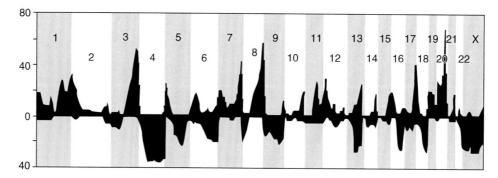

Figure 5.1 Genome distribution showing the frequencies of copy number gains (positive values) and losses (negative values) in human ovarian cancers. The bands indicate chromosome locations. Chromosomes are identified along the top of the graph. Reproduced from Gray et al. Gynecol Oncol 2003;88:516–21[3] with permission from Academic Press.

Recent advances have allowed genomic segments spotted on arrays to be substituted for the metaphase spreads in the CGH technique (Figure 5.2).[7] This allows significant improvement in resolution, as well as the potential to improve efficiency and reproducibility. The first of these platforms utilized bacterial artificial chromosomes (BACs) as large inserts. Investigators then used the cDNA microarrays originally designed for expression profiling for CGH. Increasingly, commercially produced oligonucleotide microarrays are being used for CGH.[8] In addition, new single-nucleotide polymorphism (SNP) arrays are now available for use.[9,10] The arrays can focus on a specific area, such as a particular chromosome or region of a chromosome known to have an oncogene of interest, or can assess the entire genome (Figure 5.3).[7] Table 5.1 summarizes some of the features of these platforms. Excellent reviews of array CGH have been produced by Albertson and Pinkel[11,12] and by Tapper et al.[13]

CGH analysis of ovarian cancer

Metaphase CGH has been utilized to evaluate copy number abnormalities in *BRCA1* and

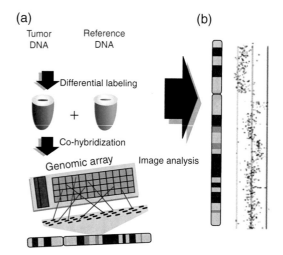

Figure 5.2 General principles of array comparative genomic hybridization. (a) Normal and tumor DNA samples are isolated and used to create fluorescently labeled probes, commonly with cyanine-3 (Cy3; green) and cyanine-5 (Cy5; red) dyes. The probes are pooled and competitively co-hybridized to a glass slide spotted with a known array of mapped genomic clones. The arrays are analyzed with a microarray scanner, producing an image that is used to assess the $\log_2$ ratios of the Cy5 to Cy3 intensities for each clone. (b) A $\log_2$ ratio profile is assembled to determine relative copy number changes between the cancer and tumor samples. Each dot on the graph represents a clone. Values to the left of the '0' line indicate a loss of a genomic region, values to the right indicate a gain or amplification, and values at '0' indicate no change. Reproduced from Davis et al. Chromosome Res 2005; 13:237–48[7] with permission from Springer.

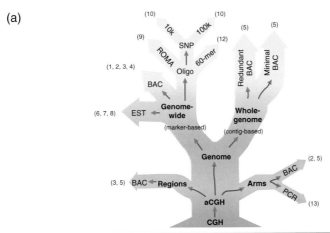

(b)

Probe type	Manufacturer	Website
(1) BAC'	Sanger	www.sanger.ac.uk/Projects/Microarrays/
(2) BAC'	UCSF	cc.ucsf.edu/microarray
(3) BAC'	DKFZ	www.dkfz.heidelberg.de/kompl_genome
(4) BAC	AFCRI	acgh.afcri.upenn.edu
(5) BAC	BCCRC	www.bccrc.ca/cg/ArrayCGH_Group.html
(6) EST	BD Biosciences	www.bdbiosciences.com
(7) EST	Bioscience Corp,	www.superarray.com
(8) EST	UHN	www.microarray.ca
(9) oligo	NimbleGen Systems	www.nimblegen.com
(10) oligo	Affymetrix	www.affymetrix.com
(11) oligo	Bioscience Corp.	www.superarray.com
(12) oligo	Agilent Technologies	we.home.agilent.com/USeng/home.html
(13) PCR'	UU	puffer.genpat.uu.se/chrom_22_array/chrom22.php

Figure 5.3 (a) 'Evolution' of array comparative genomic hybridization (CGH) technologies. (b) Examples of current array platforms. Each platform corresponds to a number in (a). Clone sets contain other large-insert clones. BAC, bacterial artificial chromosome; EST, expressed sequence tag; UCSF, University of California, San Francisco; DKFZ, Deutsches Krebsforschungszentrum; AFCRI, Abramson Family Cancer Research Institute; BCCRC, British Columbia Cancer Research Centre; UHN, University Health Network; UU, Uppsala Universitet. Reproduced from Davies et al. Chromosome Res 2005;13:237–48[7] with permission from Springer.

Table 5.1 Platforms for array comparative genomic hybridization(CGH)[7–10]

Array platform	Spatial resolution	Weaknesses	Strengths
Bacterial artificial chromosome (BAC)	Limited	• Large amounts of DNA or amplification required • Inclusion of redundant sequences	• Precision • Ability to customize
cDNA	Moderate	• Low signal-to-noise ratio • Microgram quantity or amplification may be required	• Can evaluate CGH and RNA expression simultaneously
Oligonucleotide	High	• Cross-hybridization to multiple targets may require complexity-reducing techniques • Microgram quantity or amplification may be required	• Commercialization is lowering cost • Can evaluate CGH, RNA expression, and allelotype simultaneously
Single-nucleotide polymorphism (SNP)	High	• Requires high-quality DNA	• Can evaluate CGH and loss of heterozygosity (LOH) simultaneously

BRCA2 mutation carriers compared with sporadic ovarian cancer cases.[13–15] Inconsistent results have been obtained so far, likely due to small sample sizes and varying inclusion of specific mutations. However, two studies have shown increased copy numbers on 2q, while two have shown losses on chromosomes 9 and 19, particularly in the *BRCA1* group, that merit further evaluation.[13–15]

Increasingly, a combination of cytogenetic techniques is employed to make the analysis as robust as possible. Schraml et al[16] evaluated the 11q13–14 amplicon, using a combination of metaphase CGH, array CGH, FISH, and immunohistochemistry (IHC) assessment. Metaphase CGH of 26 ovarian carcinomas and three cell lines revealed frequent abnormalities on 2q, 3q, 5p, 8q, 11q, 12p, 17q, and 20q. Array CGH confirmed copy number gains for *PIK3CA* on 3q and *PAK1* on 11q, among others. A tissue microarray including 268 ovarian tumors was used to perform FISH and IHC, confirming *PAK1* copy number gains in 30% of the tumors and increased protein expression in 85%, while *CCND1* copy numbers and protein expression were aberrant less often. Schraml et al[16] concluded that *PAK1* may be the critical oncogene in the amplicon.

Brown et al[17] further examined the 11q13 locus. Based on findings in breast cancer, they evaluated the novel oncogene *EMSY* in ovarian cancer using FISH, array CGH, and real-time quantitative polymerase chain reaction (PCR). *EMSY* encodes a protein that interacts with *BRCA2* and could be a mechanism for *BRCA2* loss in sporadic cancer. Brown et al[17] observed *EMSY* amplification in approximately 18% of high-grade serous carcinomas, along with lower rates in other histologic subtypes. Array CGH localized the area of highest copy number gain to *EMSY* rather than *CCDN1*. *EMSY*, *PAK1*, and *CCDN1* gene amplification and RNA expression were significantly correlated. These results suggest that multiple oncogenes may be located in the 11q13 region.

Chemoresistant tumors

Array CGH has been used to assess chromosomal aberrations associated with chemotherapy response. Wang et al[18] used CGH, PCR, and western blotting to identify a novel role for the protein TWIST in acquired resistance to paclitaxel and other microtubule-disrupting drugs. CGH was also used to assess the differences between platinum-sensitive cell lines and platinum-resistant sublines.[19] A host of chromosomal gains and deletions were observed, suggesting that acquired resistance was associated with substantial genomic instability. Subsequent work by Takano et al[20,21] identified specific gains of 1q21–22 in platinum resistance, which includes *MUC1*. Copy number abnormalities as well as expression levels of MUC1 were significantly higher in platinum-resistant tumors compared with platinum-sensitive ones.[20] Recent work combining array CGH with extreme drug resistance assays has allowed preliminary identification of an amplicon on chromosome 1 that seems to correlate highly with paclitaxel resistance.[22]

Prognosis

Other studies have evaluated the impact of cytogenetic abnormalities on prognosis. Hu et al[23] compared CGH analysis of 10 primary and 10 recurrent serous ovarian carcinomas; they found widespread copy number aberrations, with 1q41–44, 2p22–25, and 3q26–29 gains and 5q14–22 losses more common in recurrent tumors. Survival correlated inversely with the number of abnormalities. Kildal et al[24] studied ovarian germ cell tumors. They determined that

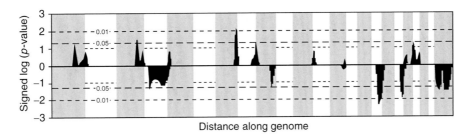

Figure 5.4 Statistical significance of associations between genomic aberrations and survival duration for aberrations detected using CGH. The aberration significance is plotted at the normal genomic location of the aberration. Significance values for aberrations present in less than 20% of the tumors are not plotted. Associations with increases in copy number are plotted as positive values and associations with deletions are plotted as negative values. Reproduced from Gray et al. Gynecol Oncol 2003;88:516–21[3] with permission from Academic Press.

all of the immature teratomas were diploid, while the endodermal sinus tumors and dysgerminomas were tetraploid, polyploid, or aneuploid. CGH revealed that DNA copy number abnormalities were more common in tetraploid and aneuploid tumors compared with diploid ones. In addition, DNA ploidy was a significant prognostic indicator for survival, along with stage and residual tumor volume. Finally, Gray et al[3] and Suzuki et al[25] subjected 60 ovarian carcinoma specimens to CGH and found that copy number abnormalities were more commonly associated with high grade than high stage, particularly loss of 4q. Patients with fewer than five aberrations lived significantly longer than those with more than five. Specifically, gains on 1q, 3q, 7q, 8, and 20 as well as losses on 4p, 9, 16q, 18q, and X were also associated with reduced survival (Figure 5.4).

EXPRESSION PROFILING

Platforms

Microarray technology has been developed as a method to evaluate the relative abundance of gene expression in tumor samples. Two different array platforms have been generated: cDNA and oligonucleotide arrays (Figure 5.5). Both platforms allow for the simultaneous analysis of a large number of genes. Although initially limited in the number of genes included, a single array now can test approximately 35000 genes, the entire human genome.

cDNA arrays were first developed at the Brown Laboratory at Stanford University.[26] To generate these arrays, cDNA clones undergo PCR amplification using vector-based primers flanking the cDNAs. The amplified products are then gel-purified and robotically printed onto glass slides. Sample RNA is then harvested from test specimen and undergoes reverse transcription and labeling with a fluorescent dye. Cyanine-3 and cyanine-5 fluorescent dyes are typically used due to their good incorporation by reverse transcription, relative photostability, and widely separated excitation/emission spectra. Hybridization of the specimen to the array is then performed. Detection of hybridized probes is achieved by laser excitation of the fluorescent markers followed by scanning using confocal laser microscopy.

In contrast, Affymetrix oligonucleotide arrays are created using photolithography and solid-phase DNA synthesis to produce specific oligonucleotide sequences.[27] Synthetic linker

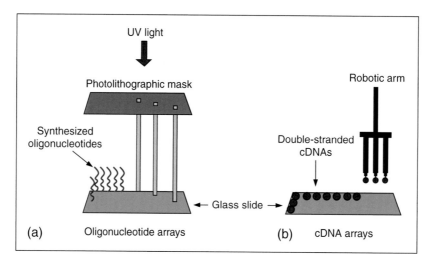

Figure 5.5 Two main microarray formats are currently available. (a) Oligonucleotide arrays, which were initially pioneered by Affymetrix, are generated using a combination of oligonucleotide synthesis and photolithography. A photolithographic mask is used to generate localized areas of photodeprotection on a glass slide that has been coated with linker molecules containing a photochemically removable protecting group. Specific deoxyribonucleotide triphosphates (dNTPs) are then chemically coupled at the deprotected site, facilitating the syntheses of specific oligonucleotide sequences. A series of different photolithographic masks are used with an intervening dNTP coupling reaction to generate the desired array. Other methods of generating oligonucleotide arrays rely on depositing a presynthesized oligonucleotide onto the array. (b) cDNA arrays are generated by robotically printing double-stranded cDNAs of known sequence onto a glass slide at a predetermined spatial orientation. The printing is achieved by a computer-controlled robot arm moving in three dimensions and containing up to 12 pen tips that deposit a precise volume of purified cDNA onto the glass, which has been coated with aminosilanes or amino-reactive silanes. Other methods of printing are also available, such as piezo or ink-jet delivery. The spotted cDNA is then crosslinked to the slide by ultraviolet irradiation. Reproduced from Harkin et al. The Oncologist 2000;5:501–7 with permission from AlphaMed Press.

molecules with a photochemically removable protecting group are attached to a solid support. A photolithographic mask is then applied, through which ultraviolet light is passed.

This generates localized areas of photodeprotection, to which deoxyribonucleotide triphosphates (dNTPs) are attached in a chemical coupling reaction. Each mask generates different areas of photodeprotection, and, with an intervening chemical coupling step, the desired probes are synthesized. Oligonucleotide arrays are therefore synthesized based on sequence information alone, without the need for physical intermediates such as clones and PCR products. Oligonucleotide probe synthesis provides

the opportunity to include internal control sequences. In the array design, multiple oligonucleotide sequences of the same parent gene are used. In addition, intentional mismatch probes containing a single-base difference are produced. These yield internal positive and negative controls within a single hybridization.

Sample preparation for oligonucleotide arrays involves reverse transcription of RNA, amplification, and labeling of the cDNA probe by in vitro transcription in the presence of biotinylated dNTP, resulting in linear amplification of the cDNA. The biotin-labeled cRNA probe is then hybridized to the oligonucleotide array, followed by binding to a streptavidin-conjugated fluorescent marker. Detection of the bound probe is performed with laser excitation and scanning of the emission spectra using confocal laser microscopy. An example of a hybridized array is shown in Figure 5.6.

Microarrays containing probes for 35 000 genes yield a substantial amount of data, even in a single hybridization experiment. The degree of fluorescence identified is recorded as an amplitude change numerically by the array scanner. Bioinformatics programs are then essential to assimilate and analyze the data. Hierarchichal clustering is one technique utilized to group samples that have relative similarity in their gene expression profiles.

Sample selection and procurement

Expression profiles can be performed on ovarian tumors and compared with expression profiles generated from normal tissues. These comparisons highlight the genes whose aberrant expression is present in the malignant cell compared

with that of its normal counterpart. The selection of the appropriate control sample is critical, as it serves as the basis for this analysis. For ovarian tumors, the control sample potentially can include RNA harvested from the whole ovary or solely from the ovarian surface epithelium. Since the majority of ovarian cancers are thought to be of epithelial origin, the surface epithelium may provide a more specific normal counterpart. Alternatively, there is the potential loss of genetic alterations in the ovarian stroma, the local host microenvironment, which may be important to the adjacent tumor cell growth. One group studied this question by evaluating the five tissues typically selected as a normal ovarian control in ovarian cancer microarray profiling.[28] The comparison of each normal tissue with ovarian cancer generated a unique set of differentially expressed genes, emphasizing the importance of the normal control when assessing the list of genes found to be up- or downregulated in an ovarian cancer profiling study. While there is no broadly accepted standard for the optimal normal ovarian control,

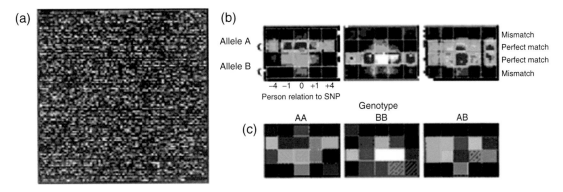

Figure 5.6 Genotyping arrays. (a) A single array with over 120 000 probes designed to determine the genotype of a sample at over 3000 biallelic loci. (b) The fluorescence intensity pattern for a set of probes designed to interrogate a single locus, showing the presence of an AA homozygote, a BB homozygote and an AB heterozygote. The upper and lower halves of the probe blocks interrogate the A and B alleles, respectively. Each half consists of pairs of probes centered on the polymorphic position and offset one and four bases to either side. The probe pairs consist of a perfect match and single-base mismatch to the reference sequence for the specific allele. For each locus, interrogation blocks are included for both the sense and the antisense strands. Reproduced from Lipshutz et al. Nature Genetics 1999;21:20–4 with permission from Nature Publishing Group.

these data indicate the potential hazards in cross-comparison between microarray studies if alternate control sample acquisition is used.

For tumors that present as small surface lesions, laser capture microdissection can be utilized to assure that an adequate proportion of tumor cells are present in the sample. Amplification of the sample RNA material prior to labeling for hybridization can be performed. Alternatively, some probes provide an amplified signal, which can be of sufficient magnitude for scan detection and avoids the potential for uneven amplification of the primary specimen. Microdissection also allows various components of a tumor to be analyzed while avoiding contamination from unwanted adjacent tissue; for example, tumor vasculature or stroma can be selectively profiled while excluding necrotic or normal tissue nearby. In laser capture microdissection, a laser microbeam adheres cells of interest to a thermoplastic membrane. This process is guided by the operator, who identifies the cells of interest and activates the laser while visualizing tissue sections under light microscopy (Figure 5.7). A representative sample of tissue prior to microdissection, following this procedure, and the resultant isolated cells of interest are shown in Figure 5.8.

Profiles in ovarian cancer

A number of investigators have utilized molecular profiling to characterize ovarian tumors, and have demonstrated distinct expression profiles based on histologic subtype, chemosensitivity, and overall survival.

Histologic subtype

Ovarian cancers of different histologic subtype have been profiled.[29–34] In each of these studies, histologic subtype was shown to correlate with

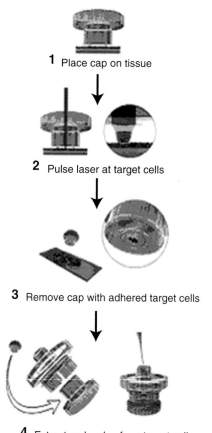

1 Place cap on tissue

2 Pulse laser at target cells

3 Remove cap with adhered target cells

4 Extract molecules from target cells

Figure 5.7 The laser capture microdissection process. Guided microscopically, the LCM cap is placed over the target tissue. A laser microbeam is then activated, which melts a thermoplastic ethyl vinyl acetate membrane on the clear plastic cap and causes adherence of the target tissue. The captured cells are then extracted from the cap surface for analysis. Reprinted courtesy of Molecular Devices, a division of MDS Analytical Technologies, available at www.moleculardevices.com.

unique gene expression patterns. The expression of these genes likely contributes to the clinical and biologic characteristics of each of these tumors and forms the basis for additional study. The following discussion reviews some of the largest studies to date, as grouped by their results for a particular histologic subtype.

Clear cell carcinoma of the ovary has traditionally been associated with chemoresistance

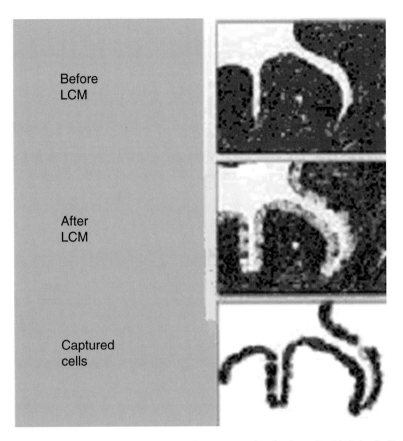

Figure 5.8 Laser capture microdissection (LCM) allows for a targeted collection of epithelial cells. Reprinted courtesy of Molecular Devices, a division of MDS Analytical Technologies, available at www.moleculardevices.com.

and an overall poor clinical outcome. Using oligonucleotide arrays, Schwartz et al[29] analyzed the four major histologic types of ovarian cancer among 113 separate tumors.[29] A unique expression profile of 73 genes was demonstrated in the clear cell ovarian cancers. Similarly, other investigators have also noted a distinct profile among clear cell ovarian cancers compared with ovarian cancers of other histologic subtype.[30] One study compared the expression profiles of ovarian cancers of different histologies with the analogous subtypes of endometrial cancer.[31] This analysis showed a strong influence of the organ of origin for papillary serous and endometrioid histologies. In contrast, tumors

of clear cell histology demonstrated a striking similarity despite different organs of origin, even when renal clear cell carcinomas were included in the analysis (Figure 5.9). Collectively, these data suggest that there may be a benefit to type-specific diagnostic and therapeutic strategies for ovarian cancer. Subsequent validation studies with clinical correlation have identified upregulation of the *ABCF2* gene in clear cell ovarian cancers (Figure 5.10).[32] The *ABCF2* gene belongs to the ATP-binding cassette gene superfamily. Currently this gene requires further characterization, as it may represent a useful prognostic marker or a potential therapeutic target in clear cell ovarian malignancy.

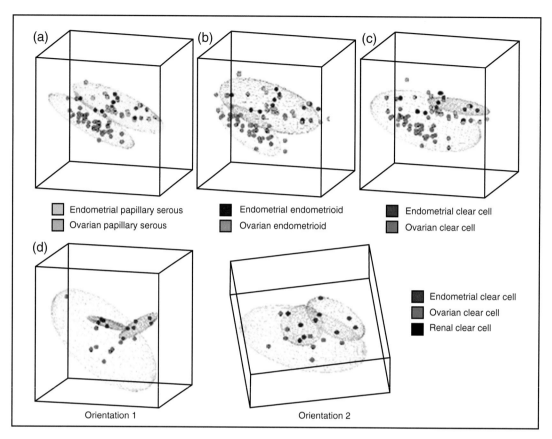

Endometrial papillary serous
Ovarian papillary serous

Endometrial endometrioid
Ovarian endometrioid

Endometrial clear cell
Ovarian clear cell

Endometrial clear cell
Ovarian clear cell
Renal clear cell

Orientation 1

Orientation 2

Figure 5.9 Graphic depiction of principal component analysis of ovarian and endometrial cancer according to histology. Principal component analysis was done after inputing values using Partek Pro 2000 software (Partek). These data were imported into Matlab software (The Mathworks) to allow depiction of the elliptical region where an additional sample of a particular group would fall with a 95% confidence interval. (a) Analysis of tumors with serous histology, showing two nonoverlapping elliptical regions separating endometrial (top) from ovarian (bottom) specimens. (b) Analysis of tumors with endometrioid histology, showing two nonoverlapping elliptical regions separating endometrial (top) from ovarian (bottom) specimens. (c) Analysis of tumors with clear cell histology, showing overlapping elliptical regions representing endometrial (top) and ovarian (bottom) specimens. (d) Analysis of tumors according to organ of origin shows three overlapping elliptical regions among ovarian, endometrial, and renal clear cell specimens; two different orientations (1 and 2) are shown. Reproduced from Zorn et al. Clin Cancer Res 2005;11:6422–30.[31] with permission from the American Association for Cancer Research.

Other investigators have focused on the molecular signature identified in mucinous ovarian tumors. Microdissected mucinous cystadenomas, tumors of low malignant potential (LMPs), and adenocarcinomas were compared with normal ovarian surface epithelium and a series of microdissected serous ovarian tumors.[33] Hierarchical clustering showed a close association of mucinous tumors. Analysis of the gene

expression profiles in mucinous tumors demonstrated upregulation of genes involved in cytoskeletal function, and confirmational analysis of these data was performed with reverse transcriptase (RT)-PCR. Other investigators have utilized whole-tissue samples, and, similarly, mucinous tumors demonstrate a distinct pattern of gene expression.[34] One gene highly overexpressed in mucinous ovarian cancers is *LGALS4*,

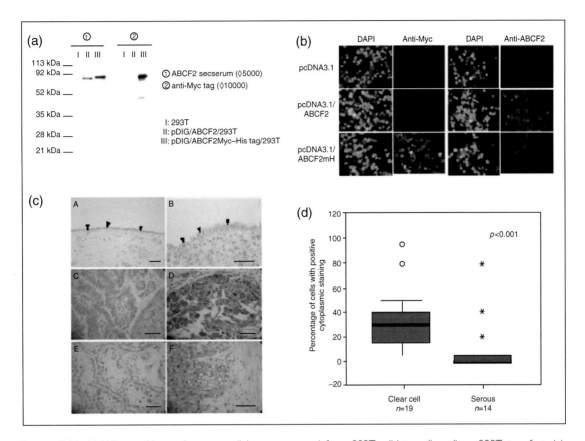

Figure 5.10 (a) Western blot analyses on cell lysates prepared from 293T wild-type (lane I) or 293T transfected by pcDNA3.1 carrying ABCF2 (lane II) or Myc–His-tagged ABCF2 (lane III) using an anti-ABCF2 polyclonal antibody or an anti-Myc tag monoclonal antibody. (b) Immunolocalization of ABCF2 and Myc tag proteins in 293T cells transfected with pcDNA3.1 vector alone or with vectors containing ABCf2 or Myc–His-tagged ABCF2. (c) Immunolocalization of ABCF2 protein in normal ovaries, endometrioid cysts, and ovarian cancer tissue: (A) negative immunostaining of ABCF2 in the surface epithelium of a normal ovary; (B) negative immunostaining of ABCF2 in the epithelial lining of an endometriotic cyst; (C) positive immunostaining of ABCF2 in serous cystadenocarcinoma; (D) negative immunostaining of ABCF2 in serous cystadenocarcinoma; (E) positive immunostaining of ABCF2 in clear cell adenocarcinoma. (d) Comparison of protein expression of ABCF2 between clear cell adenocarcinoma and serous cystadenocarcinoma. The box is bounded abouve and below by the 75th and 25th percentiles, and the median is the line in the box. Whiskers are drawn to the nearest value not beyond a standard span from the quartiles; points beyond outliers are drawn individually, where the standard span is 1.5× (interquartile range). Reproduced from Tsuda et al. Clin Cancer Res 2005;11:6880–8[32] with permission from the American Association for Cancer Research.

which encodes an intestinal cell surface molecule. Interestingly, *LGALS4* is located at 19q13.3, a region previously identified as harboring a high frequency of loss of heterozygosity (LOH) in mucinous ovarian cancers.[35]

Other research has focused on clarifying whether a continuum from normal to premalignant to malignant tissue exists for ovarian cancer as it does for other malignancies such as colorectal and cervical cancers. For instance, LMPs also known as borderline tumors of the ovary, have metastatic potential and some histologic features similar to those of invasive ovarian cancers; however, LMPs generally demonstrate a slow growth rate and an indolent clinical course. Gene expression profiling has been applied to define the relationship between LMPs and invasive ovarian cancers.[36] Microdissected LMPs and invasive ovarian cancer of both serous and mucinous histology were compared with normal ovarian surface epithelium. Unsupervised clustering of the expression profiles demonstrated that the serous LMPs cluster separately from high-grade tumors and closer to normal epithelial cells (Figure 5.11). Interestingly, the majority of low-grade serous

invasive tumors clustered with serous LMP tumors, with p53-dependent genes prominently represented on the gene lists. The high-grade invasive tumors showed enhanced expression of genes linked to proliferation, chromosomal instability, and epigenetic silencing compared with the low-grade tumors and LMPs. These findings strongly support the concept that serous LMPs develop via a pathway that includes the low-grade tumors,

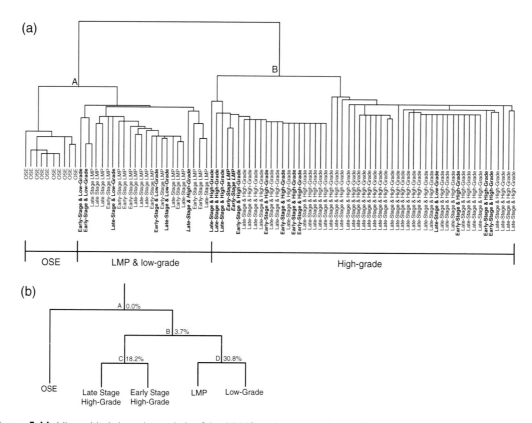

Figure 5.11 Hierarchical clustering analysis of the 14 119 probe sets passing the filtering criteria for tumors of low malignant potential (LMP), low-grade and high-grade tumors, and normal ovarian serous epithelium (OSE) specimens and binary tree validation. (a) Clustering analysis was completed using the 1-correlation metric with centroid linkage. The overall tree structure was retained, despite the association of low-grade tumors with LMPs and the grouping of early-stage and late-stage high-grade lesions. Low-grade and early-stage high-grade samples are indicated in bold. Misclassified specimens are bold italicized. (b) Binary tree analysis confirmed the hierarchical clustering results. The diagram was generated using binary tree prediction followed by leave-one-out cross-validation to estimate the error associated with the tree building process. OSE samples were classified as base to the ovarian cancer specimens. LMPs and low-grade cancer were more closely aligned to each other, as were early-stage and late-stage high-grade tumors. Percentages indicate the misclassification error associated with each node. Reproduced from Bonome et al. Cancer Res 2005;65:10602–12[36] with permission from the American Associated for Cancer Research.

whereas high-grade tumors develop along an independent route. In contrast, analysis of mucinous tumors revealed a much closer relationship between LMPs and their invasive counterparts. In fact, a molecular continuum from benign mucinous cystadenoma to mucinous LMPs to invasive cancer seems to exist. This supports the idea that a benign mucinous cyst can progress via a borderline lesion to an invasive tumor, whereas a serous cyst typically will not undergo transformation to a high-grade ovarian cancer. Additional insights from profiling research such as this may identify the specific molecular events involved in the etiology of each type of ovarian tumor. These molecular events can then be utilized as targets for screening strategies or for therapeutic intervention.

Clinical outcomes

Gene expression profiling has been used to identify patterns of gene expression in ovarian cancer that correlate with important clinical outcomes.[37] One study employed an oligonucleotide array with over 40 000 features to achieve a whole-genome assessment, in which 1191 genes demonstrated differential expression when compared with normal ovarian surface epithelium. RT–PCR was utilized as a confirmatory analysis on 14 randomly selected genes. The differentially expressed genes include those associated with cell growth, differentiation, adhesion, apoptosis, and migration. Further investigation into the role of these genes specifically in ovarian cancer provides a fertile ground for future study. With regard to other known clinical prognostic markers, unique gene expression profiles have been demonstrated for early-versus late-stage disease, tumor grade, surgical resectability, and overall survival.[38–40]

Recently, correlation of gene expression profiles with ovarian cancer chemoresistance has been defined.[41–44] Unique profiles are associated with primary ovarian cancers that subsequently demonstrate either sensitivity or resistance to chemotherapy. Intrinsic and acquired chemoresistance yield different patterns of gene expression. Further, gene expression profiles have been used to predict early recurrence and positive second-look surgical findings, which are clinical markers of chemoresistant disease.[45,46] Other investigators have studied the molecular changes in ovarian cancer cells treated with cytotoxic agents in vitro in order to characterize the mechanism of drug activity and drug resistance.[47,48] The opportunity to define changes in gene activity associated with chemoresistance provides an opportunity to target the involved pathways and improve response to chemotherapy. For example, groups of genes with an altered expression profile may point to an upregulated molecular signaling pathway that correlates with a tumor's resistance to chemotherapy. The mechanism of this candidate pathway can then be further explored in vitro to identfy a useful target and thereby prevent or reduce chemoresistance. Alternatively, identification of aberrant expression profiles could be prognostic of a patient's likelihood for resistance to a particular chemotherapy program and thereby have an impact on treatment selection. This area of study requires further investigation and an exploration of these datasets in comparison to genes, such as *MDR1*, that are already known to play a role in drug resistance.

PROTEOMICS

Following the advent of genomics, proteomics has surfaced as the large-scale study of cellular protein expression and function.[49,50] The protein complement of the cell, the proteome, is more dynamic and variable than the genome due to its multitude of potential interactions and secondary modifications. Proteomic technologies consist of a protein separation phase and a detection phase. The classic approach of two-dimensional gel electrophoresis consists of protein separation first based on charge and then on mass, followed by detection using specific protein stains. Mass spectrometry (MS) plays an important role in proteomics due to its ability to perform protein separation based on a mass/charge ratio as well as protein detection.

One method of protein expression profiling is electrospray ionization (ESI), which ionizes analysates out of a solution. Protein samples flow into a high-voltage electric field and are received on an ion detector. In contrast, matrix-assisted laser desorption/ionization time-of-flight MS (MALDI-TOF-MS) involves mixing a protein sample with an energy-absorbing organic molecule called the matrix. The proteins are crystallized within the matrix, placed on a metal probe, and irradiated with a laser. The matrix facilitates energy transfer from the laser to the proteins, causing the proteins to ionize and desorb for detection by the analyzer (Figure 5.12).

Surface-enhanced laser desorption/ionization time-of-flight MS (SELDI-TOF-MS) is an improved approach that uses arrays of distinct chromatographic surfaces to selectively bind and retain proteins. After washing with buffers, the mass and amount of each protein is measured

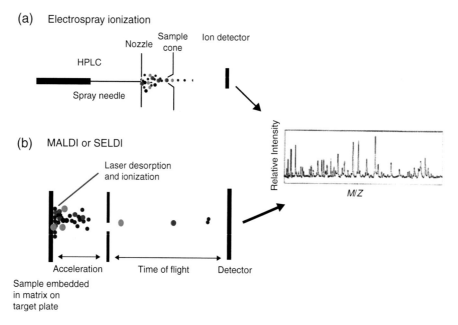

Figure 5.12 The essential components of mass spectrometry are the ionization source, the mass analyzer, and the detector. (a) Electrospray ionization produces ions when protein samples in a solvent flow through a fine needle in a high-voltage electric field. The technique is often coupled with prior separation by high-performance liquid chromatography (HPLC). (b) Matrix-assisted laser desorption/ionization (MALDI) creates ions by mixing a protein sample with an energy-absorbing organic molecule to both ionize and desorb from the surface. Surface-enhanced laser desorption/ionization (SELDI) uses the same principle as MALDI but employs arrays of distinct chromatographic surfaces to selectively bind and retain proteins. After peptides are ionized by either the electrospray or MALDI or SELDI methods, they are accelerated from the ion source and guided into an analyzer that separates the molecules according to their mass-to-charge (M/Z) ratios. Reproduced from Hoehn and Suffredini, Proteomics, Crit Care Med 2005;33:S444–8 with permission from Lippincott Williams & Wilkins.

by irradiating the surface with a laser and measuring the time of flight. Bound proteins are thereby detected by low-resolution TOF-MS and the expression of each retained protein can be compared among clinical samples. In addition to protein separation, the chromatographic surface used in SELDI binds proteins more homogeneously compared with the inert MALDI plate and leads to more reproducible protein expression profiling.

SELDI-TOF-MS has become popular for examining protein expression differences in clinical samples. This technology was utilized to identify serum protein expression profiles in ovarian cancer patients and tested as a putative novel screening technique for ovarian cancer by Petricoin et al.[51] In this study, protein expression profiles from 50 patients with ovarian cancer and 50 unaffected women were generated using SELDI-TOF-MS. Distinct protein profiles were identified for each of these groups of patients. This profile was then used on a test set of 116 masked samples comprising 50 ovarian cancer cases and 66 unaffected cases. The authors reported 100% sensitivity and 95% specificity and a 94% positive predictive value (PPV) in the correct identification of ovarian cancer and unaffected cases in the test set.

Despite initial enthusiasm, there were several limitations of this study. It is the relative low prevalence of ovarian cancer that is the major challenge in the identification of a useful screening technique. From a statistical standpoint, the study by Petricoin et al[51] used a test set of cases that had an arbitrarily high (close to 50%) prevalence of ovarian cancer. Ovarian cancer prevalence, however, is closer to 1 in 2500 in the general population. Since PPV is largely dependent on disease prevalence, the profiling results actually yield a PPV <1% when real-world prevalence is applied. The PPV is similarly low when statistically applied with disease prevalence in high-risk populations. Another limitation of this study is the emphasis on protein profiling without the identification of specific discriminatory proteins. The possibility therefore exists that the protein spectral changes identified in this study represent secondary changes rather than protein events specific to ovarian cancer. Further, the study results could not be replicated by other investigators.[52] Despite several limitations, this study was a novel utilization of developing molecular techniques and importantly raised awareness with regard to molecular profiling and its potential for application in the clinical setting.

Subsequently, a multi-institutional case–control study was performed in which serum proteomic expressions were analyzed on patients with invasive ovarian cancer, patients with benign pelvic masses, and healthy women without any known pelvic pathology.[53] Cross-validation between participating centers was performed. Three biomarkers were identified, including apolipoprotein A1, a truncated form of transthyretin, and a cleavage fragment of inter-α-trypsin inhibitor.

Other investigators have studied ovarian surface epithelium from ovaries removed prophylactically in high-risk patient groups. He et al[54] studied ovarian surface epithelium obtained from patients in the general population undergoing a benign gynecologic procedure. This was compared with expression profiles generated from ovarian surface epithelium harvested from women undergoing prophylactic oophorectomy due to a strong family history of breast/ovarian cancer (at least two first-degree relatives with such cancer and/or testing positive for BRCA1 mutations). A predominance of sequences related to the stress response pathway was identified in the ovarian epithelium of high-risk patients and confirmed by western blotting and RT–PCR. These protein alterations require further characterization, as they may represent potential early markers for the diagnosis of ovarian cancer.

Reverse-phase protein microarray technology is being evaluated as a new means to track biologic response to therapy through measurement of post-translational phosphorylation events and thereby track the protein function in their signaling pathways. Since protein expression is the downstream event of the genomic complement, protein expression profiling provides a unique perspective on active cellular processes.

CONCLUSIONS

Molecular profiling at the genomic and proteomic levels has become available due to recent advances in molecular technologies. The current challenge is to harness the broad scope of information acquired with molecular profiling. The opportunity to understand the molecular profile of ovarian cancer may unlock meaningful information about the basis of ovarian cancer cell growth and thereby provide an opportunity to develop more precise screening techniques and targeted molecular therapeutics.

REFERENCES

1. Shayesteh L, Lu Y, Kuo WL, et al. PIK3CA is implicated as an oncogene in ovarian cancer. Nat Genet 1999;21:99–102.

2. Kallioniemi A, Kallioniemi OP, Sudar D, et al. Comparative genomic hybridization for molecular cytogenetic analysis of solid tumors. Science 1992;258:818–21.

3. Gray J, Suzuki S, Kuo WL, et al. Genome copy number abnormalities in ovarian cancer. Gynecol Oncol 2003;88:S16–21.

4. Snijders A, Nowee M, Fridlyand J, et al. Genome-wide-array-based comparative genomic hybridization reveals genetic homogeneity and frequent copy number increases encompassing CCNE1 in fallopian tube carcinoma. Oncogene 2003;22:4281–6.

5. Pere H, Tapper J, Seppala M, et al. Genomic alterations in fallopian tube carcinoma: comparison to serous uterine and ovarian carcinomas reveals similarity suggesting likeness in molecular pathogenesis. Cancer Res 1998;58:4274–6.

6. Heselmeyer K, Hellstrom AC, Blegen H, et al. Primary carcinoma of the fallopian tube: comparative genomic hybridization reveals high genetic instability and a specific, recurring pattern of chromosomal aberrations. Int J Gynecol Pathol 1998;17:245–54.

7. Davies J, Wilson I, Lam W. Array CGH technologies and their application to cancer genomes. Chromosome Res 2005;13:237–48.

8. Ylstra B, van den Ijssel P, Carvalho B, et al. BAC to the future! or oligonucleotides: a perspective for microarray comparative genomic hybridization. Nucleic Acids Res 2006;34:445–50.

9. Zhou X, Rao N, Cole S, et al. Progress in concurrent analysis of loss of heterozygosity and comparative genomic hybridization utilizing high density single nucleotide polymorphism arrays. Cancer Genet Cytogenet 2005;159:53–7.

10. Matsuzaki H, Loi H, Dong S, et al. Parallel genotyping of over 10,000 SNPs using a one-primer assay on a high-density oligonucleotide array. Genome Res 2004;14:414–25.

11. Pinkel D, Albertson D. Array comparative genomic hybridization and its applications in cancer. Nat Genet 2005;37:S11–17.

12. Albertson D, Pinkel D. Genomic microarrays in human genetic disease and cancer. Hum Mol Genet 2003;12:R145–52.

13. Tapper J, Sarantaus L, Vahteristo P, et al. Genetic changes in inherited and sporadic ovarian carcinomas by comparative genomic hybridization: extensive similarity except for a difference at chromosome 2q24–q32. Cancer Res 1998;58:2715–19.

14. Patael-Karasik Y, Daniely M, Gotlieb WH, et al. Comparative genomic hybridization in inherited and sporadic ovarian tumors in Israel. Cancer Genet Cytogenet 2000;121:26–32.

15. Israeli O, Gotlieb WH, Friedman E, et al. Familial vs sporadic ovarian tumors: characteristic genomic alterations analyzed by CGH. Gynecol Oncol 2003;90:629–36.

16. Schraml P, Schwerdtfeger G, Burkhalter F, et al. Combined array comparative genomic hybridization and tissue microarray analysis suggest *PAK1* at 11q13.5–q14 as a critical oncogene target in ovarian cancer. Am J Pathol 2003;163:985–92.

17. Brown L, Irving J, Parker R, et al. Amplification of *EMSY*, a novel oncogene on 11q13, in high grade ovarian surface epithelial carcinomas. Gynecol Oncol 2006;100:264–70.

18. Wang X, Ling MT, Guan XY, et al. Identification of a novel function of TWIST, a bHLH protein, in the development of acquired Taxol resistance in human cancer cells. Oncogene 2004;23:474–82.

19. Wasenius VM, Jekunen A, Monni O, et al. Comparative genomic hybridization analysis of chromosomal changes occurring during development of acquired resistance to cisplatin in human ovarian carcinoma cells. Genes Chromosomes Cancer 1997;18:286–91.

20. Takano M, Fujii K, Kita T, et al. Amplicon profiling reveals cytoplasmic overexpression of MUC1 protein as an indicator of resistance to platinum-based chemotherapy in patients with ovarian cancer. Oncol Rep 2004;12:1177–82.

21. Takano M, Kudo K, Goto T, et al. Analyses by comparative genomic hybridization of genes relating with cisplatin resistance in ovarian cancer. Hum Cell 2001;14:267–71.

22. Smith D, Shahbahrami B, Kerfoot C, et al. Identification of amplifications and deletions in Taxol-resistant ovarian cancer by comparative genomic hybridization screening. Gynecol Oncol 2006;101:S92.

23. Hu J, Khanna V, Jones M, et al. Comparative study of primary and recurrent ovarian serous carcinomas: comparative genomic hybridization analysis with a potential application for prognosis. Gynecol Oncol 2002;89:369–75.

24. Kildal W, Kaern J, Kraggerud SM, et al. Evaluation of genomic changes in a large series of malignant germ cell tumors – relation to clinicopathologic variables. Cancer Genet Cytogenet 2004;155:25–32.

25. Suzuki S, Moore DH, Ginzinger DG, et al. An approach to analysis of large-scale correlations between genome changes and clinical endpoints in ovarian cancer. Cancer Res 2000;60: 5382–5.

26. Schena M, Shalon D, Davis RW, et al. Quantitative monitoring of gene expression patterns with complimentary DNA microarray. Science 1995;270:467–70.

27. Lockhart DJ, Dong H, Mittman M, et al. Expression monitoring by hybridization to high density oligonucleotide arrays. Nat Biotechnol 1996;14:1675–80.

28. Zorn K, Jazaeri AA, Awtrey CS, et al. Choice of normal ovarian control influences determination of differentially expressed genes in ovarian cancer expression profiling studies. Clin Cancer Res 2003;9:4811–18.

29. Schwartz DR, Kardia SL, Shedden KA, et al. Gene expression in ovarian cancer reflects both morphology and biological behavior, distinguishing clear cell from other poor-prognosis ovarian carcinomas. Cancer Res 2002;62:4722–9.

30. Schaner ME, Ross DT, Ciaravino G, Sorlie T, et al. Gene expression patterns in ovarian carcinomas. Mol Biol Cell 2003;14:4376–86.

31. Zorn K, Bonome T, Gangi L, et al. Gene expression profiles of serous, endometrioid,

and clear cell subtypes of ovarian and endometrial cancer. Clin Cancer Res 2005;11:6422–30.

32. Tsuda H, Ito YM, Ohashi Y, et al. Identification of overexpression and amplification of *ABCF2* in clear cell ovarian adenocarcinomas by cDNA microarray analyses. Clin Cancer Res 2005;11:6880–8.

33. Wamunyokoli FW, Bonome T, Lee JY, et al. Expression profiling of mucinous tumor of the ovary identifies genes of clinicopathologic importance. Clin Cancer Res 2006; 12:690–700.

34. Heinzelmann-Schwartz VA, Gardiner-Garden M, Henshall SM. A distinct molecular profile associated with mucinous epithelial ovarian cancer. Br J of Cancer 2006;94:904–13.

35. Felmate CM, Lee KR, Johnson M, et al. Whole-genome allelotyping identified distinct loss-of-heterozygosity patterns in mucinous ovarian and appendiceal carcinomas. Clin Cancer Res 2005;11:7651–7.

36. Bonome T, Lee JY, Park DC, et al. Expression profiling of serous low malignant potential, low-grade, and high-grade tumors of the ovary. Cancer Res 2005;65:10602–12.

37. Donninger H, Bonome T, Radonovich M, et al. Whole genome expression of profiling of advance stage papillary serous ovarian cancer reveals activated pathways. Oncogene 2004;23:8065–77.

38. Berchuck A, Iversen ES, Lancaster JM, et al. Patterns of gene expression that characterize long-term survival in advanced stage serous ovarian cancers. Clin Cancer Res 2005;11:3686–96.

39. Shridhar V, Lee J, Pandita A, Iturria S, et al. Genetic analysis of early- versus late-stage ovarian tumors. Cancer Res 2001;61:5895–904.

40. Berchuck A, Iversen ES, Lancaster JM, et al. Prediction of optimal versus suboptimal cytoreduction of advanced-stage serous ovarian cancer with the use of microarrays. Am J Obstet Gynecol 2004;190:910–25.

41. Jazaeri AA, Lu K, Schmandt R, et al. Molecular determinants of tumor differentiation in papillary serous ovarian carcinoma. Mol Carcinog 2003;36:53–9.

42. Jazaeri AA, Awtrey CS, Chandramouli GV, et al. Gene expression profiles associated with response to chemotherapy in epithelial ovarian cancers. Clin Cancer Res 2005;11:6300–10.

43. Helleman J, Jansen MP, Span PN, et al. Molecular profiling of platinum resistant ovarian cancer. Int J Cancer 2006;118:1963–71.

44. Selvanayagam ZE, Cheung TH, Wei N, et al. Prediction of chemotherapeutic response in ovarian cancer with DNA microarray expression profiling. Cancer Genet Cytogenet 2004; 154:63–6.

45. Hartmann LC, Lu KH, Linette GP, et al. Gene expression profiles predict early relapse in ovarian cancer after platinum-paclitaxel chemotherapy. Clin Cancer Res 2005;11:2149–55.

46. Spentzos D, Levine DA, Kolia S, et al. Unique gene expression profile based on pathologic response in epithelial ovarian cancer. J Clin Oncol 2005;23:7911–18.

47. Khabele D, Lopez-Jones M, Yang W, et al. Tumor necrosis factor-alpha related gene response to epothilone B in ovarian cancer. Gynecol Oncol 2004;93:19–26.

48. Wang TH, Chan YH, Chen CW, et al. Paclitaxel (Taxol) upregulates expression of functional interleukin-6 in human ovarian cancer cells through multiple signaling pathways. Oncogene 2006;25:4857–66.

49. Aebersold R, Mann M. Mass spectrometry-based proteomics. Nature 2003;422:198–207.

50. Sellers TA, Yates JR. Review of proteomics with applications to genetic epidemiology. Genet Epidemiol 2003;24:83–98.

51. Petricoin EF, Ardekani AM, Hitt BA, et al. Use of proteomic patterns in serum to identify ovarian cancer. Lancet 2002;359:572–7.

52. Baggerly KA, Morris JS, Edmonson SR, Coombes KR. Signal in noise: evaluating

reported reproducibility of serum proteomic tests for ovarian cancer. J Natl Cancer Inst 2005;97:307–9.

53. Zhang Z, Bast RC, Yu Y, et al. Three biomarkers identified from serum proteomic analysis for the detection of early stage ovarian cancer. Cancer Res 2004;64:5882–90.

54. He QY, Zhou Y, Wong E, et al. Proteomic analysis of a preneoplastic phnotype in ovarian surface epithelial cells derived from prophylactic oophorectomies. Gynecol Oncol 2005;98:68–76.

Angiogenesis and epithelial ovarian carcinoma

6

Yvonne G Lin, Robert B Jaffe, and Anil K Sood

INTRODUCTION

Progressive angiogenesis and tumor metastasis characterize advanced-stage ovarian cancer and ultimately lead to poor outcome, with 5-year survival rates <30%.[1] A better understanding of the biologic mechanisms by which ovarian cancer grows and metastasizes is paramount to improving this dismal outcome. Cancer metastasis requires a sequential cascade of interrelated events between the cancer cell and its microenvironment.[2] Following transformation into a malignant phenotype and evasion of the body's immune and nonimmune defenses, tumor cells will grow to a critical mass of about $1\,mm^3$.[2] Growth beyond this size and subsequent metastasis depend on the ability of the tumor to initiate and maintain a sufficient vascular network (angiogenesis).

This chapter will focus on some of the key factors, both structural and biochemical, associated with angiogenesis in ovarian carcinoma. The prognostic relevance of each of these factors will also be discussed.

MECHANISMS AND STEPS IN ANGIOGENESIS

Angiogenesis occurs by either sprouting or nonsprouting processes.[3] Sprouting angiogenesis occurs by branching (true sprouting) of new capillaries from preexisting vessels.

Nonsprouting angiogenesis results from enlargement, splitting, and fusion of preexisting vessels produced by the proliferation of endothelial cells within the wall of a vessel.[3,4] However, tumor vascularization is a complex process and likely involves multiple mechanisms (Table 6.1). For example, in certain tumors, malignant cells may attach to preexisting blood vessels in a process called vessel cooption.[5,6] As the distance between tumor cells and the preexisting blood

Table 6.1 Mechanisms of tumor vascularization

Mechanism	Definition
Angiogenesis	Formation of new blood vessels by proliferation and migration of endothelial cells from preexisting vessels into tubular vascular structures
Vasculogenesis	Formation of new blood vessels from progenitor cells
Vessel cooption	Process by which tumor cells surround preexisting vessels, thus recruiting them during early tumor vascularization
Mosaic vessels	Localization and integration of tumor cells into luminal walls of blood vessels
Vasculogenic mimicry	Ability of aggressive tumor cells to express endothelium-associated genes and to form extracellular matrix-rich vasculogenic-like networks in 3-dimensional cultures

vessel extends beyond 100–200 µm, oxygen supplied via simple diffusion becomes insufficient to maintain further growth.[7] As the tumor becomes hypoxic due to the decreased oxygen gradient, expression of proangiogenic factors such as vascular endothelial growth factor (VEGF) is upregulated, leading to subsequent angiogenesis. Additional features of the developing tumor vasculature include vasculogenic mimicry,[8,9] mosaic vessels,[10] and mobilization of latent blood vessels.[11] The assessment of tumor vasculature and associated factors offers opportunities for their use as potential prognostic and predictive markers.

STRUCTURAL ASPECTS OF TUMOR BLOOD VESSELS

The three main components of a blood vessel are endothelial cells, vascular smooth muscle cells, and pericytes (Figure 6.1).[4] Endothelial cells line the inner aspect of the blood vessel, and the outermost aspect of the blood vessel is covered by pericytes, which are mural cells of mesenchymal origin. Pericytes support the endothelium and play a key role in the structural integrity of normal vasculature.

To date, most studies have focused on the role of endothelial cells in ovarian cancer vasculature. Early evidence describing the role of angiogenesis in ovarian cancer used CD34 as an endothelial cell marker to calculate microvessel counts, and demonstrated their correlation with disease-free survival and overall survival.[12] Subsequent studies utilized von Willebrand factor (vWF); also known as factor VIII-related antigen) immunohistochemistry to show that microvessel counts, or microvessel density (MVD), for metastatic ovarian carcinoma implants in the omentum correlated with CA-125 levels and were independent prognostic indicators of survival.[13] In a larger series using primarily vWF immunohistochemistry, patients with a tumor microvessel count >10 microvessels/high-power field (HPF) had a significantly shorter median survival compared with those with microvessel counts ≤10 microvessels/HPF (2.7 years vs 7.9 years; $p = 0.03$).[14] After controlling for disease stage, 5-year survival rates were significantly lower for those patients with higher tumor

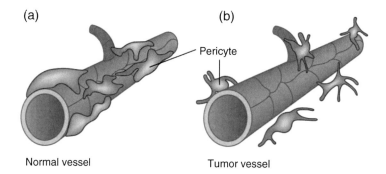

(a)   (b)

Pericyte

Normal vessel   Tumor vessel

Figure 6.1 Structural alterations in tumor vasculature. (reproduced with permission from A.A. Kamat and A.K. Sood, *Current Oncology Reports*, Volume 7, Philadelphia, Current Medicine Group, LLC. 2005.) (a) Mature blood vessels have endothelial cells with tight gap junction and uniform pericyte coverage. (b) Tumor blood vessels are leaky. Although pericytes are present, they are poorly attached to the endothelial cells and have processes projecting toward the abluminal surface or into the tumor stroma.

MVD counts.[14] Taken together, these and additional studies of quantitative analyses of tumor angiogenesis provide relatively consistent evidence that vessel density can be used as an angiogenic prognosticator (Table 6.2).

Recent studies have also demonstrated that blood vessels within tumors actually possess different structural characteristics than traditional blood vessels, such as alterations in pericyte coverage.[4,15–17] Pericytes are stromal (mesenchymal) in origin and are essential for proper vascular development. In murine breast, lung, and pancreatic cancer models, pericytes were identified on most blood vessels; however,

Table 6.2 Prognostic value of angiogenesis markers in ovarian carcinoma

Endothelial cell marker	Associated outcome	Ref
CD34	OS, DFS	12
	OS	98
	Age at diagnosis	99
	PFS	26
	OS	100
	Response to chemotherapy	101
	OS	102
	OS	103
	No association	104
	No association	105
	OS	106
CD31	Response to chemotherapy	107
	OS, stage	14
	OS	108
	OS, stage, grade	109
	Response to chemotherapy	101
	Recurrence, distant metastasis, disease-specific survival	110
	OS	58
von Willebrand factor (factor VIII-related antigen)	OS, preoperative CA-125	13
	No association	27
	Stage	111

OS, overall survival; DFS, disease-free survival; PFS, progression-free survival.

pericytes on tumor vessels were noted to be vastly different from those on normal blood vessels.[18] Specifically, tumor-associated pericytes were loosely associated with endothelial cells, formed cytoplasmic processes projecting into the tumor parenchyma, and formed a sleeve extending beyond the endothelial sprouts.[18] Moreover, 20–50% of the endothelial surface was not covered by pericytes.[17,18] The microvessel pericyte coverage index (MPI), defined as the percentage of microvessels co-localizing endothelial cell staining and pericyte staining over 5 microscopic fields per section, has been used to quantify pericyte coverage. MPI has been found to be heterogeneous, depending on the type of human tumor.[17] For example, MPI has been found to be as low as 12% for gliomas and as high as 67% for breast cancers.[17] Recently, Yonenaga et al[19] reported on the correlation between the MPI and clinicopathologic factors, including survival. Using anti-α-smooth muscle actin (α-SMA) antibody to identify pericytes, they quantified pericyte coverage or vessel maturation. Furthermore, a low MPI, representing poor pericyte coverage and a larger fraction of immature microvessels, was significantly associated with poor histologic subtype as well as the presence of distant metastases at the time of initial surgery. In addition, a low MPI was associated with lower survival rates ($p = 0.04$).[19] While MVD was associated with survival, it was not found to be associated with poor histologic subtype or distant metastases, thus highlighting the importance of also assessing maturity of the vasculature in predicting clinical outcome.

BIOCHEMICAL FACTORS ASSOCIATED WITH ANGIOGENESIS

Based on a growing understanding of angiogenic mechanisms, significant strides have been made in identifying key regulators of angiogenesis. These regulators include both pro- and antiangiogenic factors (Table 6.3). In normal physiologic processes such as embryogenesis, these factors are balanced, whereas in tumor angiogenesis, dysregulation of this balance results in a relative increase in proangiogenic factors. The best studied of these proangiogenic factors include VEGF, basic fibroblast growth factor (bFGF), and interleukin-8 (IL-8).[3]

Table 6.3 Pro- and antiangiogenic factors in ovarian carcinoma[a]

Activators of angiogenesis	Inhibitors of angiogenesis
Vascular endothelial growth factor (VEGF)	Angiostatin
Acidic and basic fibroblast growth factor (aFGF, bFGF)	Endostatin
Platelet-derived growth factor (PDGF)	Thrombospondin-1
Matrix metalloproteinases (MMPs)	Interleukin-12 (IL-12)
Tumor necrosis factor α (TNF-α)	Interferon-α (INF-α)
Transforming growth factor β (TGF-β)	Tissue inhibitors of metalloproteinases (TIMPs)
Interleukin-8 (IL-8)	Dopamine
Interleukin-6 (IL-6)	Vasculostatin
Cyclooxygenase-2 (COX-2)	Platelet factor 4 (PF4)
Hypoxia-inducible factor 1α (HIF-1α)	
Ephrins/Eph	
Epidermal growth factor (EGF)	
Lysophosphatic acid (LPA)	
Angiopoietin-1 and -2	
Catecholamines (norepinephrine, epinephrine)	

[a]This list is meant to be illustrative and not comprehensive.

Vascular endothelial growth factor

VEGF, originally called vascular permeability factor (VPF), is a 35–43 kDa homodimer with multiple isoforms, as a result of alternative splicing of a single gene. As its original name implies, VEGF plays a critical role in cellular permeability and ascites development. In tumor angiogenesis, the most widely studied VEGF, VEGF-A, appears to be the most relevant to tumor angiogenesis in its interactions with at least two transmembrane tyrosine kinase receptors – VEGFR-1 (Flt-1) and VEGFR-2 (KDR/Flk-1) – which are expressed on the surface of tumor vascular endothelial cells.[20] VEGF stimulates the proliferation and migration of endothelial cells and induces metalloproteinase expression and plasminogen activity,[3,21–23] both of which are important in angiogenesis as well as metastasis. Furthermore, VEGF serves as an antiapoptotic or survival factor for endothelial cells in newly formed blood vessels.[20] Many types of tumor cells overexpress VEGF, which stimulates vascularization, thereby producing more VEGF and perpetuating vascularization and progressive tumor growth.[20]

VEGF levels within the tumor are significantly higher in invasive ovarian tumors compared with benign ovarian neoplasms.[24] Furthermore, increased VEGF levels are also associated with advanced stage of disease and decreased survival.[24] Using reverse transcriptase polymerase chain reaction (RT–PCR), western blotting, and immunohistochemistry, several investigators have shown that VEGF levels in ovarian tumors also have prognostic value.[24,25] Patients with high levels of VEGF were found to have shortened median disease-free survival (<30 months) compared with patients with low levels of VEGF (>60 months).[24,25] However, others have not found significant associations between VEGF levels, as determined by immunohistochemistry, and clinical outcomes, after controlling for other variables.[26,27]

In addition to in situ angiogenic markers, circulating markers of angiogenesis that predict clinical outcome may prove relevant and practical. Preoperative serum VEGF levels were found to be useful in differentiating between benign and malignant adnexal masses; furthermore, these levels were significantly higher in women with even stage I invasive epithelial ovarian cancer compared with women with low-malignant-potential (LMP) or benign ovarian tumors. In a multivariate analysis of patients with invasive ovarian cancer, a serum VEGF level ≤380 pg/ml was an independent predictor of survival ($p = 0.02$), even after controlling for traditional covariates representing aggressive disease (e.g. stage, grade, and ascites).[28] The use of plasma versus serum levels of VEGF has also been considered. Serum VEGF levels comprise circulating VEGF as well as VEGF released from platelets upon activation after venipuncture, and are higher than plasma VEGF levels in matched samples.[29,30] Because of the potential for confounding results based on serum VEGF levels, some investigators contend that plasma VEGF levels better reflect circulating tumor-associated VEGF.[29,30] However, due to the role of platelets in tumor metastasis, platelet-derived VEGF may be as important as tumor-derived VEGF, and therefore should be accounted for by using serum measurements.[28]

Fibroblast growth factor

The role of bFGF (also known as FGF-2) was initially reported by Shing et al[31] in chondrosarcoma. Since then, the FGF family of proteins has expanded to include 20 members, of which bFGF appears to be the main player in angiogenesis.[32] Basic FGF appears to function as a tumor-derived capillary growth factor and stimulates angiogenesis in models such as granulation tissue formation.[33] Also known as a heparin-binding growth factor, bFGF is activated when tumors secrete heparin-degrading enzymes.[34]

In vitro assays have shown that bFGF can promote tumor growth in ovarian cancer cell lines.[35] The clinical utility of bFGF has also been explored in ovarian cancer,[34] as well as in other tumor sites, such as endometrial, lung, breast and oropharyngeal carcinomas;[36–38] however, its role as a prognostic marker is not clear.[38] Most studies have shown a significant association between high bFGF expression and clinicopathologic factors such as advanced stage, poor histologic grade, increased invasiveness, and poor clinical outcome.[38] However, others have reported that low levels of bFGF are associated with more invasive tumors and lower survival rates.[34,38] Specifically, some studies have reported that lower levels of intratumoral bFGF conferred a statistically significant nearly threefold greater risk of death compared with patients with higher levels, even after controlling for other variables such as stage, volume of residual disease after surgery, and grade.[34,38] Additional studies delineating the prognostic utility of bFGF are needed to clarify its role in ovarian carcinoma.

The predictive role of circulating bFGF as a surrogate marker of angiogenesis has also been examined. Plasma bFGF could have some clinical utility, given that plasma bFGF levels were found to be elevated in colorectal cancer patients with metastatic spread 1 year after treatment.[39] Conversely, plasma bFGF levels were found to be significantly decreased in colorectal cancer patients who were disease-free 1 year after completing treatment, compared with matched preoperative bFGF levels.[39] In addition, plasma levels were elevated among patients with metastatic spread of their disease,[39] thus supporting the clinical use of plasma bFGF levels in the assessment of disease status. In a limited sample population, circulating bFGF levels were measured at different areas of the tumor vasculature in patients with colorectal, ovarian, and cervical cancers, and tumor cells were not the only cell type responsible for the elevated levels of circulating bFGF. Rather, platelets and white blood cells were also thought to contribute to serum bFGF levels.[40]

Interleukin-8

IL-8, an 8.6 kDa cytokine, was originally identified as a chemotactic factor for leukocytes; however, significant evidence has since surfaced implicating it as a key factor in angiogenesis. In vitro experiments in ovarian cancer cell lines demonstrate that the IL-8 receptors, CXCR1 and CXCR2, are highly expressed.[41] Furthermore, exogenously administered IL-8 elicited increased ovarian cancer cell proliferation, which may represent a more aggressive phenotype.[41] Upregulation of IL-8 expression appears to be mediated by nuclear factor κB (NF-κB) activation.[42,43] Increased IL-8 expression has been documented in several tumors, such as breast,[44] prostate,[45] and bladder.[42] High levels of IL-8 in human ovarian carcinomas have also been noted using RT–PCR,[24] and were predictive of poor survival. Additionally, increased IL-8 in ovarian neoplasms has also been associated with VEGF overexpression.[24] Both factors are associated with decreased survival, which is believed to be secondary to increased tumor growth due to greater angiogenesis.[24]

Some chemotherapeutic agents transiently increase the production of angiogenic factors. For example, paclitaxel increases VEGF and IL-8 transcription in ovarian carcinoma as well as IL-8 secretion by ovarian cancer cell lines,[46] probably reflecting the transient activation of survival factors. Therefore, monitoring of serum IL-8 levels has been proposed as a prognostic marker for tumor volume and responsiveness to paclitaxel therapy.[47] As rapidly as 8 days after paclitaxel and cisplatin therapy, patients with advanced stage disease or with tumor volume precluding optimal surgical cytoreduction were found to have significantly higher serum IL-8 levels after chemotherapy than before chemotherapy.[47] However, among patients with optimal surgical cytoreduction of tumors, no significant difference was found between the pre- and post-paclitaxel serum IL-8 levels. While serum IL-8 appears to correlate with paclitaxel response, additional studies are needed to determine its relevance for predicting survival or recurrence.

Recent advances in therapeutic targeting using small molecule inhibitors have generated interest in disrupting aberrantly expressed pathways such as the Src family kinases in order to decrease downstream angiogenic factors.[48–50] Known downstream events of Src kinase activation include increased VEGF and IL-8 expression; therefore, optimizing a means of quantifying VEGF and IL-8 may provide clinically useful biomarkers for some of these novel targeted therapies.[49,51]

EphA2

The Eph receptors comprise a large family of receptor tyrosine kinases divided into two subclasses based on their interactions with the ligands, ephrin A and ephrin B.[52–54] Increasing evidence supports the important role that EphA2 plays in cancer cell growth, survival, invasion, and angiogenesis.[54,55] For example, EphA2 receptor activation can mediate in vitro endothelial cell network formation and vascular endothelial growth factor (VEGF)-dependent endothelial cell migration, sprouting, and survival.[54,56,57] In vivo studies support an important role for EphA2 receptor tyrosine kinase activation in VEGF-mediated angiogenesis as well as invasion.[54] Moreover, EphA2 may directly regulate tumor VEGF levels, thereby affecting the tumor microenvironment. EphA2 is overexpressed in the majority of epithelial ovarian cancers and is independently associated with aggressive tumor characteristics such as high histologic grade and advanced stage.[54] EphA2 overexpression has also been associated with poor clinical outcome.[54] The median survival rates among patients with high levels of EphA2 expression was significantly lower compared with those with low expression (3 years vs >12 years, $p = 0.004$).

While the molecular pathways underlying these associations are still being characterized, the potential role of EphA2 in tumorigenesis includes regulation of angiogenesis.[54,55] In vitro studies have demonstrated that EphA2 receptor activation mediates endothelial cell network formation and (VEGF)-dependent endothelial cell migration, sprouting, and survival.[56,57] In vivo studies support an important role for EphA2 receptor tyrosine kinase activation in VEGF-mediated angiogenesis as well as invasion.[54] Moreover, EphA2 may directly regulate tumor VEGF levels, thereby affecting the tumor microenvironment. In clinical samples, our laboratory has recently demonstrated that EphA2 overexpression in ovarian carcinoma is associated with increased angiogenesis and markers of invasion such as matrix metalloproteinases, further supporting EphA2 as an emerging target for antiangiogenesis-based therapies.[58] Emerging data suggest that other Eph receptors and their ligands, notably EphB4 and ephrin B2, play important roles in vascular development and arteriovenous differentiation.[59] Ephrin B2 is upregulated in ovarian tumors;[60] however,

the precise function of the EphB receptors and their clinical relevance have yet to be elucidated.

Tissue factor

Tissue factor (TF), a 47 kDa transmembrane receptor for factor VII, is expressed by smooth muscle cells in and around blood vessels, as well as by activated endothelial cells.[61] Moreover, TF is the primary initiator of coagulation.[61] Two primary pathways in which TF contributes to angiogenesis have been proposed: a clot-dependent pathway and a clot-independent pathway.[61] For the clot-dependent pathway, after TF activates factor VII, the clotting cascade commences, generating thrombin and activating platelets, which secrete VEGF. The VEGF from the platelets, in turn, stimulates endothelial cells, exposing TF, which further promotes thrombin formation and subsequent fibrin clot scaffolding for new vasculature.[61] The clotting-independent pathway involves the protease-activated receptors (PARs), a four-member family of seven-transmembrane-domain surface receptors that mediate cell activation via G-proteins and contribute to inflammation, angiogenesis, metastasis, and cell migration.[61,62] In addition to its role in coagulation, TF can also activate PAR-2 via its cytoplasmic domain. The effects of PAR-2 activation are synergistically enhanced with platelet-derived growth factor (PDGF)-BB from sprouting endothelial cells and platelets,[61,63] and this enhanced TF/PAR-2 complex comprises the clot-independent pathway to promote angiogenesis.[61]

Immunohistochemical studies have demonstrated elevated levels of TF in several tumor types, including breast cancer, lung cancer, and colorectal cancer.[61] TF has also been positively associated with increased parameters of angiogenesis such as MVD and VEGF, as well as poor clinical outcome in several solid tumors, including breast cancer, prostate cancer, and hepatocellular carcinoma.[61] In a pancreatic cancer study, high tumor TF, as determined by immunohistochemistry, resulted in a statistically significant hazard ratio of 2.01 compared with those with low tumor TF.[64] Serum TF levels have also been proposed to be of prognostic value in ovarian carcinoma. Patients with invasive ovarian carcinoma exhibited significantly higher levels of preoperative serum TF compared with those with benign and LMP ovarian neoplasms. Furthermore, a preoperative serum TF level ≥190 pg/ml was an independent prognostic factor for death due to disease, with a hazard ratio of 3.5.[65] These findings provide additional support for the development of serum TF as part of a panel of clinical biomarkers for managing or monitoring invasive disease.

CIRCULATING ENDOTHELIAL CELLS

Levels of circulating endothelial cells (CECs) are increased in cancer patients, likely due to mobilization from the bone marrow or displacement from the vessel wall.[4,66] CECs are typically found in adult blood and are mobilized in response to VEGF in both murine models and humans.[66] Two subpopulations of CECs have been identified: circulating endothelial precursors (CEPs), a subset of CECs derived from the bone marrow that can differentiate into mature endothelial cells and contribute to pathologic neovascularization in murine models and in humans,[67,68] and mature CECs, believed to be derived from mature vasculature (Figure 6.2).[69] CECs and CEPs can be identified on the basis of their expression of endothelial markers such as VEGFR-2 (KDR/Flk-1), AC133, and CD 34.[70,71] CECs have been used as surrogate angiogenesis markers in preclinical studies using murine models of cancer as well as in several clinical studies of angiogenesis inhibitors.[72–74] An increase in mature CECs during the first cycle of therapy is believed to directly reflect damage to or apoptosis of the vessel wall-derived endothelial cells, possibly in

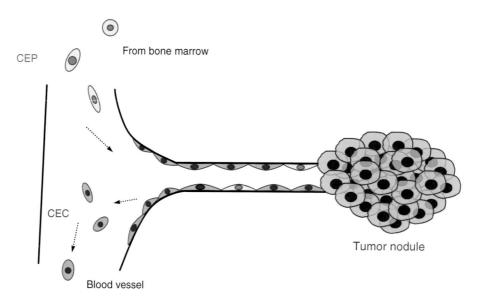

Figure 6.2 Relationship of mature circulating endothelial cells (CECs) and circulating endothelial precursors (CEPs) in tumor vasculature. CEPs are derived from the bone marrow and contribute to the tumor neovascularization. Mature CECs shed from the tumor vasculature into the circulation.

response to therapy.[38,66] Metronomic cytotoxic chemotherapy (i.e. administering lower doses of cytotoxic agents at more frequent, regular intervals) is also associated with consistently lower than expected CEP numbers and viability,[75,76] thus supporting its potential clinical use as an angiogenesis marker.

THERAPEUTIC IMPLICATIONS OF ANGIOGENESIS

A comparison of antiangiogenesis strategies against VEGF receptors (Figure 6.3), including neuropilin, indicated that anti-VEGF approaches were the most efficacious, decreasing tumor growth by about 80%, versus about 20% for the other approaches.[77] Bevacizumab, a recombinant fully humanized immunoglobulin G (IgG) monoclonal antibody targeting VEGF-A, is the first approved antiangiogenic drug for cancer therapy. After obtaining initial US Food and Drug Administration (FDA) approval in 2004 for front-line therapy for metastatic colorectal cancer, bevacizumab has also demonstrated efficacy in overall and progression-free survival in advanced non-small cell lung cancer and in progression-free survival in advanced breast cancer. Preclinical studies in ovarian cancer indicate encouraging activity of bevacizumab monotherapy in reducing ascites.[78] A phase II trial of bevacizumab monotherapy in patients with relapsed ovarian cancer demonstrated an 18% response rate by RECIST criteria.[79] Additional randomized phase III trials for advanced-stage ovarian cancer are currently ongoing to evaluate its efficacy in combination with paclitaxel and carboplatin chemotherapy.[79]

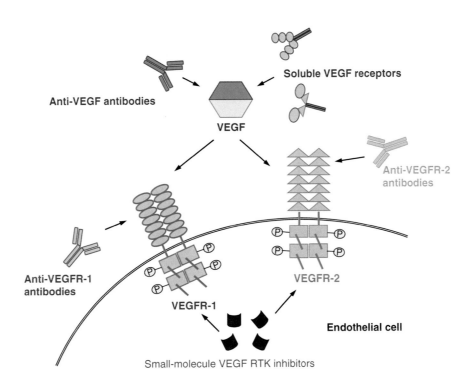

Figure 6.3 VEGF/VEGFR-targeted therapies.

Another approach for interfering with VEGF signaling is to use small peptides that inhibit the tyrosine kinase catalytic domain of the VEGF receptors,[80–83] and many of these agents are currently being evaluated in clinical trials. Other methods for disrupting the VEGF pathway include VEGF-Trap, which is a fully humanized soluble VEGF receptor fusion protein.[84] This agent binds VEGF with significantly higher affinity than previously reported VEGF antagonists, thus preventing VEGF from stimulating its native receptor. This VEGF-blocker has been tested using in vivo models and has been shown to effectively suppress the growth and neovascularization of various tumor types.[84] In a murine model of ovarian cancer, VEGF-Trap prevented ascites accumulation and inhibited tumor growth.[85] In addition, the combination of VEGF-Trap with paclitaxel reduced tumor burden by about 98% and blocked the development of ascites.[86] Clinical trials with VEGF-Trap alone and in combination with chemotherapy are ongoing.

A growing area of interest in antiangiogenic therapy development lies in the angiopoietin family of ligands and receptors, which are involved in the secondary stages of blood vessel formation during angiogenesis. While the exact role of the angiopoietin system in ovarian cancer angiogenesis remains unclear, preclinical murine models have demonstrated that acute administration of angiopoietin-1 protects the adult vasculature from leakage, effectively counteracting the detrimental effects of VEGF.[87,88] Conversely, angiopoietin-2, which is strongly upregulated at sites of active vessel remodeling, inhibits angiopoietin-1-induced phosphorylation and destabilizes blood vessels.[89] The ability of angiopoietin-1 to reestablish vascular integrity in the setting of leaky vessels, as found in the tumor vasculature, and the inhibition of VEGF-stimulated neovascularization

by angiopoietin-2-selective inhibitors, support further investigation of angiopoietins as a potential antiangiogenic therapy.[90]

As additional mechanisms involved in tumor angiogenesis and vasculogenesis are elucidated, new and more efficacious therapeutics and combinations of novel therapies are likely to evolve. For example, therapeutic strategies aimed at targeting EphA2 using either short interfering RNA (siRNA) delivered via a neutral liposome or an agonistic antibody have demonstrated therapeutic efficacy in preclinical models, especially in combination with traditional chemotherapy.[54,91] This area is currently the focus of growing clinical interest as a rational and highly specific approach for targeted therapy.

In addition to the biotechnological advances in vascular targeting, increasing evidence suggests that natural compounds such as curcumin, the rhizome of the plant *Curcuma longa*, may have antiangiogenic properties.[92] Preliminary in vitro assays have demonstrated suppression of proangiogenic factors by curcumin in ovarian cancer cell lines, and in vivo data support decreased tumor growth, proliferation, and angiogenesis. At present, we are actively investigating the mechanisms by which curcumin may inhibit tumor growth and angiogenesis.[93]

While chemotherapy has been traditionally administered based on the concept of maximally tolerated doses (MTDs), growing evidence suggests that alternative dosing schedules may be as efficacious, with lower toxicities. Metronomic chemotherapy entails the frequent administration of chemotherapeutic agents at doses below the traditional MTD without prolonged drug-free intervals. The basis for metronomic dosing stems from the differential therapeutic sensitivity of endothelial cells versus tumor cells. For example, endothelial cells of newly forming capillaries appear to be highly and selectively sensitive (10–100 000-fold) to very low doses of chemotherapy such as paclitaxel, docetaxel, cyclophosphamide, or vinblastine.[15,94] Endothelial cells in newly formed tumor vasculature proliferate and divide more frequently than endothelial cells on mature blood vessels; therefore, they are more sensitive to traditional cytotoxic agents.[95] Folkman and colleagues showed that as chemotherapy is currently delivered on an MTD schedule, the long breaks between doses also reduce the antiangiogenic effects of the drugs by allowing time for the damaged tumor vasculature to repair itself.[94]

In addition to its effects on the tumor vasculature, metronomic dosing also appears to have significant efficacy in inhibiting the growth of tumors that have acquired resistance to conventional dosing.[15] In ovarian carcinoma patients, a significant proportion of tumors with acquired taxane resistance during the MTD dosing schedule were subsequently found to respond to the same drug on a semimetronomic schedule at a significantly lower dose than the MTD.[96] These encouraging results provide justification for continued development of new dosing schedules and identification of other cytotoxic agents with metronomic activity. The biomarkers discussed in this chapter may be valuable in following patients undergoing treatment with antiangiogenic approaches.

CONCLUDING REMARKS

The last few decades have witnessed a surge in research trying to delineate the mechanisms and factors involved in tumor neovascularization. Not only has characterization of the VEGF family and its corresponding receptors led to significant strides in the development of targeted antiangiogenic therapies for human malignancies, but in addition new pathways and potential targets are continuously being explored. In fact, compelling preclinical data describe the putative adrenergic-mediated effects of chronic stress in tumor angiogenesis.[97] An improved understanding and appreciation of the differences between normal vasculature and tumor-associated blood vessels has also provided additional insight in identifying novel targets. As the development of new antiangiogenic therapeutics advances, the ability to monitor the effects of such therapies remains of utmost importance. Identifying pro- and antiangiogenic factors, as well as other serum markers for aberrant angiogenic processes, can aid physicians in both monitoring therapeutic effects and, more importantly, potentially detecting malignancies at an earlier stage. Furthermore, the clinical development of angiogenic markers may be useful for determining the optimal biologic dose of novel agents. Such approaches indeed offer hope for improving the clinical outcome of patients with ovarian and other cancers.

ACKNOWLEDGMENT

YGL is supported by an NCI/DHHS/NIH Training of Academic Gynecologic Oncologists Grant (T32-CA101642). Portions of work in this chapter were supported by NIH Grants (CA 11079301 and CA 10929801), the UT MD Anderson Ovarian Cancer SPORE (P50 CA083639), a Program Project Development Grant from the Ovarian Cancer Research Fund, Inc., and The Marcus Foundation.

REFERENCES

1. Ries LAG, Eisner MP, Kosary CL, et al., eds. SEER Cancer Statistics Review, 1975–2002. Bethesda, MD: National Cancer Institute, 2005.

2. Fidler IJ. Critical factors in the biology of human cancer metastasis: twenty-eighth G.H.A. Clowes memorial award lecture. Cancer Res 1990;50:6130–8.

3. Risau W. Mechanisms of angiogenesis. Nature 1997;386:671–4.

4. Kamat AA, Sood AK. The merits of vascular targeting for gynecologic malignancies. Curr Oncol Rep 2005;7:444–50.

5. Yancopoulos GD, Davis S, Gale NW, et al. Vascular-specific growth factors and blood vessel formation. Nature 2000;407:242–8.

6. Kim ES, Serur A, Huang J, et al. Potent VEGF blockade causes regression of coopted vessels in a model of neuroblastoma. Proc Natl Acad Sci USA 2002;99:11399–404.

7. Fidler IJ. The organ microenvironment and cancer metastasis. Differentiation 2002;70:498–505.

8. Maniotis AJ, Folberg R, Hess A, et al. Vascular channel formation by human melanoma cells in vivo and in vitro: vasculogenic mimicry. Am J Pathol 1999;155:739–52.

9. Sood AK, Seftor EA, Fletcher MS, et al. Molecular determinants of ovarian cancer plasticity. Am J Pathol 2001;158:1279–88.

10. Chang YS, di Tomaso E, McDonald DM, et al. Mosaic blood vessels in tumors: frequency of cancer cells in contact with flowing blood. Proc Natl Acad Sci USA 2000;97:14608–13.

11. Lu W, Schroit AJ. Vascularization of melanoma by mobilization and remodeling of preexisting latent vessels to patency. Cancer Res 2005;65:913–18.

12. Hollingsworth HC, Kohn EC, Steinberg SM, et al. Tumor angiogenesis in advanced stage ovarian carcinoma. Am J Pathol 1995;147:33–41.

13. Abulafia O, Triest WE, Sherer DM. Angiogenesis in primary and metastatic epithelial ovarian carcinoma. Am J Obstet Gynecol 1997; 177:541–7.

14. Alvarez AA, Krigman HR, Whitaker RS, et al. The prognostic significance of angiogenesis in epithelial ovarian carcinoma. Clin Cancer Res 1999;5:587–91.

15. Kerbel RS, Kamen BA. The anti-angiogenic basis of metronomic chemotherapy. Nat Rev Cancer 2004;4:423–36.

16. Hellstrom M, Gerhardt H, Kalen M, et al. Lack of pericytes leads to endothelial hyperplasia and abnormal vascular morphogenesis. J Cell Biol 2001;153:543–53.

17. Eberhard A, Kahlert S, Goede V, et al. Heterogeneity of angiogenesis and blood vessel maturation in human tumors: implications for antiangiogenic tumor therapies. Cancer Res 2000;60:1388–93.

18. Morikawa S, Baluk P, Kaidoh T, et al. Abnormalities in pericytes on blood vessels and endothelial sprouts in tumors. Am J Pathol 2002;160:985–1000.

19. Yonenaga Y, Mori A, Onodera H, et al. Absence of smooth muscle actin-positive pericyte coverage of tumor vessels correlates with hematogenous metastasis and prognosis of colorectal cancer patients. Oncology 2005;69:159–66.

20. Kerbel RS. Tumor angiogenesis: past, present and the near future. Carcinogenesis 2000;21:505–15.

21. Harris AL. Anti-angiogenesis therapy and strategies for integrating it with adjuvant therapy. Recent Results. Cancer Res 1998;152: 341–52.

22. Ferrara N, Henzel WJ. Pituitary follicular cells secrete a novel heparin-binding growth factor specific for vascular endothelial cells. Biochem Biophys Res Commun 1989;161:851–8.

23. Unemori EN, Ferrara N, Bauer EA, et al. Vascular endothelial growth factor induces interstitial collagenase expression in human endothelial cells. J Cell Physiol 1992;153: 557–62.

24. Kassim SK, El-Salahy EM, Fayed ST, et al. Vascular endothelial growth factor and interleukin-8 are associated with poor prognosis in epithelial ovarian cancer patients. Clin Biochem 2004;37:363–9.

25. Garzetti GG, Ciavattini A, Lucarini G, et al. Vascular endothelial growth factor expression as a prognostic index in serous ovarian cystoadenocarcinomas: relationship with MIB1 immunostaining. Gynecol Oncol 1999;73: 396–401.

26. Ogawa S, Kaku T, Kobayashi H, et al. Prognostic significance of microvessel density, vascular cuffing and vascular endothelial growth factor expression in ovarian carcinoma: a special review for clear cell adenocarcinoma. Cancer Lett 2002;176:111–18.

27. Sonmezer M, Gungor M, Ensari A, et al. Prognostic significance of tumor angiogenesis in epithelial ovarian cancer: in association with transforming growth factor beta and vascular endothelial growth factor. Int J Gynecol Cancer 2004;14:82–8.

28. Cooper BC, Ritchie JM, Broghammer CL, et al. Preoperative serum vascular endothelial growth factor levels: significance in ovarian cancer. Clin Cancer Res 2002;8:3193–7.

29. Adams J, Carder PJ, Downey S, et al. Vascular endothelial growth factor (VEGF) in breast cancer: comparison of plasma, serum, and tissue VEGF and microvessel density and effects of tamoxifen. Cancer Res 2000;60:2898–905.

30. Banks RE, Forbes MA, Kinsey SE, et al. Release of the angiogenic cytokine vascular endothelial growth factor (VEGF) from platelets: significance for VEGF measurements and cancer biology. Br J Cancer 1998;77: 956–64.

31. Shing Y, Folkman J, Sullivan R, et al. Heparin affinity: purification of a tumor-derived capillary endothelial cell growth factor. Science 1984;223:1296–9.

32. Huang Z, Bao SD. Roles of main pro- and anti-angiogenic factors in tumor angiogenesis. World J Gastroenterol 2004;10:463–70.

33. Folkman J, Klagsbrun M. Angiogenic factors. Science 1987;235:442–7.

34. Obermair A, Speiser P, Reisenberger K, et al. Influence of intratumoral basic fibroblast growth factor concentration on survival in ovarian cancer patients. Cancer Lett 1998;130:69–76.

35. Crickard K, Gross JL, Crickard U, et al. Basic fibroblast growth factor and receptor expression in human ovarian cancer. Gynecol Oncol 1994;55:277–84.

36. Stefansson IM, Salvesen HB, Akslen LA. Vascular proliferation is important for clinical progress of endometrial cancer. Cancer Res 2006;66:3303–9.

37. Iwasaki A, Kuwahara M, Yoshinaga Y, et al. Basic fibroblast growth factor (bFGF) and vascular endothelial growth factor (VEGF) levels, as prognostic indicators in NSCLC. Eur J Cardiothorac Surg 2004;25:443–8.

38. Poon RT, Fan ST, Wong J. Clinical implications of circulating angiogenic factors in cancer patients. J Clin Oncol 2001;19:1207–25.

39. George ML, Tutton MG, Abulafi AM, et al. Plasma basic fibroblast growth factor levels in colorectal cancer: a clinically useful assay? Clin Exp Metastasis 2002;19:735–8.

40. Salgado R, Benoy I, Vermeulen P, et al. Circulating basic fibroblast growth factor is partly derived from the tumour in patients with colon, cervical and ovarian cancer. Angiogenesis 2004;7:29–32.

41. Xu L, Yoneda J, Herrera C, et al. Inhibition of malignant ascites and growth of human ovarian carcinoma by oral administration of a potent inhibitor of the vascular endothelial growth factor receptor tyrosine kinases. Int J Oncol 2000;16:445–54.

42. Karashima T, Sweeney P, Kamat A, et al. Nuclear factor-kappaB mediates angiogenesis and metastasis of human bladder cancer through the regulation of interleukin-8. Clin Cancer Res 2003;9:2786–97.

43. Brown MR, Blanchette JO, Kohn EC. Angiogenesis in ovarian cancer. Baillieres Best

Pract Res Clin Obstet Gynaecol 2000; 14:901–18.

44. Lin Y, Huang R, Chen L, et al. Identification of interleukin-8 as estrogen receptor-regulated factor involved in breast cancer invasion and angiogenesis by protein arrays. Int J Cancer 2004;109:507–15.

45. Konig JE, Senge T, Allhoff EP, et al. Analysis of the inflammatory network in benign prostate hyperplasia and prostate cancer. Prostate 2004;58:121–9.

46. Lee LF, Schuerer-Maly CC, Lofquist AK, et al. Taxol-dependent transcriptional activation of IL-8 expression in a subset of human ovarian cancer. Cancer Res 1996;56: 1303–8.

47. Uslu R, Sanli UA, Dikmen Y, et al. Predictive value of serum interleukin-8 levels in ovarian cancer patients treated with paclitaxel-containing regimens. Int J Gynecol Cancer 2005;15:240–5.

48. Han LY, Landen CN, Trevino JG, et al. Antiangiogenic and antitumor effects of SRC inhibition in ovarian carcinoma. Cancer Res 2006;66:8633–9.

49. Summy JM, Trevino JG, Lesslie DP, et al. AP23846, a novel and highly potent Src family kinase inhibitor, reduces vascular endothelial growth factor and interleukin-8 expression in human solid tumor cell lines and abrogates downstream angiogenic processes. Mol Cancer Ther 2005;4:1900–11.

50. Trevino JG, Summy JM, Gallick GE. SRC inhibitors as potential therapeutic agents for human cancers. Mini Rev Med Chem 2006; 6:681–7.

51. Trevino JG, Summy JM, Gray MJ, et al. Expression and activity of SRC regulate interleukin-8 expression in pancreatic adenocarcinoma cells: implications for angiogenesis. Cancer Res 2005;65:7214–22.

52. Murai KK, Pasquale EB. 'Eph'ective signaling: forward, reverse and crosstalk. J Cell Sci, 2003; 116:2823–32.

53. Pasquale EB. Eph receptor signalling casts a wide net on cell behaviour. Nat Rev Mol Cell Biol 2005;6:462–75.

54. Landen CN, Kinch MS, Sood AK. EphA2 as a target for ovarian cancer therapy. Expert Opin Ther Targets 2005;9:1179–87.

55. Kinch MS, Carles-Kinch K. Overexpression and functional alterations of the EphA2 tyrosine kinase in cancer. Clin Exp Metastasis 2003;20:59–68.

56. Ojima T, Takagi H, Suzuma K, et al. EphrinA1 inhibits vascular endothelial growth factor-induced intracellular signaling and suppresses retinal neovascularization and blood-retinal barrier breakdown. Am J Pathol 2006;168: 331–9.

57. Brantley-Sieders DM, Fang WB, Hicks DJ, et al. Impaired tumor microenvironment in EphA2-deficient mice inhibits tumor angiogenesis and metastatic progression. Faseb J 2005; 19:1884–6.

58. Lin YG, Han LY, Kamat AA, et al. EphA2 over-expression is associated with angiogenesis in ovarian cancer. Cancer 2007;109:332–40.

59. Heroult M, Schaffner F, Augustin HG. Eph receptor and ephrin ligand-mediated interactions during angiogenesis and tumor progression. Exp Cell Res 2006;312:642–50.

60. Lugli A, Spichtin H, Maurer R, et al. EphB2 expression across 138 human tumor types in a tissue microarray: high levels of expression in gastrointestinal cancers. Clin Cancer Res 2005;11:6450–8.

61. Forster Y, Meye A, Albrecht S, et al. Tissue factor and tumor: clinical and laboratory aspects. Clin Chim Acta 2006;364:12–21.

62. Pawlinski R, Mackman N. Tissue factor, coagulation proteases, and protease-activated receptors in endotoxemia and sepsis. Crit Care Med 2004;32:S293–7.

63. Belting M, Dorrell MI, Sandgren S, et al. Regulation of angiogenesis by tissue factor cytoplasmic domain signaling. Nat Med 2004;10:502–9.

64. Nitori N, Ino Y, Nakanishi Y, et al. Prognostic significance of tissue factor in pancreatic ductal adenocarcinoma. Clin Cancer Res 2005;11:2531–9.

65. Han LY, Landen CN Jr, Kamat AA, et al. Preoperative serum tissue factor levels are an independent prognostic factor in patients with ovarian carcinoma. J Clin Oncol 2006;24:755–61.

66. Rafii S, Circulating endothelial precursors: mystery, reality, and promise. J Clin Invest 2000;105:17–19.

67. Asahara T, Murohara T, Sullivan A, et al. Isolation of putative progenitor endothelial cells for angiogenesis. Science 1997;275:964–7.

68. Asahara T, Takahashi T, Masuda H, et al. VEGF contributes to postnatal neovascularization by mobilizing bone marrow-derived endothelial progenitor cells. Embo J 1999;18:3964–72.

69. Beaudry P, Force J, Naumov GN, et al. Differential effects of vascular endothelial growth factor receptor-2 inhibitor ZD6474 on circulating endothelial progenitors and mature circulating endothelial cells: implications for use as a surrogate marker of antiangiogenic activity. Clin Cancer Res 2005;11:3514–22.

70. Peichev M, Naiyer AJ, Pereira D, et al. Expression of VEGFR-2 and AC133 by circulating human CD34(+) cells identifies a population of functional endothelial precursors. Blood 2000;95:952–8.

71. Reyes M, Dudek A, Jahagirdar B, et al. Origin of endothelial progenitors in human postnatal bone marrow. J Clin Invest 2002;109:337–46.

72. Bertolini F, Mingrone W, Alietti A, et al. Thalidomide in multiple myeloma, myelodysplastic syndromes and histiocytosis. Analysis of clinical results and of surrogate angiogenesis markers. Ann Oncol 2001;12:987–90.

73. Monestiroli S, Mancuso P, Burlini A, et al. Kinetics and viability of circulating endothelial cells as surrogate angiogenesis marker in an animal model of human lymphoma. Cancer Res 2001;61:4341–4.

74. Schuch G, Heymach JV, Nomi M, et al. Endostatin inhibits the vascular endothelial growth factor-induced mobilization of endothelial progenitor cells. Cancer Res 2003;63:8345–50.

75. Bertolini F, Paul S, Mancuso P, et al. Maximum tolerable dose and low-dose metronomic chemotherapy have opposite effects on the mobilization and viability of circulating endothelial progenitor cells. Cancer Res 2003;63:4342–6.

76. Shaked Y, Emmenegger U, Man S, et al. Optimal biologic dose of metronomic chemotherapy regimens is associated with maximum antiangiogenic activity. Blood 2005;106:3058–61.

77. Kuo CJ, Farnebo F, Yu EY, et al. Comparative evaluation of the antitumor activity of antiangiogenic proteins delivered by gene transfer. Proc Natl Acad Sci USA 2001;98:4605–10.

78. Mesiano S, Ferrara N, Jaffe RB. Role of vascular endothelial growth factor in ovarian cancer: inhibition of ascites formation by immunoneutralization. Am J Pathol 1998;153:1249–56.

79. Aghajanian C. The role of bevacizumab in ovarian cancer – an evolving story. Gynecol Oncol 2006;102:131–3.

80. Drevs J, Hofmann I, Hugenschmidt H, et al. Effects of PTK787/ZK 222584, a specific inhibitor of vascular endothelial growth factor receptor tyrosine kinases, on primary tumor, metastasis, vessel density, and blood flow in a murine renal cell carcinoma model. Cancer Res 2000;60:4819–24.

81. Drevs J, Muller-Driver R, Wittig C, et al. PTK787/ZK 222584, a specific vascular endothelial growth factor-receptor tyrosine kinase inhibitor, affects the anatomy of the tumor vascular bed and the functional vascular properties as detected by dynamic enhanced magnetic resonance imaging. Cancer Res 2002;62:4015–22.

82. Wood JM, Bold G, Buchdunger E, et al. PTK787/ZK 222584, a novel and potent

inhibitor of vascular endothelial growth factor receptor tyrosine kinases, impairs vascular endothelial growth factor-induced responses and tumor growth after oral administration. Cancer Res 2000;60:2178–89.

83. Pandya NM, Dhalla NS, Santani DD. Angiogenesis – a new target for future therapy. Vascul Pharmacol 2006;44:26S–74.

84. Holash J, Davis S, Papadopoulos N, et al. VEGF-Trap: a VEGF blocker with potent antitumor effects. Proc Natl Acad Sci USA 2002; 99:11393–8.

85. Byrne AT, Ross L, Holash J, et al. Vascular endothelial growth factor-trap decreases tumor burden, inhibits ascites, and causes dramatic vascular remodeling in an ovarian cancer model. Clin Cancer Res 2003;9:5721–8.

86. Hu L, Hofmann J, Holash J, et al. Vascular endothelial growth factor trap combined with paclitaxel strikingly inhibits tumor and ascites, prolonging survival in a human ovarian cancer model. Clin Cancer Res 2005; 11:6966–71.

87. Holash J, Thurston G, Rudge JS, et al. Inhibitors of growth factor receptors, signaling pathways and angiogenesis as therapeutic molecular agents. Cancer Metastasis Rev 2006;25:243–52.

88. Thurston G, Rudge JS, Ioffe E, et al. Angiopoietin-1 protects the adult vasculature against plasma leakage. Nat Med 2000;6: 460–3.

89. Thurston G. Role of Angiopoietins and Tie receptor tyrosine kinases in angiogenesis and lymphangiogenesis. Cell Tissue Res 2003; 314:61–8.

90. Oliner J, Min H, Leal J, et al. Suppression of angiogenesis and tumor growth by selective inhibition of angiopoietin-2. Cancer Cell 2004;6:507–16.

91. Landen CN, Jr., Lu C, Han LY, et al. Efficacy and antivascular effects of EphA2 reduction with an agonistic antibody in ovarian cancer. J Natl Cancer Inst 2006;98:1558–70.

92. Sharma RA, Gescher AJ, Steward WP. Curcumin: the story so far. Eur J Cancer 2005;41:1955–68.

93. Lin YG, Kunnumakkara AB, Nair A, et al. Curcumin inhibits tumor growth and angiogenesis in ovarian carcinoma by targeting the NF-kB pathway. Clin Cancer Res 2007. In press.

94. Folkman J. Angiogenesis. Annu Rev Med 2006;57:1–18.

95. Bergers G, Benjamin LE. Tumorigenesis and the angiogenic switch. Nat Rev Cancer 2003;3:401–10.

96. Kikuchi Y, Kita T, Takano M, et al. Treatment options in the management of ovarian cancer. Expert Opin Pharmacother 2005;6: 743–54.

97. Thaker PH, Han LY, Kamat AA, et al. Chronic stress promotes tumor growth and angiogenesis in a mouse model of ovarian carcinoma. Nat Med 2006;12:939–44.

98. Heimburg S, Oehler MK, Papadopoulos T, et al. Prognostic relevance of the endothelial marker CD 34 in ovarian cancer. Anticancer Res 1999;19:2527–9.

99. Obermair A, Wasicky R, Kaider A, et al. Prognostic significance of tumor angiogenesis in epithelial ovarian cancer. Cancer Lett 1999;138:175–82.

100. Chan JK, Loizzi V, Magistris A, et al. Differences in prognostic molecular markers between women over and under 45 years of age with advanced ovarian cancer. Clin Cancer Res 2004;10:8538–43.

101. Ferrero A, Zola P, Mazzola S, et al. Pretreatment serum hemoglobin level and a preliminary investigation of intratumoral microvessel density in advanced ovarian cancer. Gynecol Oncol 2004;95:323–9.

102. Chan JK, Magistris A, Loizzi V, et al. Mast cell density, angiogenesis, blood clotting, and prognosis in women with advanced ovarian cancer. Gynecol Oncol 2005; 99:20–5.

103. Raspollini MR, Castiglione F, Garbini F, et al. Correlation of epidermal growth factor receptor expression with tumor microdensity vessels and with vascular endothelial growth factor expression in ovarian carcinoma. Int J Surg Pathol 2005;13:135–42.

104. Ino K, Shibata K, Kajiyama H, et al. Angiotensin II type 1 receptor expression in ovarian cancer and its correlation with tumour angiogenesis and patient survival. Br J Cancer 2006;94:552–60.

105. Karavasilis V, Malamou-Mitsi V, Briasoulis E, et al. Clinicopathologic study of vascular endothelial growth factor, thrombospondin-1, and microvessel density assessed by CD34 in patients with stage III ovarian carcinoma. Int J Gynecol Cancer 2006;16:241–6.

106. Solomon LA, Munkarah AR, Schimp VL, et al. Maspin expression and localization impact on angiogenesis and prognosis in ovarian cancer. Gynecol Oncol 2006;101:385–9.

107. Gasparini G, Bonoldi E, Viale G, et al. Prognostic and predictive value of tumour angiogenesis in ovarian carcinomas. Int J Cancer 1996;69:205–11.

108. Goodheart MJ, Vasef MA, Sood AK, et al. Ovarian cancer p53 mutation is associated with tumor microvessel density. Gynecol Oncol 2002;86:85–90.

109. Stone PJ, Goodheart MJ, Rose SL, et al. The influence of microvessel density on ovarian carcinogenesis. Gynecol Oncol 2003;90:566–71.

110. Goodheart MJ, Ritchie JM, Rose SL, et al. The relationship of molecular markers of p53 function and angiogenesis to prognosis of stage I epithelial ovarian cancer. Clin Cancer Res 2005;11:3733–42.

111. Wang Z, Wang H, Lin M. Study on tumor angiogenesis in epithelial ovarian carcinoma. J Tongji Med Univ 2000;20:172–4.

Cell adhesion and matrix-associated proteins in ovarian carcinoma

7

Ben Davidson, Claes G Tropé, and Reuven Reich

INTRODUCTION

Ovarian carcinoma and the closely linked serous carcinomas of the fallopian tube and peritoneum (together with the rare diffuse peritoneal mesothelioma) exhibit a unique pattern of invasion and metastasis, with widespread dissemination within the serosal (peritoneal and pleural) cavities and a far lower degree of distant metastasis to parenchymal organs. The ability of more than two-thirds of ovarian carcinomas to metastasize prior to detection is primarily related to the late appearance of symptoms. However, this aggressive clinical behavior also depends on the presence of highly efficient cellular mechanisms that mediate profound changes in the expression of key molecules in cancer biology as functions of anatomic site and the changing microenvironment. These molecular differences are exemplified in the alterations undergone by cancer cells in effusions compared with primary tumors and solid metastases – differences that are also relevant in terms of predictive and prognostic value. Chemotherapy produces further molecular changes in ovarian carcinoma cells, requiring further stratification of tumor samples obtained at various stages of the clinical course. The dynamic molecular profile of ovarian cancer cells is complemented by their ability to cross-talk with stromal and endothelial cells in solid tumors and with mesothelial cells in effusions. This chapter will detail current data related to the expression, diagnostic role, and predictive/prognostic value of adhesion molecules and proteolytic enzymes in primary and metastatic ovarian carcinoma.

ADHESION MOLECULES

Cadherins

Cadherins, a family of calcium-dependent integral membrane glycoproteins, are located at the cell–cell adherens junctions, where they mediate homophilic contact with neighboring cells.[1] Cadherins interact through their C-terminal intracytoplasmic domain with p120 catenin, β-catenin (88 kDa), and γ-catenin (80 kDa). These in turn bind to α-catenin, a 102 kDa protein linking actin molecules.[2] Cadherins play a central role in differentiation and tissue organization during embryonic development and in maintaining the tissue structure of the mature organism. E-cadherin, the major cadherin molecule in epithelial cells, has been shown to be an inhibitor of invasion and is regarded as a tumor suppressor molecule.[3] Inactivation and downregulation of E-cadherin expression have been shown to be associated with tumor progression in various cancers and occur through genetic (mutations) and epigenetic (CpG promoter hypermethylation, transcriptional regulation, and post-translational modification) mechanisms.[4,5] Loss of E-cadherin may be accompanied by expression of pro-invasive N-cadherin, a molecule that is normally expressed in neural and mesenchymal cells, a process representing a pathologic version of the epithelial-to-mesenchymal transition (EMT) during embryogenesis.[5] There is growing evidence that epigenetic silencing of the E-cadherin promoter by transcription factors is a central mechanism in EMT. The main negative transcriptional regulators of E-cadherin in human cancer are Snail and Slug, which are members of the Snail superfamily,[6] and Smad interacting protein 1 (Sip1), which is a member of the crystallin enhancer-binding factor 1 family.[7]

Downregulation of β- and γ-catenin, often through mutation, leads to impaired cell–cell adhesion and affects signal transduction pathways, resulting in an oncogenic effect.[4,5] Under normal conditions, the degradation of β-catenin involves its phosphorylation, through the formation of a complex with the tumor suppressor adenomatous polyposis coli (APC) protein, glycogen synthase kinase 3β (GSKβ), and Axin. Mutations in the genes encoding these proteins abolish this process, leading to accumulation of β-catenin and activation of the Wnt pathway. The association of β-catenin with the transcription factors lymphoid enhancer factor 1/T-cell factor (LEF-1/TCF) in the cell nucleus results in loss of cell growth control and mediates an oncogenic effect.[4,5]

Ovarian carcinomas differ from other epithelial cancers with respect to E-cadherin and catenin expression. E-cadherin mutations are rare[8] and mutations in β-catenin, APC, and Axin are largely limited to endometrioid

carcinomas.[9,10] E-cadherin is absent in normal ovarian surface epithelium with flat morphology, but has been detected in benign invaginations of the ovarian surface epithelium, metaplastic and dysplastic lesions, and primary and metastatic carcinomas.[11,12] We have previously reported on the downregulation of E-cadherin and catenins in primary ovarian (predominantly serous) carcinomas, with subsequent upregulation in effusions and solid metastases, showing that the loss of E-cadherin is of a transient nature in this tumor (Figure 7.1).[13] A similar association with disease progression has been shown for P-cadherin,[14] a finding that we have confirmed by showing frequent coexpression of E-, N-, and P-cadherin in ovarian carcinoma effusions (Figure 7.1).[15] The upregulation of cadherin and catenin expression in effusions is morphologically reflected in the tendency of ovarian carcinoma cells in effusions to form cohesive cell aggregates in all but the most poorly differentiated tumors. In the diagnostic setting, cadherin expression aids in differentiating ovarian carcinoma cells from benign mesothelial cells – but not from malignant mesotheliomas, the main differential diagnosis in the serosal cavities, since both tumors coexpress E- and N-cadherin.[16]

The prognostic role of E-cadherin and catenins in ovarian cancer has been investigated mainly using immunohistochemistry (Table 7.1). Loss of E-cadherin protein expression correlated with poor survival in two series of 20 and 104 primary carcinomas, but the number of negative specimens was small in both series (6 and 7 tumors, respectively).[17,18] We did not detect differences in E-cadherin protein expression in primary and metastatic tumors obtained from ovarian cancer patients with short-term versus long-term survival.[19] We did find that lower E-cadherin mRNA expression in ovarian carcinoma effusions correlated with

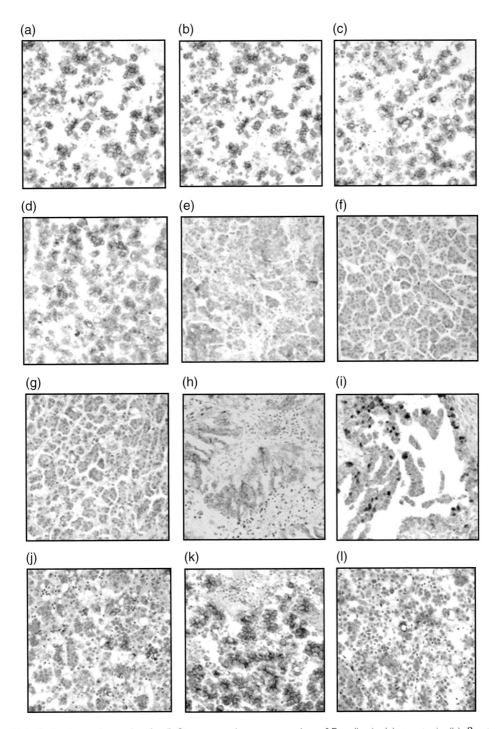

Figure 7.1 Cadherins and catenins. (a–d) Strong membrane expression of E-cadherin (a), α-catenin (b), β-catenin (c), and γ-catenin (d) in carcinoma cells in a peritoneal effusion. (e–g) Reduced expression of E-cadherin (e), β-catenin (f), and γ-catenin (g) in a primary carcinoma. (h) Partially restored expression of E-cadherin in an omental metastasis. (i) Nuclear β-catenin expression in a primary carcinoma – a rare finding in our cohort. (j–l) Coexpression of E-cadherin (j), N-cadherin (k) and P-cadherin (l) in carcinoma cells in a pleural effusion.

Table 7.1 The prognostic role of the E-cadherin complex and E-cadherin regulators in ovarian carcinoma

Ref	Molecule	Method[a]	Material	n	Univariate[b]	Multivariate[b]	Prognosis
17	E-cadherin	IHC	Primary	20	$p<0.05$	NP	Good
18	E-cadherin	IHC	Primary	104	$p=0.006$ (OS)	$p=0.014$	Good
19	E-cadherin	IHC	Primary + metastases	45	NS	NS	—
20	E-cadherin	RT–PCR	Effusions	70	$p=0.023$ (PFS)	NP	Good
19	α-catenin	IHC	Primary + metastases	45	NS	NS	—
21	α-catenin	IHC	Primary	86	$p=0.035$	$p=0.025$	Good
19	β-catenin	IHC	Primary + metastases	45	NS	NS	—
22	β-catenin	IHC	Primary	69	$p=0.016$ (PFS), $p=0.009$ (OS)	$p=0.003$ (PFS), $p=0.003$ (OS)	Good
23	β-catenin	IHC	Primary	104	$p=0.022$	$p=0.003$	Good
19	γ-catenin	IHC	Primary + metastases	45	$p=0.002$ (OS)[c]	NS	Poor
20	Snail	RT–PCR	Effusions	70	NS	NS	—
20	Slug	RT–PCR	Effusions	70	NS	NS	—
20	Sip1	RT–PCR	Effusions	70	NS[d]	NS	—

[a]IHC, immunohistochemistry; RT–PCR, reverse transcriptase polymerase chain reaction.
[b]NP, not performed; NS, not significant; OS, overall survival PFS, progression-free survival (in some studies, the terms relapse-free survival or disease-free survival are used).
[c]In primary tumors.
[d]Higher Sip1/E-cadherin ratio correlated with worse OS ($p=0.018$).

poor survival.[20] Analysis of the clinical role of negative E-cadherin regulators in effusions showed that the Sip1/E-cadherin ratio was higher in primary diagnosis compared with postchemotherapy effusions, in stage IV compared to stage III tumors, and in pleural compared to peritoneal effusions. A high Sip1/E-cadherin ratio predicted poor overall survival in univariate survival analysis (Figure 7.2 and Table 7.1).[20]

The prognostic role of catenins is documented in only a few studies (Table 7.1). Reduced expression of α-catenin correlated with poor outcome in stage I carcinomas, but not in tumors at International Federation of Gynecology and Obstetrics (FIGO) stages II–IV.[21] Favorable disease outcome (measured as disease relapse and eventual death of disease) was reported for patients with stage I–II tumors showing nuclear immunoreactivity for β-catenin

compared with patients whose tumors showed exclusively membrane localization.[22] However, the status of membrane immunostaining (preserved vs reduced) showed no association with disease relapse or survival.[23] The latter finding is in agreement with our findings in solid tumors.[19] In a study of 104 primary carcinomas, loss of β-catenin was an independent prognostic

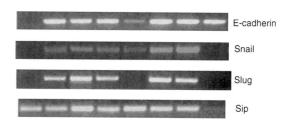

Figure 7.2 E-cadherin and its transcriptional repressors. Reverse transcriptase polymerase chain reaction (RT–PCR) analysis of eight effusions, showing expression of E-cadherin, Snail, Slug, and Sip1 in the majority of specimens.

marker of poor survival.[23] Loss of γ-catenin in primary tumors correlated with poor overall survival in univariate, although not in multivariate, analysis in our cohort of short-term and long-term survivors,[19] but did not correlate with clinical outcome in the study of Faleiro-Rodrigues et al.[23]

While some of the above-mentioned studies suggest a clinical role for E-cadherin and catenins in ovarian cancer, the overall data need to be interpreted as inconclusive. Understanding cellular events that occur along with tumor progression in ovarian carcinoma may be more relevant in terms of understanding the biology of this tumor and devising the appropriate therapeutic approaches in order to defeat it. Our data regarding the expression of transcriptional regulators of E-cadherin in effusions,[20] and the anatomic site-related differences in their expression,[24] together with data regarding cadherin and APC methylation in ovarian carcinomas,[25] may aid in expanding our knowledge regarding the regulation and role of cadherin-mediated adhesion in ovarian carcinoma.

Integrins

The unique pattern of metastasis that characterizes ovarian carcinoma requires the expression of receptors that are able to bind cells or extracellular matrix (ECM) molecules that are prevalent in the serosal cavities. The main candidates for this role are the integrins, a family of heterodimeric glycoproteins composed of α and β subunits that are involved in invasion, metastasis, angiogenesis, and intracellular signaling, with resulting proliferation, apoptosis, and synthesis of cancer-associated molecules in response to cues originating from other cells (e.g. stromal myofibroblasts) or different ECM proteins, including laminin, fibronectin, collagen, vitronectin, entactin, tenascin, and fibrinogen.[26]

To date, 18 α and 8 β subunits are known, forming 25 different combinations.[26] Most α subunits associate with a single β subunit, the largest family being the very late-activating (VLA) β_1 family, which includes the $\alpha_5\beta_1$ fibronectin receptor, the $\alpha_v\beta_1$ fibronectin receptor, and the $\alpha_6\beta_1$ laminin receptor.[27] This limitation does not apply to some α subunits, such as α_4, α_6, and α_v, which are able to bind more than one β subunit. For example, α_v integrin is a component of the receptors for fibronectin, vitronectin, fibrinogen, and several other proteins.[27] Some of the biologic roles of integrins that are essential for tumor progression, including angiogenesis, migration, invasion, and metastasis, are closely linked to the activation of metastasis-associated molecules, such as matrix metalloproteinases (MMPs).[28] Altered expression of integrins (down- or upregulation) has been detected in the majority of malignant tumors, but varies considerably, depending to the origin of the neoplasm.[27]

In vitro studies have characterized many of the interactions between integrins and ECM molecules in ovarian cancer. The α_2 and β_1 integrin subunits mediate adhesion of ovarian carcinoma cells to collagen type I,[29] and are involved in the attachment of ovarian carcinoma cells to the peritoneal mesothelium and the invasion of a mesothelial monolayer,[30–32] while $\alpha_v\beta_3$ integrin mediates binding to vitronectin in both cancer and ovarian surface epithelial cells.[33,34] Attachment to the peritoneal mesothelium via the β_1 integrin subunit may involve CD44, an adhesion molecule of the immunoglobulin superfamily, as detailed below.[31] Fibronectin and peritoneal conditioned media enhance the activity of MMP-9 in the NOM-1 cell line, an effect that is blocked by antibodies directed against the α_5 integrin subunit that forms part of the $\alpha_5\beta_1$ fibronectin receptor.[35] In support of this finding, formation of spheroids mimicking the clusters of tumor cells in effusion by the NIH:OVCAR-3 line is increased by stimulating antibodies against the β_1 integrin subunit and exogenous fibronectin.[36] Proliferation is regulated by $\alpha_v\beta_3$ integrin in IGROV1 cells and by both $\alpha_v\beta_3$ and $\alpha_v\beta_5$ integrins in SKOV-3 cells through activation of the integrin-linked kinase (ILK).[37]

As with cadherins, integrins are widely expressed in tumor samples from ovarian carcinoma patients, but their diagnostic and clinical role is undecided. The α_v and β_3 subunits and their ligand vitronectin were detected on normal ovarian epithelium and carcinomas of all grades, with more frequent loss of expression in grade 2 and 3 carcinomas.[38] However, comparative analysis of $\alpha_v\beta_3$, $\alpha_5\beta_1$, and $\alpha_2\beta_1$ integrin protein expression in invasive carcinomas and borderline tumors showed significantly higher expression of the $\alpha_v\beta_3$ receptor in carcinomas – results that were also confirmed by mRNA in situ hybridization and northern blotting for the β_3 integrin subunit.[39] Analysis of the α_6, β_4 and β_1 subunits that form the $\alpha_6\beta_4$, and $\alpha_6\beta_1$ laminin receptors in cell lines and two ascites specimens showed maximal expression of the α_6 and β_4 subunits in contact points between cancer cells in cohesive groups, with expression being detected along the entire membrane. In solid lesions, benign tumors and well-differentiated carcinomas showed polarized basolateral α_6 subunit expression, with weaker and fragmented labeling in poorly differentiated tumors.[40] These data are supported by an additional study showing that polarized α_6 and β_4 subunit expression in benign epithelium is replaced by irregular expression and loss of laminin in carcinomas, with conserved expression of the α_2, α_1 and β_1 subunits.[41]

The above studies suggest that loss of the $\alpha_6\beta_4$ laminin receptor is the main cellular event with respect to integrin expression in the transition from benign ovarian epithelium to invasive carcinoma. While studying the changes in integrin expression that occur when ovarian carcinomas metastasize, we detected the α_v and β_1 integrin subunit protein in >90% of specimens in an analysis of 121 effusions (Figure 7.3). The α_v subunit was widely expressed in corresponding solid tumors, with less frequent (50%) expression of the β_1 subunit.[42] In this study, reactive mesothelial cells were frequently β_1-positive, while α_v protein expression was cancer-specific.[42] However, an analysis using flow cytometry showed expression of both subunits in benign and malignant mesothelial cells, possibly due to the higher sensitivity of this method and the analysis of fresh-frozen tumor cells, suggesting that these proteins have limited diagnostic value.[43] In a study of laminin receptors, we analyzed the expression of the α_6 subunit and the non-integrin 67 kDa laminin receptor in 88 effusions and 116 corresponding solid tumors.[44] We found higher rather than lower expression of α_6 subunit mRNA in effusions compared to corresponding solid tumors (41% vs 26%: Figures 7.4 and 7.5), with confirmed protein expression in 17 of 27 effusions using flow cytometry.[44] These results differ from those reported in a limited analysis that included six effusion specimens, where decreased expression of α_6 and β_4, and similar expression of α_2, β_3 and β_1 integrin subunits was found compared with solid lesions.[41] The 67 kDa receptor was the more frequently expressed receptor in our series (>75% of both effusions and solid lesions, on both mRNA and protein levels: Figures 7.4 and 7.5). The frequent expression of ECM receptors of both integrin and nonintegrin type in ovarian cancer cells in effusions and solid metastases suggests that these molecules play a central role in tumor dissemination within the body cavities.

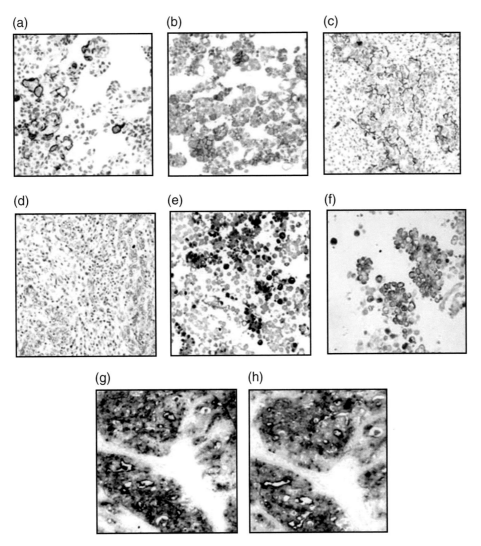

Figure 7.3 Integrins. (a–d) Protein expression: α_V integrin is expressed in carcinoma cells in effusion (a) and solid carcinoma (b); the β_1 integrin subunit is expressed in tumor cells in effusion (c), but is absent from solid carcinoma (d). (e–h) mRNA expression: the α_V (e) and β_1 (f) integrin subunit mRNA is expressed in carcinoma cells in effusion; carcinoma cells in a solid tumor from a short-term survivor (see text) similarly express both subunits: α_V in (g), β_1 in (h). (In situ hybridization: NBT-BCIP stain; counterstain with nuclear fast red.)

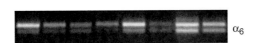

α_6

Figure 7.4 Laminin receptors. Variable expression of the two α_6 integrin isoforms is shown in seven effusion specimens.

The prognostic role of integrin expression in ovarian cancer has been investigated in several studies (Table 7.2). We found more frequent α_V integrin subunit mRNA in carcinoma cells in tumors of short-term survivors compared with long-term survivors, with correlation between α_V subunit expression and poor survival

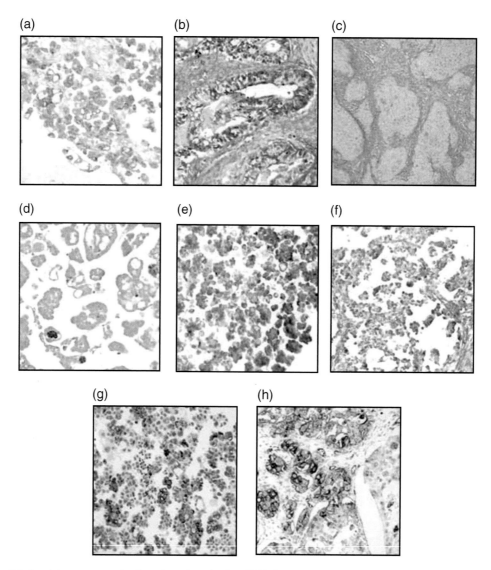

Figure 7.5 Laminin receptors. (a–c) α_6 integrin subunit mRNA is expressed in carcinoma cells in effusion (a) and in both carcinoma and stromal cells in solid carcinoma (b, c); in (c), expression is more pronounced in stromal cells. (d) An α_6 integrin-negative pleural effusion, counterstained in nuclear fast red. (e, f) mRNA for the 67 kDa nonintegrin receptor is expressed in tumor cells in a pleural effusion (e) and solid carcinoma (f). (g, h) There are similar findings for the 67 kDa protein expression. (In situ hybridization: NBT-BCIP stain; counterstain with nuclear fast red.)

in univariate and multivariate survival analyses.[45] In our cohort of patients with effusions, protein or mRNA expression of the α_v or β_1 integrin subunits did not correlate with disease outcome.[42] However, α_6 integrin mRNA expression in tumor cells of the corresponding solid lesions in the same cohort was significantly lower in FIGO stage IV compared with stage III carcinomas ($p = 0.004$), and its absence predicted significantly shorter overall survival (OS) in univariate analysis ($p = 0.018$).[44] Absence of the α_6 integrin subunit protein in carcinoma

Table 7.2 The prognostic role of the integrin subunits, the 67 kDa laminin receptor (LR), and Ets transcription factors in ovarian carcinoma

Ref	Molecule	Method[a]	Material	n	Univariate[b]	Multivariate[b]	Prognosis
42	α_v integrin	IHC	Effusions	107	NS	NP	—
42	β_1 integrin	IHC	Effusions	107	NS	NP	—
42	α_v integrin	ISH	Effusions	58	NS	NP	—
42	β_1 integrin	ISH	Effusions	58	NS	NP	—
45	α_v integrin	ISH	Primary + metastases	34	$p=0.012$ (OS)	$p=0.031$	Poor
45	β_1 integrin	ISH	Primary + metastases	34	NS	NP	—
44	α_6 integrin	ISH	Effusions	78	NS	NP	—
44	α_6 integrin	ISH	Primary + metastases	116	$p=0.018$ (OS)	NP	Good
44	67 kDa LR	ISH	Effusions	78	NS	NP	—
44	67 kDa LR	ISH	Primary + metastases	116	NS	NP	—
46	Ets-1	ISH	Primary + metastases	41	Tumor: $p=0.018$ (OS) Stroma: $p=0.026$ (OS)	Tumor: NS Stroma: $p=0.007$	Poor
47	PEA3	ISH	Primary + metastases	36	Tumor: $p=0.049$ (OS) Stroma: $p=0.019$ (DFS), $p=0.029$ (OS)	Tumor: NS Stroma: $p=0.015$ (OS)	Poor
48	Ets-1	ISH	Effusions	63	$p=0.003$ (OS)	NP	Poor
49	PEA3	ISH	Effusions	75	$p=0.03^c$	NP	Poor

[a]IHC, immunohistochemistry; ISH, mRNA in situ hybridization.

[b]NS, not significant; NP, not performed; OS, overall survival; DFS, disease-free survival (in some studies, the terms relapse-free survival or progression-free survival are used).

[c]For 41 patients with pre-chemotherapy effusions.

cells in effusions was associated with a median OS of 12 months, compared with 26 months for patients with tumors expressing the protein, although this finding did not reach significance.[44] Notably, mRNA expression of Ets-1 and PEA3, two members of the Ets family of transcription factors that are involved in activation of integrin, protease and angiogenic molecule synthesis, predicted poor survival in both cohorts (Table 7.2).[46–49] A recent report in which the expression of focal adhesion kinase (FAK), a nonreceptor tyrosine kinase that is involved in integrin signaling, was shown to be an independent marker of poor survival further supports the clinical role of integrins in ovarian cancer.[50]

Other adhesion molecules

Another group of cell membrane molecules that play a significant role in cancer is the immunoglobulin superfamily. Two members of this family – EMMPRIN (extracellular matrix metalloproteinase inducer) and CD44 – merit attention in the context of ovarian cancer.

EMMPRIN (CD147), previously known as cell-derived collagenase stimulatory factor (TCSF), is a 58 000 kDa glycoprotein that mediates signaling events leading to MMP synthesis.[51] EMMPRIN is able to bind MMP-1 on the surface of tumor cells[52] and associates with the $\alpha_3\beta_1$ and $\alpha_6\beta_1$ integrins at the cell membrane.[53] We have shown that EMMPRIN mRNA and protein are widely expressed on ovarian carcinoma cells in effusions and solid tumors (Figure 7.6), and that its presence is associated with MMP and integrin subunit expression and with activation of the mitogen-activated protein kinase (MAPK) signaling pathway.[54,55] EMMPRIN was less frequently expressed on peritumoral stromal and endothelial cells in solid tumors, but its presence on these cells correlated with poor overall survival in univariate survival analysis (Table 7.3).[54]

CD44 is an additional adhesion receptor that is member of the immunoglobulin superfamily. It is a transmembrane glycoprotein that functions as the receptor for hyaluronic acid and is expressed on cells of various lineages.[56] The CD44 gene is located on chromosome 11 and contains 20 axons. Alternative splicing of exons 5–16 generates 10 variant forms of the protein (v1–v10).[57] CD44 mediates cell–cell and cell–matrix interactions that affect lymphocyte trafficking, as well as adhesion, migration and invasion of other cells, including cancer cells.[58] Ovarian carcinoma cells expressing CD44 are able to bind hyaluronic acid on mesothelial cells, and inhibition of that interaction results in reduced peritoneal metastasis in mouse models.[30,31,59,60]

The diagnostic role of CD44 is uncertain. Both mesothelial cells and ovarian carcinoma cells express the standard form of this receptor (CD44s), which contains no variant exons, although we found higher CD44s expression on mesothelial cells, with higher CD44v3–10 expression on carcinoma cells (Figure 7.6).[61] The prognostic role of CD44 in ovarian cancer has been similarly equivocal, in part due to the use of different antibodies (Table 7.3).[62–67] Cannistra et al.[62] found no correlation between CD44s or CD44v9 expression and survival in primary tumors. We found upregulation of CD44s in carcinoma cells in effusions compared with the corresponding solid tumors.[63] However, both

CD44s and CD44v3–10 expression had no impact on disease outcome.[63] Kayastha et al[64] reported a direct correlation between CD44s and poor survival while opposite results were found by Ross et al[65] and Sillanpaa et al.[66] Serum levels of CD44s were higher in ovarian carcinoma patients compared with healthy controls, while levels of CD44v5 were lower, and higher CD44v5 levels correlated with better overall survival.[67]

PROTEASES

Matrix metalloproteinases

Invasion and metastasis are critical events in a multistep process that requires degradation of the subepithelial and subendothelial basement membranes, ECM modification, the ability to enter and exit the circulation, and the establishment of metastases in distant organs. MMPs, a family of more than 20 zinc- and calcium-dependent enzymes, are central mediators of these processes, owing to their ability to degrade basement membrane and ECM components.[68] MMPs have been previously divided into subfamilies based on substrate specificity. However, due to the overlapping substrate range between different members, MMP are currently classified into eight classes based on domain structure.[67] These domains mediate protease secretion (predomain), latency (prodomain), enzyme activity (catalytic domain), homodimerization and interactions with tissue inhibitors of metalloproteinases (TIMPs) (hemopexin/vitronectin-like domain), and membrane anchoring (transmembrane domain).[68] MMP-2 (gelatinase A, 72 kDa type IV collagenase) and MMP-9 (gelatinase B, 92 kDa type IV collagenase), the only enzymes with a gelatin-binding domain, are crucial for tumor metastasis due to their ability to degrade collagen type IV,

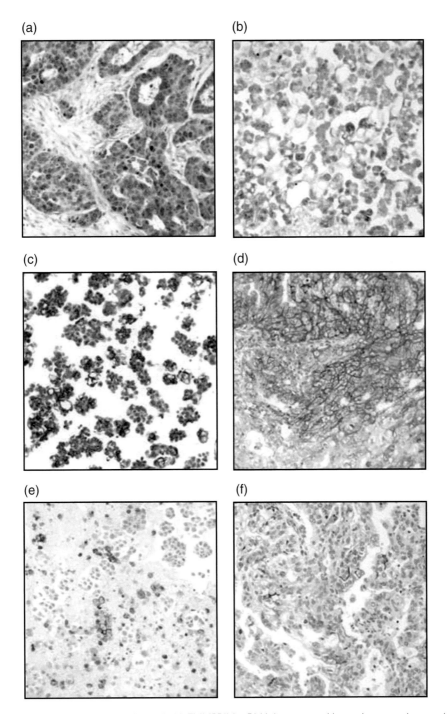

Figure 7.6 The immunoglobulin superfamily. (a, b) EMMPRIN mRNA is expressed in carcinoma and stromal cells in solid carcinomas (a), and in carcinoma cells in effusion (b). (c, d) EMMPRIN protein is similarly expressed at both anatomic sites. (e) CD44s protein expression in a peritoneal effusion. Reactive mesothelial cells express the receptor, while carcinoma cells are negative. (f) CDv3–10 expression in solid carcinoma. (In situ hybridization: NBT-BCIP stain; counterstain with nuclear fast red.)

Table 7.3 The prognostic role of CD44 and EMMPRIN in ovarian carcinoma

Ref	Molecule	Method[a]	Material	n	Univariate[b]	Multivariate[b]	Prognosis
54	EMMPRIN	IHC + ISH	Effusions	74	NS	NP	—
54	EMMPRIN	IHC + ISH	Primary + metastases (tumor cells)	28	NS	NP	—
54	EMMPRIN	IHC	Primary (stroma and vessels)	28	Stroma: $p=0.012$ Vessels: $p=0.023$ (OS)	NP	Poor
62	CD44 (different isoforms)	IHC + RT–PCR	Primary	31	NS	NP	—
63	CD44s	IHC	Effusions	58	NS	NP	—
63	CD44v3–10	IHC	Effusions	58	NS	NP	—
64	CD44s	IHC	Primary	56	$p=0.003$ (OS)	$p=0.006$ (OS)	Poor
65	CD44s	IHC	Primary	64	$p=0.04$	NS	Good
66	CD44 (all forms)	IHC	Primary	307	$p<0.001$ (OS and RFS)	OS: NS RFS: $p=0.04$	Good
67	CD44s + v6	ELISA	Serum	96	NS	NP	—
67	CD44v5	ELISA	Serum	96	$p<0.01$	$p<0.05$	Good

[a]IHC, immunohistochemistry; ISH, mRNA in situ hybridization; RT–PCR, reverse transcriptase polymerase chain reaction; ELISA, enzyme-linked immunosorbent assay.

[b]NS, not significant; NP, not performed; OS, overall survival; RFS, relapse-free survival (in some studies, the terms progression-free survival or disease-free survival are used).

a component of all basement membranes.[69] In addition to ECM molecules, MMP substrates include other MMP members, other proteases (e.g. plasminogen), growth factors (transforming growth factor, TGF), tyrosine kinase receptors (HER2/neu and FGFR1), adhesion molecules (CD44, E-cadherin, and α_v integrin), and numerous other molecules.[68,69] MMP activity is negatively regulated in a reversible manner by TIMP1–4 through the formation of a 1:1 stoichiometric binding, as well as by α_2-macroglobulins, thrombospondins, and the membrane-bound RECK protein.[68] However, cell surface-mediated activation of MMP-2 requires the formation of a complex with TIMP-2 and membrane-type-1 MMP (MT1-MMP, MMP-14).[68] Different ECM proteins, growth factors, and cytokines activate MMP synthesis (e.g. via integrin receptors), with transcriptional regulation mediated through binding of Ets family members, AP-1 and AP-2, and additional factors.[68,69]

Studies of MMP expression and activation in ovarian carcinoma have predominantly focused on the gelatinases (MMP-2 and MMP-9), their inhibitors TIMP-1 and TIMP-2, and MT1-MMP (MMP-14), the latter being a coactivator of MMP-2 at the cell membrane. MMPs are produced by ovarian carcinoma cell lines, and their synthesis is stimulated by fibroblasts.[70–72] MMP-2, MMP-9, MT1-MMP, and TIMP-2 are expressed in short-term cultures from peritoneal effusions and solid tumors,[73,74] and increased expression of MMP-9 is found when ovarian carcinoma cells are cultured in a medium containing human peritoneal tissue, an effect that is mediated by fibronectin.[35,75]

Several studies of clinical material have demonstrated MMP and TIMP protein and/or mRNA expression in ovarian carcinoma.[76–85]

Some investigators have argued that mRNA expression and thereby synthesis are limited to myofibroblasts.[77,78] However, in our two cohorts, MMP-2, MMP-9, and TIMP-2 mRNA were found in both tumor and stromal cells, while MT1-MMP was predominantly expressed in tumor cells, suggesting that ovarian cancer cells are able to produce MMP-2 and its coactivators TIMP-2 and MT1-MMP in an autonomous manner (Figure 7.7).[82,83] Similar results were reported in an additional study of MMP-9 and TIMP-1.[84] In two studies, MMP and TIMP expression has been shown to be upregulated in invasive ovarian carcinomas compared with benign tissue, with levels in borderline tumors being higher than in benign lesions but lower than in invasive carcinoma.[84,85] In one of these studies, MMP-2 activation was highest in omental metastases.[85] We found upregulated expression of MMP-2 in effusions compared with primary tumors.[83] We additionally showed that MT1-MMP and MT2-MMP, but not MT3-MMP, mRNA is expressed in ovarian carcinoma effusions.[86] MMP showed coexpression with Ets transcription factors (Figure 7.7), integrins, and angiogenic molecules, suggesting that these molecules are biologically linked in ovarian carcinoma.[87]

A number of studies have investigated the prognostic role of MMPs and TIMPs in ovarian carcinomas (Table 7.4). Two studies from the same group analyzing the prognostic role of MMP-2 protein expression in ovarian carcinomas using immunohistochemistry were inconclusive.[88,89] In an additional report, patients with carcinoma-positive stroma-negative tumors showed more frequent disease recurrence and poor survival,[81] although a more recent report found correlation between stromal MMP-2 protein expression and poor recurrence-free survival in endometrioid carcinomas.[90] In our series of patients with a follow-up period of up to 20 years, TIMP-2 mRNA expression in stromal cells and MMP-9 and TIMP-2 mRNA expression in carcinoma cells of primary tumors correlated with poor outcome in univariate analysis. In metastatic lesions, the presence of TIMP-2 mRNA in stromal cells and of MMP-2 and MT1-MMP mRNA in tumor cells correlated with poor outcome. In a multivariate analysis, TIMP-2 mRNA expression in stromal cells and MMP-9 mRNA expression in tumor cells were independent predictors of poor survival.[82]

More recent studies have documented a clinical role for at least some MMPs and TIMPs in ovarian cancer. Plasma levels of pro-MMP-9, TIMP-1, and TIMP-2 were shown to be significantly higher in patients with ovarian carcinoma compared with patients diagnosed with benign gynecologic diseases or healthy women, and higher TIMP-1 levels correlated with poor survival.[91] Gelatinolytic activity of pro-MMP-9 and active MMP-2 was found in ovarian carcinomas, but not in benign ovaries, and high pro-MMP-9 activity correlated with short overall survival in univariate and multivariate analysis.[92] MMP-8 protein expression was found to correlate with tumor grade, FIGO stage, and poor prognosis in an additional study.[93] Kamat et al[94] recently reported that high tumor and stromal expression of MMP-2, MMP-9, and MT1-MMP are significantly associated with advanced stage, the presence of ascites and lymph node metastases, and shorter disease-specific survival. Expression of MT1-MMP in both cellular compartments and of MMP-9 in stromal cells retained its significance in multivariate analysis.[94]

Plasminogen activator system

Urokinase-type plasminogen activator (uPA) is a serine protease that is synthesized as a

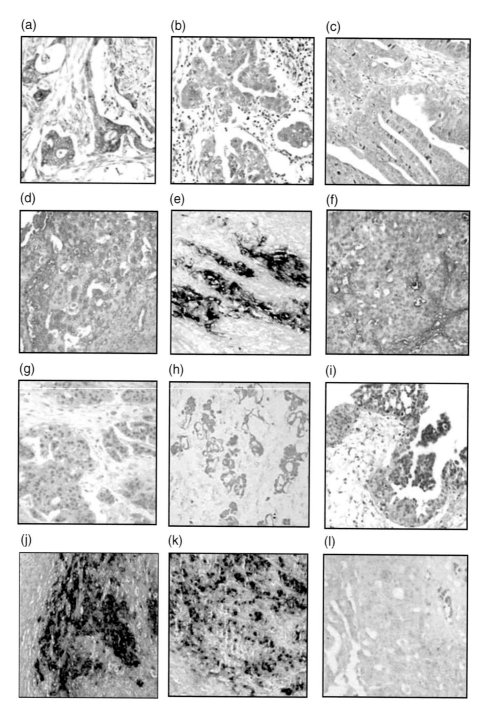

Figure 7.7 MMP, TIMP and Ets transcription factors. (a–c) Protein expression of MMP-1 (a), MMP-2 (b), and MMP-9 (c) in tumor cells from solid ovarian carcinoma. (d–f) mRNA expression of MMP-2 (d), MT1-MMP (e), and TIMP-2 (f) in carcinoma cells, with stromal cells expressing MMP-2 and TIMP-2, but not MT1-MMP. (g,h) Ets-1 mRNA expression in a solid tumor (g) and effusion (h); Ets-1 expression is also seen in stromal cells in (g). Similar localization is seen for PEA3 mRNA (i), while Ets-2 (j) and Erg (k) are localized to carcinoma cells only. (l) Hybridization with a PEA3 sense probe, with tumor cells counterstained with nuclear fast red. (In situ hybridization: NBT-BCIP stain; counterstain with nuclear fast red.)

Table 7.4 The prognostic role of matrix metalloproteinases (MMPs) and their inhibitors (TIMPs) in ovarian carcinoma

Ref	Molecule	Method[a]	Material	n	Univariate[b]	Multivariate[b]	Prognosis
81	MMP-2	IHC	Primary	33	NS	NP	—
82	MMP-2	ISH	Metastases	34	$p = 0.027$ (OS) (tumor)	NP	Poor
82	MMP-9	ISH	Primary	36	$p = 0.012$ (OS) (tumor)	$p = 0.011$	Poor
82	MT1-MMP	ISH	Metastases	34	$p = 0.008$ (OS) (tumor)	NP	Poor
82	MT1-MMP	ISH	Metastases	34	$p = 0.025$ (OS) (stroma)	NP	Good
82	TIMP-2	ISH	Primary	36	Stroma: $p < 0.001$ Tumor: $p = 0.02$	Stroma: $p = 0.006$ Tumor: NS	Poor
82	TIMP-2	ISH	Metastases	34	Stroma: $p = 0.031$	NP	Poor
88	MMP-2	IHC	Primary	18	NP	NS	-
89	MMP-2	IHC	Primary	21	$p = 0.004$ (DFS)	NP	Poor
89	MMP-2	ELISA	Serum	21	$p = 0.002$ (DFS)	NP	Poor
90	MMP-2	IHC	Primary	84	$p = 0.003$ (DFS) $p = 0.029$ (OS)[c]	NS	Poor
91	TIMP-1	ELISA	Serum	40[d]	$p = 0.017$ (OS)	NP	Poor
92	pro-MMP-9	Zymography	Primary	84	$p = 0.019$ (OS)[e]	$p = 0.023$	Poor
93	MMP-8	IHC	Primary	243	$P < 0.05$ (OS)[f]	NS	Poor
94	MMP-2	IHC	Primary	90	Tumor and stroma: $p < 0.01$ (DSS)	NS	Poor
94	MMP-9	IHC	Primary	90	Tumor and stroma: $p < 0.01$ (DSS)	Stroma: $p = 0.01$ Tumor: NS	Poor
94	MT1-MMP	IHC	Primary	90	Tumor and stroma: $p < 0.01$ (DSS)	Stroma: $p = 0.04$ Tumor: $p = 0.01$	Poor

[a]IHC, immunohistochemistry; ISH, mRNA in situ hybridization; ELISA enzyme-linked inmunosorbent assay.

[b]NS, not significant; NP, not performed; OS, overall survival; DFS, disease-free survival (in some studies, the terms relapse-free survival or progression-free survival are used); DSS, disease-specific survival.

[c]For stromal expression in 35 endometrioid tumors.

[d]Assumed to have been performed only for patients with carcinomas. MMP-2, MMP-9 and TIMP-2 levels did not correlate with survival.

[e]MMP-2 and pro-MMP-2 activity using ELISA and TIMP-1 and TIMP-2 levels using western blotting did not correlate with survival.

[f]MMP-3, MMP-7, MMP-9, MT3-MMP, TIMP-1, TIMP-2, and TIMP-3 expression did not correlate with survival.

single-chain latent proenzyme containing three functional domains: an N-terminal growth factor domain, a kringle domain of unknown function, and a C-terminal catalytic domain. uPA activation is achieved by the formation of a two-chain enzyme and is mediated by several proteases, including plasmin, cathepsins B and L, and kallikreins. uPA and its homolog tissue-type PA (tPA) cleave plasminogen to plasmin, thereby activating the degradation of fibrin and other ECM proteins and the activation of several MMPs (including MMP-9) and growth factors that are known to play a role in ovarian carcinoma, such as bFGF, insulin-like growth factor (IGF) and TGF-β. This system is negatively regulated by the plasminogen activator inhibitors PAI-1 and PAI-2 and the plasmin inhibitor α_2 antiplasmin.[95,96]

The uPA receptor uPAR is a glycosylphosphatidylinositol (GPI)-anchored protein with three domains (D1, D2, and D3) that is additionally able to bind vitronectin. uPAR is cleaved to yield a soluble form (suPAR). PAI-1 can mediate internalization of the uPA–uPAR complex, but the recycled receptor is able to return to the cell membrane.[96] In addition to its ability to bind uPA, uPAR has been shown to interact with different integrins (primarily with the $\alpha_3\beta_1$ and $\alpha_5\beta_1$ fibronectin receptors), G-coupled proteins, and caveolin. These interactions trigger the activation of major intracellular signaling pathways, including the MAPK and phosphatidylinositol 3′-kinase (PI3K) pathways.[96]

uPA levels, as measured by ELISA, have been shown to be higher in invasive carcinomas compared with borderline tumors and in high-grade carcinomas compared with more differentiated ones.[97] A similar finding was reported

in three additional studies.[98–100] van der Burg et al[98] found increasing uPA and PAI-1 levels in tissue extracts from normal ovaries through benign tumors, and borderline tumors, primary and metastatic carcinomas. Increased uPA activity was reported in grade 3 compared with grade 1–2 carcinomas, borderline tumors, benign tumors, and normal tissue.[99] An additional study showed higher plasma and tissue PAI-1 levels, higher uPA and PAI-2 tissue levels, and lower tPA tissue levels in patients with carcinomas compared with healthy controls using ELISA.[100]

The relationship between the PA system and disease outcome in ovarian carcinoma is not entirely clear, although uPA itself appears to correlate with more aggressive disease (Table 7.5). Konecny et al[101] reported correlation between higher uPA and PAI-1 primary

Table 7.5 The prognostic role of the plasminogen activator system in ovarian carcinoma

Ref	Molecule	Method	Material	n^a	Univariate[c]	Multivariate	Prognosis
101	uPA	ELISA	Primary	82	$p=0.003$ (PFS)[b] $p<0.001$ (OS)	$p=0.037$ (PFS) $p=0.006$ (OS)	Poor
101	PAI-1	ELISA	Primary	82	$p=0.039$ (PFS) $p=0.007$ (OS)	NS[c]	Poor
102[d]	uPA	ELISA	Primary	51	$p=0.02$ (OS)	NP[e]	Poor
102	uPAR	ELISA	Primary	51	$p=0.01$ (OS)	NS	Good
103	uPA	ELISA	Primary	86	$p=0.003$ (OS)	NS	Poor
103	PAI-1	ELISA	Primary	86	$p=0.012$ (OS)	$p<0.001$	Poor
105	uPAR/uPA ratio	ELISA	Ascites	36	$p<0.05$ (OS and DFI[f])	NS	Good
105	PAI-1	ELISA	Ascites	36	$p=0.03$ (DFI)	$p=0.007$	Good
105	PAI-2	ELISA	Ascites	36	$p=0.049$ (DFI) $p=0.047$ (OS)	$p=0.002$ (DFI)	Poor
106	PAI-1	IHC[g]	Primary	95	$p=0.04$ (OS)	$p=0.003$	Poor
107	PAI-2	IHC	Metastases	93	$p=0.006$ (DFS) $p=0.021$(OS)	$p=0.04$ (DFS) $p=0.03$(OS)[h]	Good

[a]n = patient number;

[b]PFS = progression-free survival. In some studies, the terms or disease-free survival or relapse-free survival are used;

[c]NS = not significant;

[d]PAI- and PAI-2 levels did not correlate with survival in this study;

[e]NP = not performed;

[f]DFI = disease-free interval;

[g]IHC = immunohistochemistry;

[h]OS = significant only for stage III patients.

tumor levels and poor progression-free and overall survival in univariate analysis, and uPA values retained their clinical role in multivariate analysis. Higher uPAR levels correlated with better survival, while higher uPA levels were associated with poor survival in univariate analysis, although none of these findings retained its significance in multivariate analysis.[102] PAI-1 and PAI-2 did not correlate with survival in this study.[102] Two studies by the same group showed correlation between uPA and PAI-1 levels and poor survival, independently for PAI-1.[103,104] A higher uPAR/uPA ratio in ascites specimens showed an inverse association with FIGO stage and residual disease, and correlated with longer overall and disease-free survival.[105] Interestingly, higher PAI-1 and lower PAI-2 levels in ascites correlated with longer DFS in univariate and multivariate analysis,[105] while opposite findings (poor prognosis for PAI-1, improved prognosis for PAI-2) were found in immunohistochemical analysis of solid tumors.[106,107]

CONCLUSIONS

As is the case in essentially any cancer type, ovarian carcinoma cells are able to proliferate, invade, and metastasize by maintaining a dynamic cellular ecosystem that allows for adaptation to different microenvironments, and by using the host cells to their advantage. These characteristics are reflected in the molecular changes affecting adhesion and proteolysis, as well as in other tumor-related aspects, such as angiogenesis, proliferation, and resistance to apoptosis, all of which are at least partly regulated by the molecules discussed in this chapter. Despite the fact that the clinical significance of these proteins has not been consistent in different studies, for reasons that may involve technical issues, case selection, and other factors, their biologic role is undisputed. Among the questions that await resolution, the regulation of these phenomena is one of the more crucial, if molecular therapy is to become a realistic goal for this disease. While no single 'master-switch' exists, the consistent expression of some regulatory molecules, such as the Ets transcription factors, in a nonredundant manner at all anatomic sites in ovarian carcinoma suggests that identifying such targets is of vital importance for future efforts to defeat ovarian cancer.

Data regarding both prognosis and prediction of treatment response are necessary for the selection of patients who would benefit from neoadjuvant or adjuvant chemotherapy or molecular therapy. Even though molecular markers cannot eliminate the stochastic uncertainties and enable us to predict outcome definitively, they will almost certainly increase our accuracy in subclassifying patients and their disease.

REFERENCES

1. Shirayoshi Y, Hatta K, Hosoda M, et al. Cadherin cell adhesion molecules with distinct binding specificities share a common structure. EMBO J 1986;5:2485–8.

2. Behrens J. Cadherins and catenins: Role in signal transduction and tumor progression. Cancer Metastasis Rev 1999;18:15–30.

3. Vleminckx K, Vakaet L Jr, Mareel M, et al. Genetic manipulation of E-cadherin expression by epithelial tumor cells reveals an invasion suppressor role. Cell 1991;66:107–19.

4. Hajra KM, Fearon ER. Cadherin and catenin alterations in human cancer. Genes Chromosomes Cancer 2002;34:255–68.

5. Van Aken E, De Wever O, Correia da Rocha AS, Mareel M. Defective E-cadherin/catenin complexes in human cancer. Virchows Arch 2001;439:725–51.

6. Nieto MA. The snail superfamily of zinc-finger transcription factors. Nat Rev Mol Cell Biol 2002;3:155–66.

7. Comijn J, Berx G, Vermassen P, et al. The two-handed E box binding zinc finger protein SIP1 downregulates E-cadherin and induces invasion. Mol Cell 2001;7:1267–78.

8. Risinger JI, Berchuck A, Kohler MF, Boyd J. Mutations of the E-cadherin gene in human gynecologic cancers. Nat Genet 1994;7: 98–102.

9. Wu R, Zhai Y, Fearon ER, Cho KR. Diverse mechanisms of β-catenin deregulation in ovarian endometrioid adenocarcinomas. Cancer Res 2001;61:8247–55.

10. Palacios J, Gamallo C. Mutations in the β-catenin gene (CTNNB1) in endometrioid ovarian carcinomas. Cancer Res 1998;58: 1344–7.

11. Sundfeldt K, Piontkewitz Y, Ivarsson K, et al. E-cadherin expression in human epithelial ovarian cancer and normal ovary. Int J Cancer 1997;74:275–80.

12. Maines-Bandiera S, Auersperg N. Increased E-cadherin expression in ovarian surface epithelium. An early step in metaplasia and dysplasia? Int J Gynecol Pathol 1997;16:250–5.

13. Davidson B, Berner A, Nesland JM, et al. E-cadherin and α-, β- and γ-catenin protein expression is up-regulated in ovarian carcinoma cells in serous effusions. J Pathol 2000; 192:460–9.

14. Patel IS, Madan P, Getsios S, et al. Cadherin switching in ovarian cancer progression. Int J Cancer 2003;106:172–7.

15. Sivertsen S, Berner A, Michael CW, Bedrossian C, Davidson S. Cadherin expression in ovarian carcinoma and malignant mesothelioma cell effusions. Acta Cytol 2006;50:603–7.

16. Davidson B, Nielsen S, Christensen J, et al. The role of desmin and N-cadherin in effusion cytology. A comparative study using established markers of mesothelial and epithelial cells. Am J Surg Pathol 2001;25:1405–12.

17. Darai E, Scoazec JY, Walker-Combrouze F, et al. Expression of cadherins in benign, borderline, and malignant ovarian epithelial tumors: A clinicopathologic study of 60 cases. Hum Pathol 1997;28:922–8.

18. Faleiro-Rodrigues C, Macedo-Pinto I, Pereira D, Lopes CS. Prognostic value of E-cadherin immunoexpression in patients with primary ovarian carcinomas. Ann Oncol 2004;15:1535–42.

19. Davidson B, Gotlieb WH, Ben-Baruch G, et al. E-cadherin complex protein expression and survival in ovarian carcinoma. Gynecol Oncol 2000;79:362–71.

20. Elloul S, Bukholt Elstrand M, Nesland JM, et al. Snail, Slug, and Smad-interacting protein 1 as novel parameters of disease aggressiveness in metastatic ovarian and breast carcinoma. Cancer 2005;103:1631–43.

21. Anttila M, Kosma V-M, Ji H, et al. Clinical significance of α-catenin, collagen IV, and Ki-67 expression in epithelial ovarian cancer. J Clin Oncol 1998;16:2591–600.

22. Gamallo C, Palacios J, Moreno G, et al. β-catenin expression pattern in stage I and II ovarian carcinomas. Relationship with β-catenin gene mutations, clinicopathological features, and clinical outcome. Am J Pathol 1999;155:527–36.

23. Faleiro-Rodrigues C, Macedo-Pinto I, Pereira D, Lopes CS. Loss of β-catenin is associated with poor survival in ovarian carcinomas. Int J Gynecol Pathol 2004;23:337–46.

24. Elloul S, Silins I, Tropé CG, et al. Expression of E-cadherin transcriptional regulators in ovarian carcinoma. Virchows Arch 2006;449: 520–8.

25. Makarla PB, Saboorian MH, Ashfaq R, et al. Promoter hypermethylation profile of ovarian

epithelial neoplasms. Clin Cancer Res 2005; 11:5365–9.

26. Hood JD, Cheresh DA. Role of integrins in cell invasion and migration. Nat Rev Cancer 2002;2:91–100.

27. Sanders RJ, Mainiero F, Giancotti FP. The role of integrins in tumorigenesis and metastasis. Cancer Invest 1998;16:329–44.

28. Heino J. Biology of tumor cell invasion: interplay of cell adhesion and matrix degradation. Int J Cancer 1996;65:717–22.

29. Moser TL, Pizzo SV, Bafetti LM et al. Evidence for preferential adhesion of ovarian epithelial carcinoma cells to type I collagen mediated by the $\alpha_2\beta_1$ integrin. Int J Cancer 1996;67:695–701.

30. Strobel T, Cannistra SA. β_1-integrins partly mediate binding of ovarian cancer cells to peritoneal mesothelium in vitro. Gynecol Oncol 1999;73:362–7.

31. Lessan K, Aguiar DJ, Oegema T, et al. CD44 and β_1 integrin mediate ovarian carcinoma cell adhesion to peritoneal mesothelial cells. Am J Pathol 1999;154:1525–37.

32. Kishikawa T, Sakamoto M, Ino Y, et al. Two distinct patterns of peritoneal involvement shown by in vitro and in vivo ovarian cancer dissemination models. Invasion Metastasis 1995;15:11–21.

33. Cruet S, Salamanca C, Mitchell GWE, Auersperg N. $\alpha_v\beta_3$ and vitronectin expression by normal ovarian surface epithelial cells: role in cell adhesion and cell proliferation. Gynecol Oncol 1999;75:254–60.

34. Cannistra SA, Ottensmeier C, Niloff J, et al. Expression and function of β_1 and $\alpha_v\beta_3$ integrins in ovarian cancer. Gynecol Oncol 1995;58:216–25.

35. Shibata K, Kikkawa F, Nawa A, et al. Fibronectin secretion from human peritoneal tissue induces Mr 92,000 type IV collagenase expression and invasion of ovarian cancer cell lines. Cancer Res 1997;57:5416–20.

36. Casey RC, Burleson KM, Skubitz KM, et al. β_1-integrins regulate the formation and adhesion of ovarian carcinoma multicellular spheroids. Am J Pathol 2001;159:2071–80.

37. Cruet-Hennequart S, Maubant S, Luis J, et al. α_v integrins regulate cell proliferation through integrin-linked kinase (ILK) in ovarian cancer cells. Oncogene 2003;22:1688–702.

38. Carreiras F, Denoux Y, Staedel C, et al. Expression and localization of α_v integrins and their ligand vitronectin in normal ovarian epithelium and in ovarian carcinoma. Gynecol Oncol 1996;62:260–7.

39. Liapis H, Adler LM, Wick MR, Rader JS. Expression of $\alpha_v\beta_3$ integrin is less frequent in ovarian epithelial tumors of low malignant potential in contrast to ovarian carcinomas. Hum Pathol 1997;28:443–9.

40. Bottini C, Miotti S, Fiorucci S, et al. Polarization of the $\alpha_6\beta_4$ integrin in ovarian carcinomas. Int J Cancer 1993;54:261–7.

41. Skubitz APN, Bast RC Jr, Wayner EA, et al. Expression of α_6 and β_4 integrins in serous ovarian carcinoma correlates with expression of the basement membrane protein laminin. Am J Pathol 1996;148:1445–61.

42. Davidson B, Goldberg I, Reich R, et al. The α_v and β_1 integrin subunits are commonly expressed in malignant effusions from ovarian carcinoma patients. Gynecol Oncol 2003;90:248–57.

43. Sigstad E, Dong HP, Nielsen S, et al. Quantitative analysis of integrin expression in effusions using flow cytometric immunophenotyping. Diagn Cytopathol 2005;33:321–31.

44. Givant-Horwitz V, Davidson B, van de Putte G, et al. Expression of the 67 kDa laminin receptor and the α_6 integrin subunit in serous ovarian carcinoma. Clin Exp Metastasis 2003;20:599–609.

45. Goldberg I, Davidson B, Reich R, et al. α_v integrin is a novel marker of poor prognosis in advanced-stage ovarian carcinoma. Clin Cancer Res 2001;7:4073–9.

46. Davidson B, Reich R, Goldberg I, et al. Ets-1 mRNA expression is a novel marker of poor survival in ovarian carcinoma. Clin Cancer Res 2001;7:551–7.

47. Davidson B, Goldberg I, Gotlieb WH, et al. PEA3 is the second Ets family transcription factor involved in tumor progression in ovarian carcinoma. Clin Cancer Res 2003;9:1412–19.

48. Davidson B, Risberg B, Goldberg I, et al. Ets-1 mRNA expression in effusions of serous ovarian carcinoma patients is a marker of poor outcome. Am J Surg Pathol 2001;25:1493–500.

49. Davidson B, Goldberg I, Reich R, et al. The clinical role of the PEA3 transcription factor in ovarian and breast carcinoma in effusions. Clin Exp Metastasis 2004;21:191–9.

50. Sood AK, Coffin JE, Schneider GB, et al. Biological significance of focal adhesion kinase in ovarian cancer: role in migration and invasion. Am J Pathol 2004;165:1087–95.

51. Kataoka H, DeCastro R, Zucker S, et al. Tumor cell-derived collagenase stimulatory factor increases expression of interstitial collagenase, stromelysin, and 72-kDa gelatinase. Cancer Res 1993;53:3154–8.

52. Guo H, Li R, Zucker S, et al. EMMPRIN (CD147), an inducer of matrix metalloproteinase synthesis, also binds interstitial collagenase to the tumor cell surface. Cancer Res 2000;60:888–91.

53. Berditchevski F, Chang S, Bodorova J, et al. Generation of monoclonal antibodies to integrin-associated proteins. J Biol Chem 1997; 272:29174–80.

54. Davidson B, Goldberg I, Berner A, et al. EMMPRIN (extracellular matrix metalloproteinase inducer) is a novel marker of poor outcome in serous ovarian carcinoma. Clin Exp Metastasis 2003;20:161–9.

55. Davidson B, Givant-Horwitz V, Lazarovici P, et al. Matrix metalloproteinases (MMP), EMMPRIN (extracellular matrix metalloproteinase inducer) and mitogen-activated protein kinases (MAPK): co-expression in metastatic serous ovarian carcinoma. Clin Exp Metastasis 2003;20:621–31.

56. Ponta H, Wainwright D, Herrlich P. The CD44 protein family. Int J Biochem Cell Biol 1998; 30:299–305.

57. Screaton GR, Bell MV, Jackson DG, et al. Genomic structure of DNA encoding the lymphocyte homing receptor CD44 reveals at least 12 alternatively spliced exons. Proc Natl Acad Sci USA 1992;89:12160–4.

58. Lesley J, Hyman R, Kincade PW. CD44 and its interaction with extracellular matrix. Adv Immunol 1993;54:271–335.

59. Gardner MJ, Catterall JB, Jones LM, Turner GA. Human ovarian tumour cells can bind hyaluronic acid via membrane CD44: a possible step in peritoneal metastasis. Clin Exp Metastasis 1996;14:325–34.

60. Strobel T, Swanson L, Cannistra SA. In vivo inhibition of CD44 limits intra-abdominal spread of a human ovarian cancer xenograft in nude mice: a novel role for CD44 in the process of peritoneal implantation. Cancer Res 1997;57:1228–32.

61. Berner HS, Davidson B, Berner A, et al. Differential expression of CD44s and CD44v3–10 in adenocarcinoma cells and reactive mesothelial cells in effusions. Virchows Arch 2000;436:330–5.

62. Cannistra SA, Abu-Jawdeh G, Niloff J, et al. CD44 variant expression is a common feature of epithelial ovarian cancer: lack of association with standard prognostic factors. J Clin Oncol 1995;13:1912–21.

63. Berner HS, Davidson B, Berner A, et al. Expression of CD44 in effusions of patients diagnosed with serous ovarian carcinoma - diagnostic and prognostic implications. Clin Exp Metastasis 2000;18:197–202.

64. Kayastha S, Freedman AN, Piver MS, et al. Expression of the hyaluronan receptor, CD44S, in epithelial ovarian cancer is an independent predictor of survival. Clin Cancer Res 1999;5:1073–6.

65. Ross JS, Sheehan CE, Williams SS, et al. Decreased CD44 standard form expression correlates with prognostic variables in ovarian carcinomas. Am J Clin Pathol 2001;116:122–8.

66. Sillanpaa S, Anttila MA, Voutilainen K, et al. CD44 expression indicates favorable prognosis in epithelial ovarian cancer. Clin Cancer Res 2003;9:5318–24.

67. Zeimet AG, Widschwendter M, Uhl-Steidl M, et al. High serum levels of soluble CD44 variant isoform v5 are associated with favourable clinical outcome in ovarian cancer. Br J Cancer 1997;76:1646–51.

68. Egeblad M, Werb Z. New functions for the matrix metalloproteinases in cancer progression. Nat Rev Cancer 2002;2:161–74.

69. Bjorklund M, Koivunen E. Gelatinase-mediated migration and invasion of cancer cells. Biochim Biophys Acta 2005;1755:37–69.

70. Westerlund A, Hujanen E, Puistola U, Turpeenniemi-Hujanen T. Fibroblasts stimulate human ovarian cancer cell invasion and expression of 72-kDa gelatinase A (MMP-2). Gynecol Oncol 1997;67:76–82.

71. Moore DH, Allison B, Look KY, et al. Collagenase expression in ovarian cancer cell lines. Gynecol Oncol 1997;65:78–82.

72. Boyd RS, Balkwill FR. MMP-2 release and activation in ovarian carcinoma: the role of fibroblasts. Br J Cancer 1999;80:315–21.

73. Fishman DA, Bafetti LM, Stack MS. Membrane-type matrix metalloproteinase expression and matrix metalloproteinase-2 activation in primary human ovarian epithelial carcinoma cells. Invasion Metastasis 1996;16:150–9.

74. Fishman DA, Bafetti LM, Banionis S, et al. Production of extracellular matrix-degrading proteinases by primary cultures of human epithelial ovarian carcinoma cells. Cancer 1997;80:1457–63.

75. Shibata K, Kikkawa F, Nawa A, et al. Increased matrix metalloproteinase-9 activity in human ovarian cancer cells cultured with conditioned medium from human peritoneal tissue. Clin Exp Metastasis 1997;15:612–19.

76. Höyhtyä M, Fridman R, Komarek D, et al. Immunohistochemical localization of matrix metalloproteinase 2 and its specific inhibitor TIMP-2 in neoplastic tissues with monoclonal antibodies. Int J Cancer 1994;56:500–5.

77. Afzal S, Lalani EN, Poulsom R, et al. MT1-MMP and MMP-2 mRNA expression in human ovarian tumors. Possible implications for the role of desmoplastic fibroblasts. Hum Pathol 1998;29:155–65.

78. Afzal S, Lalani EN, Foulkes WD, et al. Matrix metalloproteinase-2 and tissue inhibitor of metalloproteinase-2 expression and synthetic matrix metalloproteinase-2 inhibitor binding in ovarian carcinomas and tumor cell lines. Lab Invest 1996;74:406–21.

79. Naylor MS, Stamp GW, Davies BD, Balkwill FR. Expression and activity of MMPs and their regulators in ovarian cancer. Int J Cancer 1994;58:50–6.

80. Autio-Harmainen H, Karttunen T, Hurskainen T, et al. Expression of 72 kDa type IV collagenase (gelatinase A) in benign and malignant ovarian tumors. Lab Invest 1993;69:312–21.

81. Westerlund A, Apaja-Sarkkinen M, Höyhtyä M, et al. Gelatinase A-immunoreactive protein in ovarian lesions − prognostic value in epithelial ovarian cancer. Gynecol Oncol 1999;75:91–8.

82. Davidson B, Goldberg I, Gotlieb WH, et al. High levels of MMP-2, MMP-9, MT1-MMP and TIMP-2 mRNA correlate with poor survival in ovarian carcinoma. Clin Exp Metastasis 1999;17:799–808.

83. Davidson B, Reich R, Berner A, et al. Ovarian carcinoma cells in serous effusions show altered MMP-2 and TIMP-2 mRNA levels. Eur J Cancer 2001;37:2040–9.

84. Huang LW, Garrett AP, Bell DA, et al. Differential expression of matrix metalloproteinase-9 and tissue inhibitor of metalloproteinase-1 protein and mRNA in epithelial ovarian tumors. Gynecol Oncol 2000;77:369–76.

85. Schmalfeldt B, Prechtel D, Harting K, et al. Increased expression of matrix metalloproteinases (MMP)-2, MMP-9, and the urokinase-type plasminogen activator is associated with progression from benign to advanced ovarian cancer. Clin Cancer Res 2001;7:2396–404.

86. Davidson B, Goldberg I, Berner A, et al. Expression of membrane-type 1, 2 and 3 matrix metalloproteinases messenger RNA in ovarian carcinoma cells in serous effusions. Am J Clin Pathol 2001;115:517–24.

87. Davidson B, Goldberg I, Gotlieb WH, et al. Coordinated expression of integrin subunits, matrix metalloproteinases (MMP), angiogenic genes and Ets transcription factors in advanced-stage ovarian carcinoma – a possible activation pathway? Cancer Metastasis Rev 2003;22:103–15.

88. De Nictolis M, Garbisa S, Lucarini G, et al. 72-kDa type IV collagenase, type IV collagen, and Ki 67 antigen in serous tumors of the ovary: a clinicopathologic, immunohisto-chemical, and serological study. Int J Gynecol Pathol 1996;15:102–9.

89. Garzetti GG, Ciavattini A, Lucarini G, et al. Tissue and serum metalloproteinase (MMP-2) expression in advanced ovarian serous cystade-nocarcinomas: clinical and prognostic implica-tions. Anticancer Res 1995;15:2799–804.

90. Torng PL, Mao TL, Chan WY, et al. Prognostic significance of stromal metalloproteinase-2 in ovarian adenocarcinoma and its relation to carcinoma progression. Gynecol Oncol 2004;92:559–67.

91. Manenti L, Paganoni P, Floriani I, et al. Expression levels of vascular endothelial growth factor, matrix metalloproteinases 2 and 9 and tissue inhibitor of metalloproteinases 1 and 2 in the plasma of patients with ovarian carcinoma. Eur J Cancer 2003;39:1948–56.

92. Lengyel E, Schmalfeldt B, Konik E, et al. Expression of latent matrix metalloproteinase 9 (MMP-9) predicts survival in advanced ovarian cancer. Gynecol Oncol 2001;82: 291–8.

93. Stadlmann S, Pollheimer J, Moser PL, et al. Cytokine-regulated expression of collagenase-2 (MMP-8) is involved in the progression of ovarian cancer. Eur J Cancer 2003;39: 2499–505.

94. Kamat AA, Fletcher M, Gruman LM, et al. The clinical relevance of stromal matrix metallo-proteinase expression in ovarian cancer. Clin Cancer Res 2006;12:1707–14.

95. Duffy MJ, Duggan C. The urokinase plas-minogen activator system: a rich source of tumour markers for the individualized man-agement of patients with cancer. Clin Biochem 2004;37:541–8.

96. Blasi F, Carmeliet P. uPAR: a versatile sig-nalling orchestrator. Nat Rev Mol Cell Biol 2002;3:932–42.

97. Gleeson NC, Hill BJ, Moscinski LC, et al. Urokinase plasminogen activator in ovarian cancer. Eur J Gynaecol Oncol 1996;17:110–13.

98. van der Burg ME, Henzen-Logmans SC, Berns EM, et al. Expression of urokinase-type plasminogen activator (uPA) and its inhibitor PAI-1 in benign, borderline, malignant primary and metastatic ovarian tumors. Int J Cancer 1996;69:475–9.

99. Ho CH, Yuan CC, Liu SM. Diagnostic and prognostic values of plasma levels of fibri-nolytic markers in ovarian cancer. Gynecol Oncol 1999;75:397–400.

100. Murthi P, Barker G, Nowell CJ, et al. Plasminogen fragmentation and increased pro-duction of extracellular matrix-degrading pro-teinases are associated with serous epithelial ovarian cancer progression. Gynecol Oncol 2004;92:80–8.

101. Konecny G, Untch M, Pihan A, et al. Association of urokinase-type plasminogen activator and its inhibitor with disease progres-sion and prognosis in ovarian cancer. Clin Cancer Res 2001;7:1743–9.

102. Borgfeldt C, Bendahl PO, Gustavsson B, et al. High tumor tissue concentration of urokinase plasminogen activator receptor is associated

with good prognosis in patients with ovarian cancer. Int J Cancer 2003;107:658–65.

103. Kuhn W, Schmalfeldt B, Reuning U, et al. Prognostic significance of urokinase (uPA) and its inhibitor PAI-1 for survival in advanced ovarian carcinoma stage FIGO IIIc. Br J Cancer 1999;79:1746–51.

104. Kuhn W, Pache L, Schmalfeldt B, et al. Urokinase (uPA) and PAI-1 predict survival in advanced ovarian cancer patients (FIGO III) after radical surgery and platinum-based chemotherapy. Gynecol Oncol 1994;55:401–9.

105. Chambers SK, Gertz RE Jr, Ivins CM, Kacinski BM. The significance of urokinase-type

plasminogen activator, its inhibitors, and its receptor in ascites of patients with epithelial ovarian cancer. Cancer 1995;75:1627–33.

106. Chambers SK, Ivins CM, Carcangiu ML. Plasminogen activator inhibitor-1 is an independent poor prognostic factor for survival in advanced stage epithelial ovarian cancer patients. Int J Cancer 1998;79: 449–54.

107. Chambers SK, Ivins CM, Carcangiu ML. Expression of plasminogen activator inhibitor-2 in epithelial ovarian cancer: a favorable prognostic factor related to the actions of CSF-1. Int J Cancer 1997;74:571–5.

Immune biomarkers in ovarian cancer

8

George Coukos, Ioannis Alagkiozidis, Sarah Kim, Mark Cadungog, Sarah Adams, Christina Chu, José Ramon Conejo-Garcia, Weiping Zou, Tyler Curiel, Dionysios Katsaros, Lin Zhang, and Phyllis Gimotty

INTRODUCTION

Emerging evidence over the past decade has revealed the significance of tumor-host interactions and of the tumor microenvironment in tumor growth and progression. Among these mechanisms, a bulk of experimental evidence in animal tumor models has clearly established that the ability of the host to recognize and attack tumors, or vice versa the ability of tumors to evade such a response, largely determines the fate of developing tumors.[1] It is now generally accepted that human tumors may be antigenic, i.e. cancer cells express unique tumor-specific antigens that, in select patients, may be recognized by the immune system. Lessons learned from melanoma indicate that such antigens may be tumor-specific proteins that are normally absent in adult normal tissues except for germline cells, tissue-specific differentiation proteins that are normally not expressed within a specific organ, mutated proteins, overexpressed proteins, or unmasked protein epitopes due to protein underglycosylation. Strong proof that spontaneously occurring tumor-reactive T cells are directed against tumor antigens and can reject tumors in the human comes from recent adoptive T-cell therapy in melanoma. Ex vivo expanded T-cell clones induced tumor regression under conditions enhancing T-cell homeostasis. A significant association has been demonstrated between tumor regression and the persistence of adoptively transferred T-cell clones in peripheral blood.[2–4]

In epithelial ovarian carcinoma, antigen characterization has not been systematic, but evidence exists that tumor-associated antigens are present. The best differentiation tumor rejection antigen identified to date is the HLA-A2-restricted onconeuronal protein cdr2, shared by ovarian cancer cells and cerebellar Purkinje cells. Its recognition by cytotoxic lymphocytes (CTL) is associated with paraneoplastic cerebellar degeneration and occult ovarian cancer.[5] Other antigens identified in ovarian cancer include the following: HER2 protein, the product of the *ERBB2* oncogene; the *TP53* tumor suppressor gene protein product p53; topoisomerase-IIα; folate-binding protein; amino enhancer of split protein; sialylated TN (sTN), a mucin antigen; MUC-1; NY-ESO-1, a testis differentiation antigen; and mesothelin (for reviews see reference 6). In addition, universal tumor antigens such as human telomerase reverse transcriptase (hTERT), cytochrome P450 CYP1B1, and surviving[7] are expressed by epithelial ovarian carcinoma cells.[8,9] Tumor-specific T cells secreting interferon-γ (IFN-γ) have been reported in the peripheral blood of patients with advanced-stage ovarian carcinoma, indicating that tumor antigens are in fact recognized spontaneously in vivo.[10]

Until recently, the role of the immune system in the natural course of ovarian cancer remained unknown. However, the evidence that ovarian cancers express antigens and that ovarian carcinoma specimens harbor a brisk leukocyte infiltrate[11–13] has suggested that immune mechanisms might affect the outcome of ovarian cancer and/or provide important biomarkers for disease classification. Below we will summarize the work to date on cellular and humoral immune biomarkers in ovarian cancer as they have been discovered in our laboratories and by other investigators.

EFFECTOR T CELLS

In the human, the dominant adaptive immune effector cells targeting tumors are T cells bearing the $\alpha\beta$ T-cell receptor. Such cells have long been detected in ovarian cancer, both in solid tumor nodules and in ascites. Various groups have shown that tumor-derived T lymphocytes exhibit an activated phenotype,[11] are oligoclonal,[14,15] recognize tumor-associated antigens,[16–22] and display antitumor activity ex vivo.[22–25] In a study involving 186 patients with stage III or IV ovarian carcinoma from a single Northern Italian institution, we reported that tumor-infiltrating T cells are detectable within tumor cell islets (named *intratumoral* or *intraepithelial* T cells), in the surrounding stroma, or in both (Figure 8.1).[26] We noted that approximately half (84/186, 45.2%) of patients with stage III or IV epithelial ovarian carcinoma lacked intraepithelial CD3+ T cells. In most of these patients, however, variable numbers of CD3+ cells were noted in the stroma surrounding tumor islets. We noted a correlation between CD4+ and CD8+ T-cell infiltrates

($r^2=0.66$, $p<0.001$; $n=30$). Accordingly, intraepithelial CD4+ and CD8+ cells were either present or absent by immunohistochemistry, similarly to total CD3+ cells. Tumors with or without intraepithelial T cells contained similar numbers of CD45+ cells (leukocytes), CD11c+ cells (monocytes/granulocytes), CD19+ cells (B lymphocytes) and CD57+ (NK) cells within tumor islets, indicating that absence from tumor islets was specific for T cells. In 10 fresh tumors analyzed by flow cytometry, CD3+ T cells comprised 30–55% of all tumor-infiltrating CD45+ leukocytes.

We classified patients according to the presence or absence of intraepithelial CD3+ T cells and examined clinical outcomes. The overall 5 year progression-free and overall survival rates for all 174 evaluable patients were 20.9% and 25.3%, respectively. In these patients, there were significant differences in progression-free survival and overall survival distributions, based on the presence or absence of intraepithelial T cells ($p<0.0001$ for both) (Figure 8.2). Patients whose tumors had intraepithelial T cells experienced 3.8-fold longer median progression-free survival and 2.8-fold longer overall survival compared with patients whose tumors lacked intraepithelial T cells. The 5-year overall survival rate was 38% in the 102 patients whose tumors had intraepithelial T cells, while it was 4.5% in the 72 patients whose tumors had no such cells. The progression-free survival rate at 4 years was 31% in patients whose tumors exhibited intraepithelial T cells and 8.7% in those whose tumors lacked such cells. In the subset of 74 evaluable patients with a complete response to therapy, there were also significant differences in progression-free survival and overall survival distributions ($p<0.0001$ for both), based on the presence or absence of intraepithelial T cells. Patients whose tumors had intraepithelial

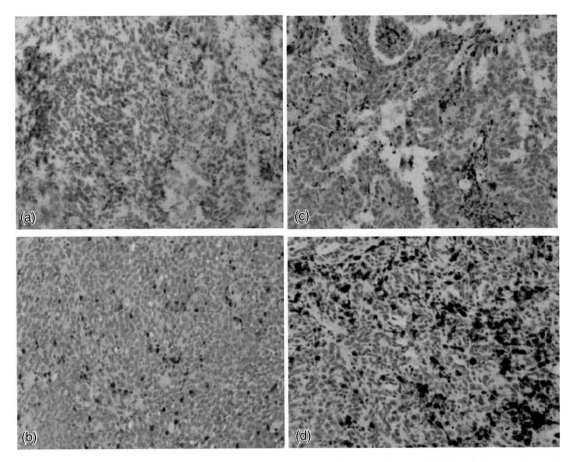

Figure 8.1 Immunohistochemistry for CD8 reveals the presence or absence of intraepithelial T cells in stage III ovarian cancer. (a) No intraepithelial T cells are seen in this tumor, but a brisk infiltrate is seen in the stroma surrounding tumor islets. (b–d) Detection of intraepithelial T cells with progressively more brisk infiltrate in these tumors. (40× magnification.)

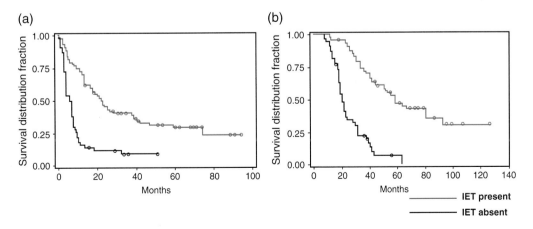

Figure 8.2 Kaplan–Meier survival curves for progression-free (a) and overall (b) survival times based on the presence or absence of intraepithelial T cells (IET) for 174 evaluable patients with stage III and IV epithelial ovarian cancer.

T cells experienced 9.8-fold longer median progression-free survival compared with patients whose tumors lacked intraepithelial T cells. The 5-year overall survival rate was 73.9% in the 43 patients whose tumors had intraepithelial T cells, while it was 11.9% in the 31 patients whose tumors had no such cells. The progression-free survival rate at 4 years was 61.4% in patients whose tumors exhibited intraepithelial T cells and 14.8% in those whose tumors lacked such cells. Among patients with a complete response, significant differences in progression-free and overall survival distributions were seen in both suboptimally and optimally debulked patients, based on the presence or absence of intraepithelial T cells ($p < 0.001$ for all). Among patients with a complete response to therapy following suboptimal debulking, the 5-year overall survival was 52.8% in the 14 patients whose tumors exhibited intraepithelial T cells and 6.5% in the 22 patients whose tumors lacked such cells. Only 29% of tumors lacking intraepithelial T cells were optimally debulked, while 67.4% of tumors having intraepithelial T cells were optimally debulked ($p = 0.001$).[26]

Among 174 evaluable patients, 159 had at least 3 years' observation time. The absence of intraepithelial T cells ($n = 66$) predicted 1.5% and 7.6% chances of progression-free and overall survival, respectively, at 3 years. Among 74 patients with a complete response, 61 had at least 3 years' of observation time. The absence of intraepithelial T cells ($n = 26$) predicted 3.9% and 19.2% chances of progression-free and overall survival, respectively, at 3 years.[26]

No association was found between intraepithelial T cells and age, histotype, or tumor grade. Univariate analysis revealed that T cells ($p < 0.0001$) and residual tumor ($p < 0.001$), but not grade ($p = 0.06$ for 1 vs 3; $p = 0.30$ for 2 vs 3), tumor histology ($p = 0.41$), inclusion of paclitaxel in chemotherapy ($p = 0.74$), or age (<55 years vs ≥ 55 years; $p = 0.25$), correlated with overall survival. The results were similar for progression free survival with the exception of grade ($p = 0.047$ for 1 vs 3; $p = 0.76$ for 2 vs 3). Intraepithelial T cells and residual tumor, but not age, tumor grade, or type of front-line chemotherapy, were independent prognosticators of progression-free survival and overall survival by multivariate analysis. Tumor histotype predicted overall but not progression-free survival.[26]

An important aspect revealed by our data is that an improved clinical outcome depends on the infiltration of tumor islets by T cells, rather than the mere presence of T cells in ovarian carcinoma specimens. Indirect evidence of T-cell activation selectively in tumors with intraepithelial T cells was provided by measurement of the mRNA levels of two cytokines associated with T-cell activation. IFN-γ and interleukin-2 (IL-2) mRNA levels were 10 ($p = 0.019$) and 26-fold ($p = 0.091$) higher in tumors with intraepithelial T cells compared with tumors lacking intraepithelial T cells, and were undetectable in 7 of 10 (70%) and 9 of 10 (90%), respectively, tumors lacking intraepithelial T cells.

Our findings were confirmed by other groups. In a study conducted on patients undergoing debulking surgery at Roswell Park Cancer Institute, patients with higher frequencies of intraepithelial CD8+ T cells demonstrated improved survival compared with patients with lower CD8+ T-cell frequencies (median survival 55 months vs 26 months; hazard ratio 0.33; $p = 0.0003$).[27] Thus, recruitment and spontaneous activation of T effector cells portends improved clinical outcome in advanced epithelial ovarian carcinoma.

REGULATORY T CELLS

A critical mechanism of peripheral immune tolerance is mediated by CD4+CD25+ regulatory

T cells (Treg), a T-cell subset endowed with powerful suppressor activity. Treg prevent specific T-cell immunity by suppressing CD8$^+$ T-cell activation and secretion of IL-2 and IFN-γ. Treg inhibit specific cytotoxicity in a contact-dependent fashion and/or through contact-independent, paracrine mechanisms.[28–30] Treg also affect the function of other immunosuppressive populations such as tolerogenic antigen-presenting cells (APC).

The first evidence of the contribution of Treg to immune dysfunction in cancer in the human was provided in patients with ovarian cancer and lung tumors by June's group[31] who identified an increased frequency of transforming growth factor β (TGF-β)-secreting CD4$^+$ CD25$^+$ Treg with potent immunosuppressive functions in tumor, ascites, and peripheral blood.[31] Tumor-derived CD4$^+$CD25$^+$ cells were shown to suppress efficiently the activation of effector cells in response to cognate antigen.[32] Ovarian cancer has been also the tumor model in which Treg were demonstrated to play an important immunopathogenetic role in the human in a study by Zou, Curiel and co-workers.[33] Tumor-infiltrating CD4$^+$CD25$^+$ T cells represented approximately 25% of tumor-infiltrating CD4$^+$ T cells, and the percentage of CD4$^+$CD25$^+$CD3$^+$ T cells in CD4$^+$CD3$^+$ T cells was higher in later disease stages (stage II–IV) than in early disease stages (stage I). In addition, approximately 75% of CD4$^+$CD25$^+$ CD3$^+$ T cells in the tumor mass were in proximity to infiltrating CD8$^+$ T cells, suggesting that physical contact between CD4$^+$CD25$^+$ T cells and CD8$^+$ cytotoxic T cells mediates regulatory functions.[33]

Treg isolated from tumor ascites shared the phenotype of blood CD4$^+$CD25$^+$ T cells. They expressed similar levels of membrane and intracellular glucocorticoid-induced tumor necrosis factor (TNF) receptor family-related gene (*GITR*) and cytolytic T-lymphocyte-associated antigen 4 (CTLA-4) as blood CD4$^+$CD25$^+$ T cells. Furthermore, CD4$^+$ CD25$^+$ T cells isolated from malignant ascites, solid tumor, and blood from individuals with epithelial ovarian carcinoma expressed the transcription factor forkhead box P3 (FoxP3), which is crucial for the differentiation and function of CD4$^+$CD25$^+$ Treg in the mouse. Treg infiltration in human ovarian cancer was shown by that study to defeat tumor antigen-specific immunity and promote tumor growth in a mouse xenograft model of ovarian cancer.

FoxP3 immunostaining reveals Treg in tissues (Figure 8.3). An increased frequency of FoxP3$^+$CD4$^+$CD25$^+$ Treg (assessed by immunohistochemistry) predicted poor patient survival in the patient group as a whole ($n = 70$; $p < 0.0001$ for all), and also for individuals in stage II ($p = 0.0362$), stage III ($p = 0.0003$), and stage IV ($p = 0.0001$). Tumor Treg were a significant predictor of death hazard ($p < 0.0001$) in a Cox proportional hazards model.[33] When stage III and IV individuals were stratified into three subgroups of low (<131 cells per high-power field (hpf)), medium (132–345/hpf), and high (>346/hpf) tumor Treg numbers, survival functions were still significantly different for the three groups in stage III ($p < 0.0003$) and stage IV ($p < 0.0001$).[33]

These findings have been confirmed by other groups. Quantification of FoxP3 mRNA was found to correlate with the frequency of Treg by immunohistochemistry in epithelial ovarian cancer patients from Innsbruck, Austria. Increased FoxP3 mRNA expression (>81th percentile) identified a patient subgroup characterized by significantly worse prognosis in terms of overall survival (27.8 months vs 77.3 months; $p = 0.0034$) and progression-free survival (18 months vs 57.5 months; $p = 0.0041$).[34]

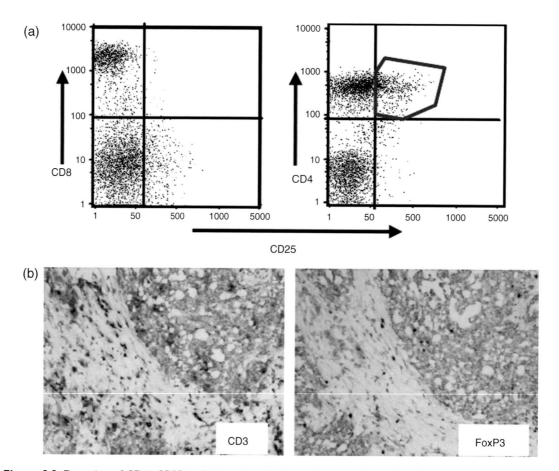

Figure 8.3 Detection of CD4$^+$ CD25$^+$ cells in ascites of a chemotherapy-naive patient with stage III ovarian cancer by flow cytometry. Note that about 20% of CD4$^+$ cells are CD25$^+$ (blue area). This coincides with suppressed phenotype of CD8$^+$ cells, less than 2% of which are CD25$^+$ (activated CTL). The gate is on CD3$^+$ cells. (b) CD3 and FoxP3 immunohistochemistry identifies total CD3$^+$ and FoxP3$^+$ (regulatory) T cells infiltrating this tumor. Note that FoxP3$^+$ T cells infiltrate both stroma and islets.

High FoxP3 expression represented an independent prognostic factor for overall survival ($p = 0.004$) and progression-free survival ($p = 0.004$). Furthermore, in a parallel study conducted on patients undergoing debulking surgery at Roswell Park Cancer Institute, a high CD8$^+$/Treg cell ratio (FoxP3$^+$ CD25$^+$) was a strong positive prognosticator. The median survival for patients with high CD8$^+$/Treg ratios was 58 months, whereas patients with low ratios had a median survival of 23 months (hazard ratio 0.31; $p = 0.0002$).[27]

B CELLS

B cells and humoral immunity are involved in antitumor immune response. Although the spontaneous induction of autoantibodies against specific tumor antigens may be ineffective in controlling tumor growth or may even promote tumor progression,[35] tumor-specific antibodies might provide sensitive biomarkers that are readily accessible in serum. It has been shown that HER2/*neu* overexpression in the primary tumor is associated with production of

HER2-specific antibodies, and that there is a strong correlation between accumulation of p53 in primary tumor cells and the presence of serum p53-specific antibodies in patients with different cancers.[36,37] In addition, there is evidence that antigen-specific antibody immunity is positively associated with antigen-specific T-cell responses, suggesting that the immunoglobulin G (IgG) immunity might develop together with T-cell immunity against the same tumor antigens.[38] If that were true, one would expect that antibody response against known tumor antigens might predict survival. Disis and co-workers[39] have recently proved just this notion: multivariate analysis showed the presence of p53 autoantibodies to be an independent variable for prediction of overall survival in patients with advanced-stage epithelial ovarian cancer. Overall survival was significantly higher for patients with antibodies to p53 compared with patients without p53 antibodies ($p = 0.01$). The median survival for p53 antibody-positive patients was 51 months (95% confidence interval (CI) 23.5–60.5 months), compared with 24 months (95% CI 19.4–28.6 months) for patients without antibodies to p53. However, previous studies failed to demonstrate a similar relationship.[40,41] Anti-p53 autoantibodies were more frequently present in patients with p53-overexpressing tumors or with moderately or poorly differentiated tumors. In univariate or bivariate analysis, p53 antibody-positive patients were at an increased risk for relapse, but not death. In multivariate analysis, the differences in disease-free and overall survival between patients who were p53 antibody-positive or -negative were not statistically significant.[40,41] Interestingly, in the former study by Disis and co-workers, there was no survival benefit related to humoral immunity to other oncogenic proteins evaluated, including HER2/ *neu* and topoisomerase IIa.

According to another study, high levels of antibodies against epithelial mucin (MUC1) were correlated with a decreased risk for ovarian cancer. These antibodies target MUC1 expressed on the surface of several types of polarized epithelial cells. Factors predicting antibodies included previous use of oral contraceptive use, history of breast mastitis, bone fracture, or osteoporosis, pelvic surgery, non-use of talc in genital hygiene, and (to a lesser extent) intrauterine device use and current smoking. There was a significantly higher incidence of anti-MUC1 antibodies in women with five or more conditions (51.4%) than in women with no or one condition (24.2%). The risk of ovarian cancer was inversely associated with number of conditions predisposing to anti-MUC1 antibodies ($p < 0.0001$).[42]

DENDRITIC CELLS

Dendritic cells (DC) are viewed as critical regulators of adaptive immune response against tumors. DC take up, process, and present antigens to naive T cells in major histocompatibility complex (MHC) class I- and/or class II-restricted fashion.[43] They are now recognized as a diverse population of cells with remarkable plasticity, exhibiting diverse phenotypes that can elicit potent type 1 T-cell stimulation, promoting type 2 responses, or inducing T-cell tolerance, with these properties, depending on lineage and level of maturation.[43–45] Both in humans and in mice, at least two DC subsets with distinct phenotypic markers and functional properties have been described: myeloid and plasmacytoid DC.

To trigger effective immune responses, DC should be recruited into solid tumors, phagocyte tumor antigen, undergo maturation, and consequently migrate to lymphoid organs, where they present antigen to lymphocytes.

Mature myeloid DC induce a potent immune response against presented antigens, and their presence has been associated with improved clinical outcome in a number of tumors. A correlative study conducted on a small number of patients suggested that a high frequency of tumor-infiltrating HLA-DR[+]CD1a[+] Langhans-type myeloid DC predict significantly better survival in ovarian cancer.[46] Most DC detected in tumors have an immature phenotype. CD83 is a marker of myeloid DC maturation. We have quantified CD83[+] cells in tumor specimens of stage III epithelial ovarian carcinoma by immunostaining. A significantly increased frequency of CD83[+] cells was seen in tumors with intraepithelial T cells and longer survival (Figure 8.4).

Plasmacytoid DC may alter suppress antitumor immunity in the steady state. Zou et al[47] identified plasmacytoid DC in ovarian cancer and showed that they are recruited to tumors by the stromal-derived factor 1 (CXCL-12) chemokine. The significance of plasmacytoid DC as biomarkers is unknown.[47]

We have identified in ovarian cancer a novel DC phenotype, called vascular leukocytes, expressing DC and endothelial markers.[48,49] These endothelial-like DC engage in vasculogenesis and function as co-conspirators of tumor progression in the mouse. We have confirmed the existence of the same population of leukocytes coexpressing endothelial and DC markers in human ovarian carcinoma, where these cells were detected at relatively high frequency in many specimens analyzed. The significance of vascular leukocytes as biomarkers remains unknown.

CYTOKINES

Cytokines are important regulators of immune development and function. Critical cytokines

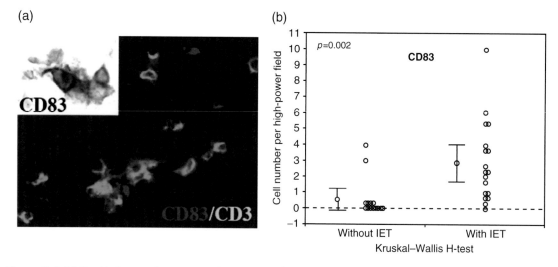

Figure 8.4 (a) Double immunofluorescence demonstrates clustering of CD3[+] T cells (green) around a CD83[+] cell (red). The insert shows immunohistochemical detection of a CD83[+] cell with morphologic features of a dendritic cell, surrounded by small mononuclear cells with scant cytoplasm compatible with lymphocytes. (b) Quantification by image analysis of CD83[+] detected by immunohistochemistry in tumors with or without intraepithelial T cells (IET). A significantly higher number of CD83[+] cells are noted in tumors harboring intraepithelial T cells compared with tumors lacking intraepithelial T cells.

produced by T helper (Th)1 cells are IFN-γ, IL-2, IL-12, and IL-18, while IL-4, IL-5, and IL-6 are associated with Th2 cells, and IL-10 with Th3 regulatory T cells. Th1 cells trigger cellular immunity to combat intracellular pathogens such as viruses, allotransplants, and tumor cells, while Th2 cells drive humoral immunity and upregulate antibody production to fight extracellular organisms. Since either pathway can downregulate the other, Th1 responses would be responsible for protective anticancer immunity, whereas Th2 responses would drive nonprotective responses. The Th1/Th2 hypothesis is a model of cellular interactions still used to understand anticancer immune response, although this model is too simplistic in human tumors, because cytokines are seldom restricted to pure Th1 or Th2 patterns and because humoral immunity may in fact cooperate with cellular immunity in coordinated immunity programs to successfully reject tumors.[50]

Tumor immune rejection and protection of the host against the growth of transplanted tumors or the formation of spontaneous or induced tumors requires release of IFN-γ in mice.[51] We have found 10-fold higher IFN-γ mRNA levels in tumors with intraepithelial T cells compared with tumors lacking such cells ($p = 0.019$). IFN-γ was, in fact, undetectable in 70% of tumors lacking intraepithelial T cells.[26] In a study from Hiroshima University,[52] IFN-γ and TNF-α mRNA expression levels were significantly higher in serous adenocarcinomas than in nonserous adenocarcinomas ($p < 0.05$), but with no difference between individual cytokine mRNA expression levels and clinical stage or histologic grade. In examining all combinations of Th1/Th2 expression cytokines, the most significant association was between high IFN-γ and IL-12p40/IL-6 expression levels and better prognosis in advanced-stage (II/III/IV) ovarian carcinomas ($p = 0.004$). In multivariate analysis, high IFN-γ × IL-12p40/IL-6 expression ($p = 0.009$) and debulking ($p = 0.011$) were significantly associated with survival.[52] Similarly, a study from Innsbruck[53] showed that patients with tumors with high levels of IFN-γ expression had significantly longer progression-free and overall survival. The median times to progression were 10 and 29 months for patients with low and high IFN-γ, respectively ($p = 0.039$). The corresponding survival times were 29 and 44 months ($p < 0.032$). Application of multivariate Cox regression analysis showed IFN-γ expression to be an independent prognostic factor for progression-free and overall survival.[53] Surprisingly, a later study by the same group reported a highly significant positive correlation between FoxP3 and IFN-γ mRNA expression ($r = 0.424$, $p < 0.001$) as well as IRF-1 ($r = 0.237$, $p < 0.018$), a central regulator of the IFN-γ pathway.[34]

Serum levels of cytokines may reflect intratumoral events. Serum IL-18 levels were significantly elevated in ovarian cancer patients (mean 229.6 pg/ml) relative to normal controls (151.3 pg/ml; $p < 0.01$). Univariate analysis showed that overall survival was affected by IL-18 serum levels, but multivariate analysis failed to demonstrate an independent prognostic significance for IL-18 serum levels.[54]

CHEMOKINES

Immune cell trafficking during the development of the lymphoid organs, immune surveillance, and the organization of inflammatory exudates are governed by chemokines, a family of more than 50 low-molecular-weight cytokine molecules, which bind to one or more of the approximately 20 Gi-protein-coupled cognate receptors identified to date.[55–58] Chemokines direct leukocytes into tissue by providing a combinatorial system of addressing signals. Emerging evidence indicates that effector cell trafficking mechanisms play a critical role in regulating immune response to tumors. Chemokines cooperate with other cytokines to establish polarity in the tumor microenvironment, and by doing so may directly contribute to tumor progression or rejection. Animal tumor models suggest that IFN-inducible chemokines play an important role in orchestrating antitumor immune response by recruiting type 1 effector cells. CXCL9/MIG (monokine induced by IFN-γ) and CXCL10/IP-10 (IFNγ-inducible protein 10), two CXCR3-ligand chemokines induced by IFN-γ attracting primarily CXCR3[+]-activated T cells,[59,60] were identified as the dominant downstream mediators of tumor regression induced by IL-12,[61] and can induce T-cell-mediated tumor rejection,[62,63] while intratumoral injection of recombinant 6Ckine/exodus-2/SLC, which in the mouse is also a CXCR3 ligand, led to accumulation of DC and CD4[+] and CD8[+] cells, increased expression of CXCL9/MIG and CXCL10/IP-10, and T-cell-mediated tumor eradication.[64]

We have previously reported on chemokine correlation with intraepithelial T cells and outcome in 26 patients with complete response to chemotherapy.[26] These included patients with progression-free survival <6 months and no intraepithelial T cells ($n=10$), progression-free survival <6 months and intraepithelial T cells present ($n=6$), or progression-free survival >30 months and intraepithelial T cells present ($n=10$). The mean observation times in the above groups were 20.8, 28.6, and 83.6 months, respectively. In the 16 tumors with intraepithelial T cells, the mean level of CXCL9/MIG mRNA was 50 times higher than that in the 10 tumors lacking intraepithelial T cells ($p = 0.049$). Strong expression of CXCL9/MIG protein was confirmed in

tumors with intraepithelial T cells by immunohistochemistry. CCL21/SLC (secondary lymphoid organ chemokine/exodus-2/6Ckine/ TCA4) and CCL22/MDC (macrophage-derived chemokine) attract naive or memory/non-effector T cells.[65,66] Tumors with intraepithelial T cells displayed 43-fold higher CCL21/SLC ($p=0.050$) and 14-fold higher CCL22/MDC ($p=0.034$) mRNA levels, compared with tumors lacking intraepithelial T cells. Neither chemokine mRNA was detectable in 5 of 10 tumors lacking intraepithelial T cells. Expression of CCL21/SLC and CCL22/MDC protein in tumor islets of tumors with intraepithelial T cells was confirmed by immunohistochemistry.[26] Logistic regression analysis and associated receiver operating curve showed that CCL22/MDC was strongly associated with late recurrence (>40 months; odds ratio 1.568; area under the curve 0.732; $p=0.082$). On the other hand, CCL22/MDC has also been shown to recruit Treg to tumors.[33] Thus, further analysis is required to define the prognostic value of these chemokines.

TUMOR CELL IMMUNOREGULATORY MOLECULES (HLA AND NKG2D LIGANDS)

Target cell recognition by effector cytotoxic CD8[+] T cells requires expression of functional MHC class I. Therefore, downregulation or genetic loss of MHC class I molecules is a common mechanism of tumor immune evasion during tumor progression or metastasis, as recently shown in HER2-positive ovarian cancer.[67] Freedman and co-workers[17] first reported the correlation between HLA class I expression by ovarian cancer cells and the frequency of tumor-infiltrating CD3[+], CD4[+], and CD8[+] T cells.[17] In a recent study,[68] HLA class I antigen downregulation was associated with increased disease stage: the odds ratio of stage III for HLA class I antigen-negative patients was 7.6 (95% CI 1.9–30.5; $p = 0.007$). However, multivariate analysis showed that HLA class I expression did not associate with survival. The likely explanation for this lack of correlation is that multiple overlapping mechanisms may account for tumor recognition, and HLA expression is not sufficient to predict activation of immune rejection mechanisms. The significance of tumor–effector molecular interactions are revealed by a recent study[69] showing that the HLA*0201 allele is a negative factor for survival in women with stage III–IV serous adenocarcinomas of the ovary. Among 88 patients evaluated, 44% had serous adenocarcinomas, and among them 73% were HLA-A2-positive. None of the HLA-A2-positive patients survived 5 years, compared with >50% of the HLA-A2-negative patients, with a multivariate hazard ratio of 6.8 by Cox analysis (95% CI 2.10–22.4; $p = 0.001$).[70]

Interestingly, a recent study examined the distribution of the HLA-DRB1*, -DQA1*, and -DQB1* class II alleles in 47 patients with epithelial ovarian carcinoma and 67 healthy Caucasian women. The prevalence of D^{70} and E^{71} polymorphic residues of the DRB1 alleles was significantly reduced in the cancer patients versus controls ($p = 0.009$), while the $Y^{11}R^{55}$ and R^{52} residues of DQα were increased in the cancer patients ($p = 0.008$ and 0.012, respectively). Furthermore, a relationship was identified between the protection and susceptibility alleles, indicating the dominant effect of susceptibility elements when in coexistence with the protection allele.

Effector cell function is positively regulated in peripheral tissues by the expression of ligands for the NKG2D immunoreceptor. In humans, the ligands for NKG2D fall into either the MIC group or the ULBP group.

We reported the discovery of a new MHC class I-related ligand for the NKG2D receptor that we named Letal, for lymphocyte effector cell toxicity activation ligand.[71,72] We found that Letal was upregulated in advanced ovarian carcinomas with intraepithelial T cells. These results suggest an important role for Letal in the homeostasis of peripheral CD8[+] effector T cells and the immune defense against tumors in the human. Thus, although Letal expression increases in advanced-stage ovarian carcinoma, the 5-year overall survival rate was 52% among patients whose tumors expressed Letal, but only 21% among patients whose tumors were Letal-negative. In multivariate analysis, the combination of Letal expression, optimal debulking, and the presence of intraepithelial T cells was found to be an independent prognosticator of prolonged overall survival in stage III ovarian cancer, indicating that Letal plays a protective role in ovarian carcinoma.[72]

CONCLUDING REMARKS

Investigation of tumor–host interactions has enhanced our understanding of immune mechanisms underlying tumor progression and outcome. This investigation promises to yield important therapeutic approaches. At the same time, it is evident that immunologic investigation has already produced important biomarkers. The clinical relevance of these biomarkers is not yet clear, but potential applications include disease prognosis and perhaps classification for selection of therapy. Additional work needs to be undertaken by cooperative groups to validate the predictive value of these biomarkers with respect to outcome in the context of phase III trials. An important direction of the near future will be to test the usefulness of these biomarkers in the selection of patients for biologic therapies, including vaccines, adoptive lymphocyte therapy, and therapy neutralizing Treg cells. It is possible that these therapies, similar to any other cancer therapy, will be useful only in a subset of patients. As clinical testing is designed to test biologic and immune therapeutics, it will be important to take advantage of the biomarkers already identified to define the populations of patients who may benefit from one or other form of therapy.

REFERENCES

1. Dunn GP, Old LJ, Schreiber RD. The immunobiology of cancer immunosurveillance and immunoediting. Immunity 2004; 21:137–48.

2. Dudley ME, Wunderlich JR, Robbins PF, et al. Cancer regression and autoimmunity in patients after clonal repopulation with anti-tumor lymphocytes. Science 2002;298:850–4.

3. Zhou J, Dudley ME, Rosenberg SA, Robbins PF. Persistence of multiple tumor-specific T-cell clones is associated with complete tumor regression in a melanoma patient receiving adoptive cell transfer therapy. J Immunother 2005;28:53–62.

4. Robbins PF, Dudley ME, Wunderlich J, et al. Cutting edge: Persistence of transferred lymphocyte clonotypes correlates with cancer regression in patients receiving cell transfer therapy. J Immunol 2004;173:7125–30.

5. Albert ML, Darnell JC, Bender A, et al. Tumor-specific killer cells in paraneoplastic cerebellar degeneration. Nat Med 1998;4: 1321–4.

6. Coukos G, Conejo-Garcia JR, Roden RB, Wu TC. Immunotherapy for gynaecological malignancies. Expert Opin Biol Ther 2005; 5:1193–210.

7. Gordan JD, Vonderheide RH. Universal tumor antigens as targets for immunotherapy. Cytotherapy 2002;4:317–27.

8. Vonderheide RH, Hahn WC, Schultze JL, Nadler LM. The telomerase catalytic subunit is a widely expressed tumor-associated antigen recognized by cytotoxic T lymphocytes. Immunity 1999;10:673–9.

9. Counter CM, Hirte HW, Bacchetti S, Harley CB. Telomerase activity in human ovarian carcinoma. Proc Natl Acad Sci USA 1994; 91:2900–4.

10. Schlienger K, Chu CS, Woo EY, et al. TRANCE- anti CD40 ligand-matured dendritic cells reveal MHC class I-restricted T cells specific for autologous tumor in late-stage ovarian cancer patients. Clin Cancer Res 2003;9:1517–27.

11. Santin AD, Hermonat PL, Ravaggi A, et al. Phenotypic and functional analysis of tumor-infiltrating lymphocytes compared with tumor-associated lymphocytes from ascitic fluid and peripheral blood lymphocytes in patients with advanced ovarian cancer. Gynecol Obstet Invest 2001;51:254–61.

12. Negus RP, Stamp GW, Hadley J, Balkwill FR. Quantitative assessment of the leukocyte infiltrate in ovarian cancer and its relationship to the expression of C-C chemokines. Am J Pathol 1997;150:1723–34.

13. Schondorf T, Engel H, Kurbacher CM, et al. Immunologic features of tumor-infiltrating lymphocytes and peripheral blood lymphocytes in ovarian cancer patients. J Soc Gynecol Invest 1998;5:102–7.

14. Halapi E, Yamamoto Y, Juhlin C, et al. Restricted T cell receptor V-beta and J-beta usage in T cells from interleukin-2-cultured lymphocytes of ovarian and renal carcinomas. Cancer Immunol Immunother 1993;36:191–7.

15. Hayashi K, Yonamine K, Masuko-Hongo K, et al. Clonal expansion of T cells that are specific for autologous ovarian tumor among

tumor-infiltrating T cells in humans. Gynecol Oncol 1999;74:86–92.

16. Kooi S, Freedman RS, Rodriguez-Villanueva J, Platsoucas CD. Cytokine production by T-cell lines derived from tumor-infiltrating lymphocytes from patients with ovarian carcinoma: tumor-specific immune responses and inhibition of antigen-independent cytokine production by ovarian tumor cells. Lymphokine Cytokine Res 1993;12:429–37.

17. Kooi S, Zhang HZ, Patenia R, et al. HLA class I expression on human ovarian carcinoma cells correlates with T-cell infiltration in vivo and T-cell expansion in vitro in low concentrations of recombinant interleukin-2. Cell Immunol 1996;174:116–28.

18. Fisk B, Blevins TL, Wharton JT, Ioannides CG. Identification of an immunodominant peptide of HER-2/*neu* protooncogene recognized by ovarian tumor-specific cytotoxic T lymphocyte lines. J Exp Med 1995;181:2109–17.

19. Dadmarz RD, Ordoubadi A, Mixon A, et al. Tumor-infiltrating lymphocytes from human ovarian cancer patients recognize autologous tumor in an MHC class II-restricted fashion. Cancer J Sci Am 1996;2:263.

20. Peoples GE, Anderson BW, Fisk B, et al. Ovarian cancer-associated lymphocyte recognition of folate binding protein peptides. Ann Surg Oncol 1998;5:743–50.

21. Peoples GE, Goedegebuure PS, Smith R, et al. Breast and ovarian cancer-specific cytotoxic T lymphocytes recognize the same HER2/*neu*-derived peptide. Proc Natl Acad Sci USA 1995;92:432–6.

22. Peoples GE, Schoof DD, Andrews JV, Goedegebuure PS, Eberlein TJ. T-cell recognition of ovarian cancer. Surgery 1993;114:227–34.

23. Santin AD, Bellone S, Ravaggi A, et al. Induction of ovarian tumor-specific CD8+ cytotoxic T lymphocytes by acid-eluted peptide-pulsed autologous dendritic cells. Obstet Gynecol 2000;96:422–30.

24. Luiten RM, Warnaar SO, Sanborn D, et al. Chimeric bispecific OC/TR monoclonal antibody mediates lysis of tumor cells expressing the folate-binding protein (MOv18) and displays decreased immunogenicity in patients. J Immunother 1997;20:496–504.

25. Bouet-Toussaint F, Genetel N, Rioux-Leclercq N, et al. Interleukin-2 expanded lymphocytes from lymph node and tumor biopsies of human renal cell carcinoma, breast and ovarian cancer. Eur Cytokine Netw 2000;11:217–24.

26. Zhang L, Conejo-Garcia JR, Katsaros D, et al. Intratumoral T cells, recurrence, and survival in epithelial ovarian cancer. N Engl J Med 2003;348:203–13.

27. Sato E, Olson SH, Ahn J, et al. Intraepithelial CD8+ tumor-infiltrating lymphocytes and a high CD8+/regulatory T cell ratio are associated with favorable prognosis in ovarian cancer. Proc Natl Acad Sci USA 2005; 102:18538–43.

28. Bluestone JA, Abbas AK. Natural versus adaptive regulatory T cells. Nat Rev Immunol 2003;3:253–7.

29. Sakaguchi S. Naturally arising CD4+ regulatory T cells for immunologic self-tolerance and negative control of immune responses. Annu Rev Immunol 2004;22:531–62.

30. Read S, Powrie F. CD4+ regulatory T cells. Curr Opin Immunol 2001;13:644–9.

31. Woo EY, Chu CS, Goletz TJ, et al. Regulatory CD4+ CD25+ T cells in tumors from patients with early-stage non-small cell lung cancer and late-stage ovarian cancer. Cancer Res 2001;61:4766–72.

32. Woo EY, Yeh H, Chu CS, et al. Cutting edge: Regulatory T cells from lung cancer patients directly inhibit autologous T cell proliferation. J Immunol 2002;168:4272–6.

33. Curiel TJ, Coukos G, Zou L, et al. Specific recruitment of regulatory T cells in ovarian carcinoma fosters immune privilege and

predicts reduced survival. Nat Med 2004; 10:942–9.

34. Wolf D, Wolf AM, Rumpold H, et al. The expression of the regulatory T cell-specific forkhead box transcription factor FoxP3 is associated with poor prognosis in ovarian cancer. Clin Cancer Res 2005;11:8326–31.

35. de Visser KE, Korets LV, Coussens LM. De novo carcinogenesis promoted by chronic inflammation is B lymphocyte dependent. Cancer Cell 2005;7:411–23.

36. Broll R, Duchrow M, Oevermann E, et al. p53 autoantibodies in sera of patients with a colorectal cancer and their association to p53 protein concentration and p53 immunohisto-chemistry in tumor tissue. Int J Colorectal Dis 2001;16:22–7.

37. Disis ML, Pupa SM, Gralow JR, et al. High-titer HER-2/*neu* protein-specific antibody can be detected in patients with early-stage breast cancer. J Clin Oncol 1997;15:3363–7.

38. Gnjatic S, Atanackovic D, Jager E, et al. Survey of naturally occurring CD4$^+$ T cell responses against NY-ESO-1 in cancer patients: correlation with antibody responses. Proc Natl Acad Sci USA 2003;100:8862–7.

39. Goodell V, Salazar LG, Urban N, et al. Antibody immunity to the p53 oncogenic protein is a prognostic indicator in ovarian cancer. J Clin Oncol 2006;24:762–8.

40. Vogl FD, Stickeler E, Weyermann M, et al. p53 autoantibodies in patients with primary ovarian cancer are associated with higher age, advanced stage and a higher proportion of p53-positive tumor cells. Oncology 1999; 57:324–9.

41. Angelopoulou K, Rosen B, Stratis M, et al. Circulating antibodies against p53 protein in patients with ovarian carcinoma. Correlation with clinicopathologic features and survival. Cancer 1996;78:2146–52.

42. Cramer DW, Titus-Ernstoff L, McKolanis JR, et al. Conditions associated with antibodies against the tumor-associated antigen MUC1

and their relationship to risk for ovarian cancer. Cancer Epidemiol Biomarkers Prev 2005;14:1125–31.

43. Banchereau J, Briere F, Caux C, et al. Immunobiology of dendritic cells. Annu Rev Immunol 2000;18:767–811.

44. Bhardwaj N. Processing and presentation of antigens by dendritic cells: implications for vaccines. Trends Mol Med 2001;7:388–94.

45. Steinman RM, Turley S, Mellman I, Inaba K. The induction of tolerance by dendritic cells that have captured apoptotic cells. J Exp Med 2000;191:411–16.

46. Eisenthal A, Polyvkin N, Bramante-Schreiber L, et al. Expression of dendritic cells in ovarian tumors correlates with clinical outcome in patients with ovarian cancer. Hum Pathol 2001;32:803–7.

47. Zou W, Machelon V, Coulomb-L'Hermin A, et al. Stromal-derived factor-1 in human tumors recruits and alters the function of plasmacytoid precursor dendritic cells. Nat Med 2001;7:1339–46.

48. Conejo-Garcia JR, Benencia F, Courreges MC, et al. Tumor-infiltrating dendritic cell precursors recruited by a β-defensin contribute to vasculogenesis under the influence of Vegf-A. Nat Med 2004;10:950–8.

49. Conejo-Garcia JR, Buckanovich RJ, Benencia F, et al. Vascular leukocytes contribute to tumor vascularization. Blood 2005; 105:679–81.

50. Kidd P. Th1/Th2 balance: the hypothesis, its limitations, and implications for health and disease. Altern Med Rev 2003;8:223–46.

51. Street SE, Trapani JA, MacGregor D, Smyth MJ. Suppression of lymphoma and epithelial malignancies effected by interferon gamma. J Exp Med 2002;196:129–34.

52. Kusuda T, Shigemasa K, Arihiro K, et al. Relative expression levels of Th1 and Th2 cytokine mRNA are independent prognostic factors in patients with ovarian cancer. Oncol Rep 2005;13:1153–8.

53. Marth C, Fiegl H, Zeimet AG, et al. Interferon-γ expression is an independent prognostic factor in ovarian cancer. Am J Obstet Gynecol 2004;191:1598–605.

54. Akahiro J, Konno R, Ito K, Okamura K, Yaegashi N. Impact of serum interleukin-18 level as a prognostic indicator in patients with epithelial ovarian carcinoma. Int J Clin Oncol 2004;9:42–6.

55. Butcher EC, Williams M, Youngman K, Rott L, Briskin M. Lymphocyte trafficking and regional immunity. Adv Immunol 1999;72:209–53.

56. Rossi D, Zlotnik A. The biology of chemokines and their receptors. Annu Rev Immunol 2000;18:217–42.

57. Sallusto F, Mackay CR, Lanzavecchia A. The role of chemokine receptors in primary, effector, and memory immune responses. Annu Rev Immunol 2000;18:593–620.

58. Campbell JJ, Butcher EC. Chemokines in tissue-specific and microenvironment-specific lymphocyte homing. Curr Opin Immunol 2000;12:336–41.

59. Loetscher M, Gerber B, Loetscher P, et al. Chemokine receptor specific for IP10 and mig: structure, function, and expression in activated T-lymphocytes. J Exp Med 1996; 184:963–9.

60. Sallusto F, Kremmer E, Palermo B, et al. Switch in chemokine receptor expression upon TCR stimulation reveals novel homing potential for recently activated T cells. Eur J Immunol 1999;29:2037–45.

61. Tannenbaum CS, Tubbs R, Armstrong D, et al. The CXC chemokines IP-10 and Mig are necessary for IL-12-mediated regression of the mouse RENCA tumor. J Immunol 1998; 161:927–32.

62. Luster AD, Leder P. IP-10, a -C-X-C- chemokine, elicits a potent thymus-dependent antitumor response in vivo. J Exp Med 1993; 178:1057–65.

63. Addison CL, Arenberg DA, Morris SB, et al. The CXC chemokine, monokine induced by interferon-γ, inhibits non-small cell lung carcinoma tumor growth and metastasis. Hum Gene Ther 2000;11:247–61.

64. Sharma S, Stolina M, Luo J, et al. Secondary lymphoid tissue chemokine mediates T cell-dependent antitumor responses in vivo. J Immunol 2000;164:4558–63.

65. Cyster JG. Chemokines and cell migration in secondary lymphoid organs. Science 1999; 286:2098–102.

66. Tang HL, Cyster JG. Chemokine up-regulation and activated T cell attraction by maturing dendritic cells. Science 1999;284:819–22.

67. Norell H, Carlsten M, Ohlum T, et al. Frequent loss of HLA-A2 expression in metastasizing ovarian carcinomas associated with genomic haplotype loss and HLA-A2-restricted HER-2/*neu*-specific immunity. Cancer Res 2006;66:6387–94.

68. Vitale M, Pelusi G, Taroni B, et al. HLA class I antigen down-regulation in primary ovary carcinoma lesions: association with disease stage. Clin Cancer Res 2005;11: 67–72.

69. Gamzatova Z, Villabona L, Dahlgren L, et al. Human leucocyte antigen (HLA) A2 as a negative clinical prognostic factor in patients with advanced ovarian cancer. Gynecol Oncol 2006;103:145–50.

70. Monos DS, Pappas J, Magira EE, et al. Identification of HLA-DQα and -DRβ residues associated with susceptibility and protection to epithelial ovarian cancer. Hum Immunol 2005;66:554–62.

71. Conejo-Garcia JR, Benencia F, Courreges C, et al. Letal, a tumor-associated NKG2D immunoreceptor ligand, induces activation and expansion of effector immune cells. Cancer Biol Ther 2003;2:446–451.

72. Conejo-Garcia JR, Benencia F, Courreges MC, et al. Ovarian carcinoma expresses the NKG2D ligand Letal and promotes the survival and expansion of CD28⁻ antitumor T cells. Cancer Res 2004;64:2175–82.

Predictive factors in germ cell and stromal tumors

9

Jubilee Brown

GERM CELL TUMORS

Clinical and pathologic features

Ovarian cancer is the most frequent cause of death from gynecologic cancer among women in the USA, accounting for an estimated 22 430 new cases and 15 280 deaths in 2007.[1] Ninety percent of these malignancies are epithelial in origin, with the remaining 10% comprising sex cord-stromal tumors, germ cell tumors, soft tissue tumors not specific to the ovary, unclassified tumors, and metastatic tumors. The classification of ovarian tumors has been formalized by the World Health Organization (WHO).[2]

Germ cell tumors arise from germ cells present in the normal ovary. These tumors comprise the second most common group of malignant ovarian neoplasms, accounting for approximately 7% of all malignant ovarian tumors and 15–20% of all ovarian neoplasms.[3] A review of the Surveillance, Epidemiology, and End Results (SEER) database from 1975 to 1998 revealed that 23% of malignancies identified in young females were gynecologic in origin, and among girls and young females aged 5–19, the majority of gynecologic cancers were germ cell tumors.[4] Germ cell tumors can be divided into three broad classes of neoplasms: benign teratomas, malignant tumors arising from teratomas, and malignant germ cell tumors. The WHO classification of this category of ovarian neoplasms is outlined in Table 9.1.[2] Except for malignant tumors arising from teratomas, which tend to occur in postmenopausal women, the neoplasms in this class occur most frequently in adolescents, so the issue of fertility preservation is of clinical importance. Understanding and treatment of this group of neoplasms has improved in the past several decades, with improved understanding of the natural history of these neoplasms and an impressive rate of cure.

In the evaluation of a patient with an adnexal mass, several features may be suggestive of a germ cell tumor. Patient age is a consideration. Benign teratomas, also known as dermoid cysts or mature cystic teratomas, occur most commonly in young women, but occasionally also in children and in postmenopausal women. Malignant transformation of dermoid cysts occurs almost exclusively in women over 40 years of age. Most malignant germ cell tumors, however, occur in adolescent girls and young women. In the series studied at the MD Anderson Cancer Center, the median age at diagnosis was 16–20 years, depending on histologic type, with a range from 6 to 31 years.[5]

Although 60–70% of malignant germ cell tumors are stage I at diagnosis, 25–30% are stage III, some of which are upstaged only because of occult metastases. Therefore, if disease appears to be confined to one or both

Table 9.1 World Health Organization classification of ovarian germ cell tumors[2]

---

1. Dysgerminoma
2. Yolk sac tumor (endodermal sinus tumor)
   a. Hepatoid glandular
3. Embryonal carcinoma
4. Polyembryoma
5. Choriocarcinoma
6. Teratomas
   a. Mature (solid/cystic)
   b. Immature
7. Monodermal and highly specialized
   a. Struma ovarii
   b. Carcinoid – insular, trabecular
   c. Strumal carcinoid
   d. Mucinous carcinoid
   e. Neuroectodermal tumors
   f. Sebaceous tumors
8. Mixed primitive germ cell tumors
9. Gonadoblastoma

---

ovaries, complete surgical staging is imperative, as staging affects treatment recommendations and prognosis.[6] Cytologic evaluation of each hemidiaphragm should be performed. Biopsies should be performed of any area with suspected tumor. If no abnormalities are identified, random peritoneal samples for biopsy should be taken of each paracolic gutter, the vesicouterine fold, and the pouch of Douglas. Bilateral pelvic and para-aortic lymph node sampling should be performed, as occult metastases involving the regional lymphatics are not uncommon. An infracolic omentectomy should also be performed.

Patients with advanced-stage disease should undergo cytoreductive surgery. Every attempt should be made to achieve optimal tumor reduction (no implant >1 cm) and, when possible, to leave no visible tumor. Response to chemotherapy and survival are significantly improved in patients who undergo optimal or complete cytoreduction.[7]

Postoperatively, patients are typically treated with three to four courses of BEP (bleomycin, etoposide, and cisplatin) chemotherapy, based on a 96% sustained response rate in patients with resected early-stage germ cell tumors of the ovary.[7,8] These outcomes represent a major improvement over previous regimens and have become the standard of care in germ cell tumors. Patients with gross residual disease or advanced-stage disease after initial surgery also receive a total of three to six courses of BEP, although there is no clear consensus on the optimal number of treatment cycles in this patient population. The only patients not treated with adjuvant chemotherapy are those with a stage IA or IB grade 1 immature teratoma or stage IA pure dysgerminoma. These patients are not given adjuvant chemotherapy and can be closely observed after surgery. There is an increasing body of literature supporting no postsurgical treatment (observation only) in patients with any stage I germ cell tumor.[9,10] Future clinical trials should address and resolve this issue. For the rare patient with a recurrent germ cell tumor, no standard treatment regimen exists.

Certain tumor markers can be helpful in diagnosing germ cell tumors preoperatively. In a premenarchal or adolescent girl or a woman of reproductive age with a solid mass, it is advisable to measure levels of human chorionic gonadotropin (hCG), α-fetoprotein (AFP), and lactate dehydrogenase (LDH) prior to surgery.[6,11] These tumor markers can provide insight into the diagnosis prior to surgery (Table 9.2), thereby facilitating counseling of the patient and her family, and can also be useful in following the patient for response or recurrence. CA-125 levels, although nonspecific, may be variably elevated in germ cell tumors and therefore may be helpful in following the progress of patients.

Table 9.2 Serum tumor markers in malignant germ cell tumors of the ovary[6]

Tumor	hCG	AFP	LDH
Dysgerminoma	+/−	−	+
Endodermal sinus tumor	−	+	+/−
Immature teratoma	−	+/−	+/−
Embryonal carcinoma	+	+	+/−
Choriocarcinoma	+	−	−
Polyembryoma	+/−	+/−	+/−
Mixed	+	+	+

hCG, human chorionic gonadotropin; AFP, α-fetoprotein; LDH, lactate dehydrogenase.

Upon the intraoperative diagnosis of dysgerminoma, the pathologist should be asked to carefully evaluate the specimen for any residual normal ovary and to look for any elements of gonadoblastoma. As the pathologist is evaluating the specimen further, the surgeon should inspect the contralateral adnexa to determine whether a normal ovary or dysgenetic gonad is present. Normal ovarian tissue excludes the possibility of dysgenetic gonads, thereby allowing the surgeon to conserve the contralateral ovary and preserve reproductive potential. Dysgerminoma is bilateral in only 15% of cases, so in most patients, one ovary can be preserved if normal ovarian tissue is present.[11,12]

Although patients with dysgerminoma have historically been noted to be sensitive to radiotherapy, chemotherapy with BEP is more effective, less toxic, and less likely to adversely affect reproductive potential than radiotherapy.[13] Therefore, BEP is recommended for adjuvant and postoperative therapy at the MD Anderson Cancer Center. Patients with dysgerminoma are followed with measurement of levels of serum lactate dehydrogenase to document serologic response and to detect subclinical recurrence. Appropriate decline to physiologic levels typically reflects disease response.

Rising levels of LDH may indicate disease recurrence, and should prompt further investigation with history, physical examination including pelvic examination, and directed imaging, such as abdominopelvic computed tomography (CT).

Nongestational, isolated choriocarcinoma of the ovary is exceedingly rare, since it usually coexists with other elements. Due to the rare nature of this tumor, there is no absolute standard treatment. However, treatment options include either BEP or EMACO (etoposide, methotrexate, dactinomycin (actinomycin D), cyclophosphamide, and vincristine (Oncovin)) after surgical resection.

Pathologic considerations are tumor-specific and are described below for the most common germ cell tumors shown in Figures 9.1–9.4.

Prognostic features: clinical, pathologic, and molecular

With standard therapy as described above, excellent outcomes can usually be obtained in patients with even advanced germ cell tumors of the ovary, with overall disease-free survival rates of >95%.[8,14,15] Certain patient characteristics appear to be important prognostic factors

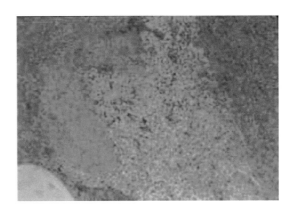

Figure 9.1 Immature teratoma.

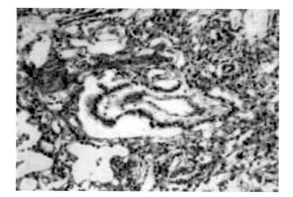

Figure 9.2 Dysgerminoma.

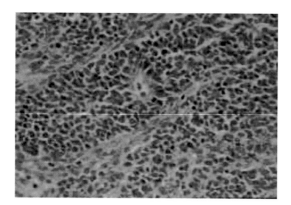

Figure 9.3 Choriocarcinoma.

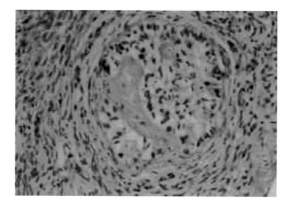

Figure 9.4 Endodermal sinus tumor.

in patients with ovarian germ cell tumors. Young age may portend a better outcome, as patients less than 22 years of age have an improved overall survival compared with their older counterparts.[14] Other investigators, however, have not found age to be a valid predictor of outcome.[16] Stage is a key prognostic factor, as patients with earlier stages do better in every histologic subgroup.[13–18] The presence of platinum in the chemotherapy regimen is an important predictor of outcome, as patients with non-platinum regimens have a lower response rate and disease-free interval. The effect of poor performance status has been noted as a poor prognostic factor,[19] but this report was published prior to current BEP chemotherapy regimens and may be less significant with modern effective chemotherapy. Also, recurrence of malignant disease represents a poor prognostic sign, with only 10% of relapsed patients achieving long-term survival.[18]

Histology is an important prognostic factor for patients with germ cell tumors of the ovary. Patients with endodermal sinus tumors, also known as yolk sac tumors, have a significantly worse outcome than those patients with other histologies.[14,20] Several poor prognostic factors have been identified specifically in patients with endodermal sinus tumor of the ovary. These include stage, response to initial chemotherapy, absence of platinum in chemotherapy, presence of ascites, and residual tumor burden.[16,17,19] The 5-year survival rate in these patients was 95% for stage I disease, 75% for stage II, 30% for stage III, and 25% for stage IV. Failure to respond to the initial chemotherapy regimen administered appeared to be a very poor prognostic factor, as no patient who failed to respond was alive at 36 months.[17] Patients who received platinum-containing regimens have a better outcome than those who receive non-platinum regimens.[16,17] Patients who had over

100 ml of ascites present at diagnosis experienced a worse prognosis.[16,17] Most importantly, patients who had ≥2 cm of residual disease at completion of surgery experienced a worse outcome than patients with <2 cm.[17] In another review, patients who had no visible residual disease at the completion of surgery did better than those with residual disease.[16] This point is key to the treating physician: one of the few ways in which the surgeon can impact the outcome of the patient with endodermal sinus tumor is by achieving optimal tumor reductive surgery. Of note, patient age, maximum tumor size, tumor weight, fertility-sparing surgery, and nodal dissection did not appear to relate to outcome. Thus, optimal tumor reductive surgery appears to be essential to the outcome of patients with even large endodermal sinus tumors, and fertility-sparing surgery remains an option for these patients.[16,17,21]

Specific histologic patterns may also be predictive factors for endodermal sinus tumors of the ovary. Those patients with intestinal or microcystic patterns have a better prognosis than those with other histologic patterns of endodermal sinus tumor.[16]

In patients with immature teratomas, grade is a predictive factor. Patients with stage I low-grade immature teratoma have such an excellent prognosis when treated with surgery alone that chemotherapy is not required. Intermediate and high-grade immature teratomas, however, still require the administration of BEP chemotherapy.[15]

Tumor markers may be important predictors of patient outcome. The presence of an elevated AFP level in germ cell tumors may indicate the presence of endodermal sinus tumor components and therefore portend a worse prognosis compared with other types of germ cell tumors.[14,18] However, within endodermal sinus tumors, the preoperative AFP level does not appear to correlate with prognosis.[16,17] Elevation of β-hCG may also be a poor prognostic factor.[18]

STROMAL TUMORS

Clinical and pathologic features

Like malignant ovarian germ cell tumors, malignant stromal tumors of the ovary account for a small proportion of ovarian neoplasms. Most studies estimate that malignant stromal tumors represent 3–10% of all malignant ovarian neoplasms.[3,22,23] The WHO classification of there tumors in shown in Table 9.3.[2] Details of histology are provided for adult granulosa cell tumor in Figure 9.5, for juvenile granulosa cell tumor in Figure 9.6, and for Sertoli–Leydig cell tumor in Figure 9.7.[2] The definitive diagnosis of a malignant stromal tumor is only made by pathologic examination of the tumor specimen, but the diagnosis can be clinically suggested by age in adolescence or young adulthood, although stromal tumors can be seen in older women. Other presenting signs and symptoms are typical for patients with a pelvic mass, with bloating, pelvic pressure or pain, increase in abdominal girth, and gastrointestinal or urinary symptoms. The physical examination, including a pelvic and rectovaginal examination, usually suggests a pelvic mass. In some patients, especially those with granulosa cell tumors, evidence of hemoperitoneum can be present, with abdominal pain and tenderness, peritoneal signs, a fluid wave, and even hemodynamic instability.[24–26]

Since these tumors may be hormonally active, physical signs of excess or inappropriate estrogen or androgen secretion may be present, such as hirsutism, virilism, isosexual precocious puberty, menorrhagia, irregular menstrual bleeding, amenorrhea, or postmenopausal bleeding.[24]

Table 9.3 World Health Organization classification of stromal tumors of the ovary[2]

1. Granulosa stromal cell tumors
   a. Granulosa cell tumors
      i. Juvenile
      ii. Adult
   b. Thecomas/fibromas
      i. Thecoma
         1. Typical
         2. Luteinized
      ii. Fibroma
   c. Cellular fibroma
   d. Fibrosarcoma
   e. Stromal tumor with minor sex cord elements
   f. Sclerosing stromal tumor
   g. Stromal luteoma
   h. Unclassified (fibrothecoma)
2. Sertoli–stromal cell tumors; androblastomas
   a. Well-differentiated
      i. Sertoli cell tumor; tubular androblastoma
      ii. Sertoli–Leydig cell tumor
      iii. Leydig cell tumor
   b. Intermediate differentiation
      i. Variant – with heterologous elements
   c. Poorly differentiated (sarcomatoid)
      i. Variant – with heterologous elements
   d. Retiform
   e. Mixed
3. Sex cord tumor with annular tubules (SCTAT)
4. Gynandroblastoma
5. Steroid (lipid) cell tumor
   a. Stromal luteoma
   b. Leydig cell tumor
Unclassified

Such menstrual abnormalities should prompt an office endometrial biopsy to exclude hyperplasia or malignancy.

General treatment guidelines for surgery follow those outlined above for germ cell tumors of the ovary. Young patients and those desiring fertility preservation should have strong consideration given to fertility-sparing surgery, as this is safe and usually feasible.[12,27,28] Postmenopausal patients and patients who have completed

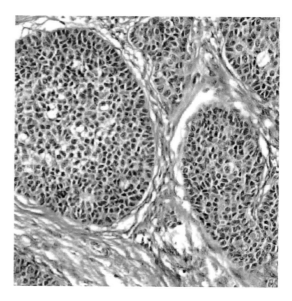

Figure 9.5 Adult granulosa cell tumor.

childbearing should have a total hysterectomy and bilateral salpingo-oophorectomy with staging procedure and optimal tumor reductive surgery, when possible. It is important to note that fertility-sparing surgery does not obviate the need for staging, and the foremost goal should be to eradicate visible tumor.

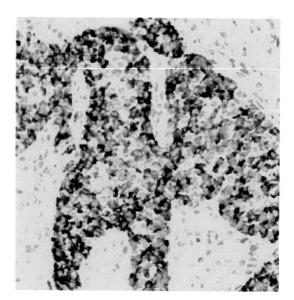

Figure 9.6 Juvenile granulosa cell tumor.

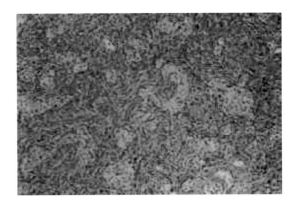

Figure 9.7 Sertoli–Leydig cell tumor.

Most patients with surgical staged stage I disease do not require adjuvant treatment.[29] Patients with stage IC disease may benefit from some adjuvant therapy. Either paclitaxel and carboplatin or hormonal therapy with leuprolide acetate have been recommended for this group of patients.[6] Patients with more advanced disease are typically treated with combination chemotherapy. In 1999, Homesley et al[30] reported on the Gynecologic Oncology Group study, GOG 115, with 57 evaluable patients with stage II–IV disease. Sixty-one percent of patients experienced grade 4 myelotoxicity, but 37% of patients had a negative second-look surgery. Thus, 69% of patients with advanced-stage primary and 51% of patients with recurrent disease remained progression-free. The progression-free interval was 24 months. As a result, many patients have been treated with three or four courses of BEP chemotherapy. However, recent reports have shown paclitaxel and carboplatin to have good results and fewer toxic effects.[31,32] Confirmation of equivalent outcomes between these two regimens awaits performance of a larger randomized trial.

Patients with recurrent disease after a long disease-free interval may undergo secondary cytoreductive surgery. In cases of widespread disease or disease refractory to surgery, chemotherapy and hormonal therapy are options for treatment.

Prognostic features: clinical, pathologic, and molecular

The clinicopathologic features of adult granulosa cell tumors have been reported in several large series, with the overall 20-year survival rate approximating 40%.[33–38] Late recurrence at 5–10 years is not unusual, and recurrence at up to 30 years from the initial diagnosis has been reported.[39] Despite an excellent prognosis for most patients with adult granulosa cell tumors, recurrence is a poor prognostic sign. Over 70% of patients with recurrent disease eventually die of their disease despite treatment regimens including chemotherapy, radiation, and surgery. This may be many years from initial diagnosis or from diagnosis of recurrence.[36]

The stage at initial presentation, however, is the strongest prognostic factor, with the 5–10-year survival rates >90% for stage I, 55% for stage II, and 25% for stage III tumors. Other clinical prognostic factors include tumor size, rupture, and bilaterality. In patients with stage I disease, recurrences are rare for tumors <5 cm in size, but recur at a rate of 20% for tumors 5–15 cm in size and over 30% for tumors >15 cm.[38]

Additional pathologic and molecular markers have emerged as potential prognostic indicators for adult granulosa cell tumors.[40–43] A high mitotic count appears to confer a worse prognosis, but the impact of atypia is less clear.[41–43] Although somewhat controversial, aneuploidy and Ki-67 expression, which are markers of cellular proliferation, appear to confer a worse prognosis.[40,42,44,45] Other molecular markers associated with poor prognosis in other tumors do not appear to play a role in granulosa cell tumors. These include p53, Myc, p21[Ras], and HER2/neu.[40,42,46]

Chromosomal abnormalities have also been recently evaluated in granulosa cell tumors. Early studies have detected trisomy 12, monosomy 22, and deletion of chromosome 6.[47–51] Most recently, monosomy 22, often in conjunction with trisomy 14, has been detected in these tumors, as have deletions in 22q and frequent microsatellite instability.[51,52]

Juvenile granulosa cell tumors are distinct from their adult counterparts, and in patients with advanced disease, the juvenile histology may portend a worse prognosis.[6] A high mitotic index may be a negative prognostic factor.[53] Cytogenetic studies have identified trisomy 12[54] and a deletion in chromosome 6q,[55] but the significance of these findings as predictors remains unknown.

Among patients with Sertoli–Leydig cell tumors, patients with stage IC disease or greater, with poorly differentiated histology of any stage, or with heterologous elements have a worse prognosis, with a 50–60% risk of recurrence. Therefore, combination chemotherapy is recommended for these patients.[6] Stage is clearly the most important prognostic factor. At the time of diagnosis, >90% of patients have stage IA disease. Stage is closely linked with grade; in one series, every patient with a well-differentiated tumor was uniformly stage IA, but only 52% of patients with poorly differentiated tumors were stage IA.[56] Only one death from disease has been reported in a patient with a well-differentiated tumor. However, 10% of intermediate, 60% of poorly differentiated, and 20% of retiform and heterologous subtypes show malignant behavior, leading to the recommendation for adjuvant treatment in these groups. Other poor prognostic factors include the presence of thyroid nodules, tumor size, mitotic activity, tumor rupture, features of rhabdomyosarcoma, and other heterologous elements, especially when containing mesenchymal elements.[57–59] Patients with recurrent disease do poorly.

In patients with steroid cell tumors not otherwise specified, negative prognostic factors include stage, age, size, increased mitotic count, and the presence of necrosis.[60] The number of mitotic figures is the strongest prognostic factor other than stage, as >90% of tumors with >2 mitoses per 10 high-power fields demonstrate malignant behavior. Although all reports are anecdotal, patients with tumors that are pleomorphic, have an increased mitotic count, are large, or are at an advanced stage may have a worse prognosis, and should be treated with additional postoperative platinum-based chemotherapy.[61]

REFERENCES

1. American Cancer Society. Cancer Facts and Figures 2007. http://www.cancer.org/docroot/stt/stt_0.asp.

2. World Health Organization. International Histologic Classification of Tumors. Geneva: WHO, 1973.

3. Koonings PP, Campbell K, Mishell DR Jr, et al. Relative frequency of primary ovarian neoplasms: a 10-year review. Obstet Gynecol 1989;74:921–6.

4. O'Leary M, Sheaffer J, Finklestein J, et al. Female genital tract cancer. In: Bleyer A, O'Leavy M, Barr R, Ries LAG, eds. Cancer Epidemiology in Older Adolescents and Young Adults 15 to 29 Years of Age, Including SEER Incidence and Survival:1975–2000. Bethesda, MD: National Institutes of Health, 2006:163–72.

5. Gershenson DM, Del Junco G, Copeland LJ, et al. Mixed germ cell tumors of the ovary. Obstet Gynecol 1984;64:200–6.

6. Brown J, Gershenson DM. Treatment of rare ovarian malignancies. In: Eifel PJ, Gershenson Don Kavanagh JJ, Silva EG, eds. Gynecologic Cancer. New York:Springer-Verlag, 2006: 207–25.

7. Williams S, Blessing JA, Liao SY, et al. Adjuvant therapy of ovarian germ cell tumors with cisplatin, etoposide, and bleomycin: a trial of the Gynecologic Oncology Group. J Clin Oncol 1994;12:701–6.

8. Gershenson DM, Morris M, Cangir A, et al. Treatment of malignant germ cell tumors of the ovary with bleomycin, etoposide, and cisplatin. J Clin Oncol 1990;8:715–20.

9. Marina NM, Cushing B, Giller R, et al. Complete surgical excision is effective treatment for children with immature teratomas with or without malignant elements: a Pediatric Oncology Group/Children's Cancer Group Intergroup Study. J Clin Oncol 1999;17:2137–43.

10. Dark GG, Bower M, Newlands ES, et al. Surveillance policy for stage I ovarian germ cell tumors. J Clin Oncol 1997;15:620–4.

11. Williams SD, Gershenson DM, Horowitz CJ, Silva E. Ovarian germ-cell tumors. In: Hoskins WJ, Perez CA, Young RC, Barakat RR, eds. Principles and Practice of Gynecologic Oncology, 3rd edn. Philadelphia: Lippincott Williams and Wilkins, 2004.

12. Gershenson DM. Fertility-sparing surgery for malignancies in women. J Natl Cancer Inst Monogr 2005;34:43–7.

13. De Palo G, Lattuada A, Kenda R, et al. Germ cell tumors of the ovary: the experience of the National Cancer Institute of Milan. I. Dysgerminoma. Int J Radiat Oncol Biol Phys 1987;13:853–60.

14. Mayordomo JI, Paz-Ares L, Rivera F, et al. Ovarian and extragonadal malignant germ-cell tumors in females: a single-institution experience with 43 patients. Ann Oncol 1994;5:225–31.

15. Lu KH, Gershenson DM. Update on the management of ovarian germ cell tumors. J Reprod Med 2005;50:417–25.

16. Kawai M, Kano T, Furuhashi Y, et al. Prognostic factors in yolk sac tumors of the ovary. A clinicopathologic analysis of 29 cases. Cancer 1991;67:184–92.

17. Nawa A, Obata N, Kikkawa F, et al. Prognostic factors of patients with yolk sac tumors of the ovary. Am J Obstet Gynecol 2001;184:1182–8.

18. Murugaesu N, Schmid P, Dancey G, et al. Malignant ovarian germ cell tumors: identification of novel prognostic markers and long-term outcome after multimodality treatment. J Clin Oncol 2006;24:4862–6.

19. Bradof JE, Hakes TB, Ochoa M, et al. Germ cell malignancies of the ovary: treatment with vinblastine, actinomycin D, bleomycin and cisplatin containing chemotherapy combinations. Cancer 1982;50:1070–5.

20. Slayton RE, Park RC, Silverberg SG, et al. Vincristine, dactinomycin, and cyclophosphamide in the treatment of malignant germ cell tumors of the ovary. A Gynecologic Oncology Group Study (a final report). Cancer 1985;56:243–8.

21. Gobel U, Schneider DT, Calaninus G, et al. Germ-cell tumors in childhood and adolescence. GPOH MAKEI and the MAHO study groups. Ann Oncol 2000;11:263–71.

22. Jacobs AJ, Deppe G, Cohen CJ. Combination chemotherapy of ovarian granulosa cell tumor with *cis*-platinum and doxorubicin. Gynecol Oncol 1982;14:294–7.

23. Gershenson DM, Copeland LJ, Kavanagh JJ, et al. Treatment of metastatic stromal tumors of the ovary with cisplatin, doxorubicin, and cyclophosphamide. Obstet Gynecol 1987; 70:765–9.

24. Young RH, Scully RE. Endocrine tumors of the ovary. Curr Top Pathol 1992;85:113–64.

25. Unkila-Kallio L, Tiitinen A, Wahlstrom T, et al. Reproductive features in women developing ovarian granulosa cell tumour at a fertile age. Hum Reprod 2000;15:589–93.

26. Gershenson DM, Hartmann LC, Young RH. Ovarian sex cord-stromal tumors. In: Hoskins WJ, Perez CA, Young RC, eds. Principles and Practice of Gynecologic Oncology, 4th edn. Philadelphia: Lippincott Williams and Wilkins, 2004.

27. Gershenson DM. Management of early ovarian cancer: germ cell and sex cord-stromal tumors. Gynecol Oncol 1994;55:S62–72.

28. Colombo N, Parma G, Lapresa MT, et al. Role of conservative surgery in ovarian cancer: the European experience. Int J Gynecol Cancer 2005;15(Suppl 3):206–11.

29. Herbst AL. Neoplastic diseases of the ovary. In: Mishell DR, Steachever MA, Droegmuller W, Herbst AL, eds. Comprehensive Gynecology. New York: Mosby-Year Book, 2006.

30. Homesley HD, Bundy BN, Hurteau JA, et al. Bleomycin, etoposide, and cisplatin combination therapy of ovarian granulosa cell tumors and other stromal malignancies: Gynecologic Oncology Group study. Gynecol Oncol 1999; 72:131–7.

31. Brown J, Shvartsman HS, Deavers MT, et al. The activity of taxanes in the treatment of sex cord-stromal ovarian tumors. J Clin Oncol 2004;22:3517–23.

32. Brown J, Shvartsman HS, Deavers MT, et al. The activity of taxanes compared with bleomycin, etoposide, and cisplatin in the treatment of sex cord-stromal ovarian tumors. Gynecol Oncol 2005;97:489–96.

33. Norris HJ, Taylor HB. Prognosis of granulosa–theca tumors of the ovary. Cancer 1968;21: 255–63.

34. Fox H, Agrawal K, Langley FA. A clinicopathologic study of 92 cases of granulosa cell tumor of the ovary with special reference to the factors influencing prognosis. Cancer 1975;35:231–41.

35. Dempster J, Geirsson RT, Duncan ID. Survival after ovarian granulosa and theca cell tumours. Scott Med J 1987;32:38–9.

36. Evans AT 3rd, Gaffey TA, Malkasian GD Jr, et al. Clinicopathologic review of 118 granulosa and 82 theca cell tumors. Obstet Gynecol 1980;55:231–8.

37. Bjorkholm E, Silfversward C. Granulosa- and theca-cell tumors. Incidence and occurrence of second primary tumors. Acta Radiol Oncol 1980;19:161–7.

38. Bjorkholm E, Silfversward C. Prognostic factors in granulosa-cell tumors. Gynecol Oncol 1981;11:261–74.

39. Bjorkholm E. Granulosa cell tumors: a comparison of survival in patients and matched controls. Am J Obstet Gynecol 1980;138:329–31.

40. Evans, MP, Webb MJ, Gaffey TA, et al. DNA ploidy of ovarian granulosa cell tumors. Lack of correlation between DNA index or proliferative index and outcome in 40 patients. Cancer 1995;75:2295–8.

41. Malmstrom H, Hogberg T, Risberg B, et al. Granulosa cell tumors of the ovary: prognostic factors and outcome. Gynecol Oncol 1994;52: 50–5.

42. King LA, Okagaki T, Gallup DG, et al. Mitotic count, nuclear atypia, and immunohistochemical determination of Ki-67, c-myc, p21-ras, c-erbB2, and p53 expression in granulosa cell tumors of the ovary: mitotic count and Ki-67 are indicators of poor prognosis. Gynecol Oncol 1996;61:227–32.

43. Miller BE, Barron BA, War JY, et al. Prognostic factors in adult granulosa cell tumor of the ovary. Cancer 1997;79:1951–5.

44. Roush GR, el-Naggar AK, Abdul-Karim FW. Granulosa cell tumor of ovary: a clinicopathologic and flow cytometric DNA analysis. Gynecol Oncol 1995;56:430–4.

45. Costa MJ, Walls J, Ames P, et al. Transformation in recurrent ovarian granulosa cell tumors: Ki67 (MIB-1) and p53 immunohistochemistry demonstrates a possible molecular basis for the poor histopathologic prediction of clinical behavior. Hum Pathol 1996;27:274–81.

46. Liu FS, Ho ES, Lai CR, et al. Overexpression of p53 is not a feature of ovarian granulosa cell tumors. Gynecol Oncol 1996;61:50–3.

47. Teyssier JR, Adnett JJ, Pigeon F, et al. Chromosomal changes in an ovarian granulosa cell tumor: similarity with carcinoma. Cancer Genet Cytogenet 1985:14:147–52.

48. Fletcher JA, Gibas Z, Donovan K, et al. Ovarian granulosa–stromal cell tumors are characterized by trisomy 12. Am J Pathol 1991;138:515–20.

49. Persons DL, Hartmann LC, Herath JF, et al. Fluorescence in situ hybridization analysis of trisomy 12 in ovarian tumors. Am J Clin Pathol 1994;102:775–9.

50. Lindgren V, Waggoner S, Rotmensch J. Monosomy 22 in two ovarian granulosa cell tumors. Cancer Genet Cytogenet 1996;89:93–7.

51. Lin YS, Eng HL, Jan YJ, et al. Molecular cytogenetics of ovarian granulosa cell tumors by comparative genomic hybridization. Gynecol Oncol 2005;97:68–73.

52. Dhillon VS, Aslam M, Husain SA. The contribution of genetic and epigenetic changes in granulosa cell tumors of ovarian origin. Clin Cancer Res 2004;10:5537–45.

53. Zaloudek C, Norris HJ. Granulosa tumors of the ovary in children: a clinical and pathologic study of 32 cases. Am J Surg Pathol 1982;6:503–12.

54. Schofield DE, Fletcher JA. Trisomy 12 in pediatric granulosa–stromal cell tumors. Demonstration by a modified method of fluorescence in situ hybridization on paraffin-embedded material. Am J Pathol 1992;141:1265–9.

55. Rodriguez E, Rao PH, Reuter V. Cytogenetic analysis of a juvenile granulosa cell tumor. Cancer Genet Cytogenet 1992;61:207–9.

56. Pankratz E, Boyes DA, White GW, et al. Granulosa cell tumors. A clinical review of 61 cases. Obstet Gynecol 1978;52:718–23.

57. Martikainen H, Penttinen J, Huhtanemi I, et al. Gonadotropin-releasing hormone agonist analog therapy effective in ovarian granulosa cell malignancy. Gynecol Oncol 1989;35:406–8.

58. Young RH, Dickersin GR, Scully RE. Juvenile granulosa cell tumor of the ovary. A clinicopathological analysis of 125 cases. Am J Surg Pathol 1984;8:575–96.

59. Lack EE, Perez-Atayde AR, Murthy AS, et al. Granulosa theca cell tumors in premenarchal girls: a clinical and pathologic study of ten cases. Cancer 1981;48:1846–54.

60. Goldstein DP, Lamb EJ. Arrhenoblastoma in first cousins. Report of 2 cases. Obstet Gynecol 1970;35:444–50.

61. Srivatsa PJ, Keeney GL, Podratz KC. Disseminated cervical adenoma malignum and bilateral ovarian sex cord tumors with annular tubules associated with Peutz–Jeghers syndrome. Gynecol Oncol 1994;53:256–64.

Section II
Endometrium

Section Editor: Karen H Lu

Rethinking traditional surgical–pathologic criteria for early endometrial cancer: studies of patterns of failure

10

Andrea Mariani, Sean C Dowdy, and Karl C Podratz

INTRODUCTION

During 2007, an estimated 39 080 new cases and 7400 deaths will be attributed to corpus cancer in the USA.[1] Of major concern is the realization that while the incidence of endometrial carcinoma has remained stable over the past decade, the annual number of deaths from this disease has more than doubled since 1987 (2900 deaths). Presumably the causes of these sobering statistics are multifactorial, but they obligate us to reassess more objectively and critically the screening, diagnostic, staging, and treatment practices that guide the overall management of this neoplasm. The variability in the staging and treatment algorithms, which are generally predicated on institutional and/or individual physician philosophies, are a noteworthy obstacle to achieving optimal management of this disease.[2]

For the above reasons, a critical reevaluation of the surgical and postoperative approaches to managing endometrial cancer at the Mayo Clinic Rochester was initiated approximately 10 years ago. Both surgical and postoperative management of endometrial cancer during a 13-year period (1984–96) were retrospectively assessed.

SURGICAL TREATMENT OF EARLY ENDOMETRIAL CANCER: PRIMARY TUMOR DIAMETER AS A RISK FACTOR FOR LYMPH NODE INVOLVEMENT

In the last two decades, many authors have attempted to identify prognostic factors for women with endometrial cancer in order to tailor surgical and adjuvant treatment on the estimated risk for recurrence.[3–5] Low-risk characteristics were defined as disease confined to the uterine corpus, histologic grade 1 or 2, endometrioid histologic subtype, and ≤50% invasion through the myometrial wall.[3] The detection of positive lymph nodes in 4–5% of patients in this low-risk group[5,6] is considered significant by some authors and worthy of a lymph node evaluation.[4] Unfortunately, we continue to lack specific tumor characteristics, evaluable before or during the operation, that can guide the decision to perform a pelvic lymphadenectomy.[7]

Tumor diameter is a well-defined predictor of lymph node involvement and prognosis in cervical[8] and breast cancers.[9] Similarly, primary tumor diameter has been described as a predictor

Table 10.1 Patients at low risk for lymph node metastasis (myometrial invasion <50%, grade 1–2, endometrioid histologic subtype, no macroscopic tumor outside the uterine corpus): stratification according to tumor diameter and pelvic lymph node metastases[11]

Tumor diameter (cm)	Patients (n)	Pelvic lymph node metastases	
		No. pelvic lymphadenectomy (%)	No. positive pelvic lymph nodes (%)
≤2	123	59 (48)	0 (0)
>2	169	107 (63)	8 (7)

of lymph node invasion[5,10] and prognosis[5] in endometrial cancer. We demonstrated that the primary tumor diameter measured at surgery, together with histologic subtype, grade, and depth of myometrial invasion, identified those 'low-risk' patients with endometrial cancer who could be managed with curative intent with a simple hysterectomy, thus avoiding the morbidity of lymphadenectomy.[11] In our series,[11] 123 patients presented with all of the following characteristics: endometrioid histologic subtype, histologic grade 1 or 2, myometrial invasion <50%, tumor diameter ≤2 cm, and absence of macroscopic tumor beyond the uterine corpus. Neither positive lymph nodes nor lymph node recurrences have been identified in this group (Tables 10.1 and 10.2). All 123 patients (100%) with the above characteristics were alive with no evidence of disease at 5 years, independent of lymphadenectomy or postoperative radiotherapy (Table 10.3).

The only recurrences were vaginal and were present in 2% of the patients (Table 10.2). These findings, which are in agreement with prior observations,[5] confirm the superiority of primary tumor diameter over grade (i.e. grade 1 vs 2) in predicting lymph node invasion in the above-defined 'low-risk' group. Patients with the above characteristics who do not require full surgical staging represent approximately 25% of the endometrial cancer patients operated on at the Mayo Clinic.

TRADITIONAL PROGNOSTIC FACTORS IN ENDOMETRIAL CANCER

Prognostic factors are usually defined as features of disease that can predict its future behavior.[12] They can be considered in five contexts: clinical, anatomic, hormonal, cellular, and molecular–genetic.[13] They are generally used

Table 10.2 Patients at low risk for lymph node metastasis (myometrial invasion <50%, grade 1–2, endometrioid histologic subtype, no macroscopic tumor outside the uterine corpus): stratification according to tumor diameter and recurrences[11]

Tumor diameter (cm)	Patients (n)	Recurrences	Sites of recurrence[a]		
			Loco-regional	Distant	Local + distant
≤2	123	3 (2%)	3 (0)[b]	0 (0)	0 (0)
>2	169	14 (8%)	3 (1)	6 (6)	5 (4)

[a]Deaths due to disease in parentheses
[b]All vaginal recurrences.

Table 10.3 Survival of the 123 patients with primary tumor diameter ≤2 cm according to definitive method of treatment[11]

Treatment	Patients (n)	5-year survival rate (%)
Hysterectomy only	59	100
Hysterectomy + LND/RT[a]	64	100
Total	123	100

[a]LND, lymphadenectomy; RT, radiotherapy (10 patients received RT: 7 for positive peritoneal cytology).

to predict prognosis,[3,6] to determine the need and type of adjuvant therapy,[2] and eventually to identify new treatment strategies.[13]

The most important traditional clinical and anatomic prognostic factors for recurrence and death in patients with endometrial cancer are advanced surgical stage, poorly differentiated histologic grade, nonendometrioid histologic subtype, deep myometrial invasion, presence of lymphovascular invasion (LVI), primary tumor diameter >2 cm, invasion of the cervical stroma, and extrauterine disease.[3,5,6,11,14–16]

IDENTIFICATION OF PREDICTORS OF DIFFERENT PATTERNS OF TUMOR DISSEMINATION IN ENDOMETRIAL CANCER

Endometrial cancer generally becomes manifest early in its natural history, such that approximately 80% of patients will present with stage I disease. Nevertheless, a proportion of nearly 1 of every 3 women who die of endometrial cancer present with presumed localized disease. The majority of treatment failures and the accompanying compromised longevity are presumably the result of the failure to recognize sites of occult extrauterine dissemination at the time of primary treatment. Furthermore, adjuvant therapy has generally been dictated by

traditional preferences (modality-based) rather than target-based algorithms as determined by patterns of recurrence. The traditional therapy (modality-based) for high-risk endometrial cancer is external radiotherapy, eventually combined with vaginal brachytherapy.[17,18] This type of approach has been demonstrated to improve local control but not survival in early-stage disease.[19–21]

The natural history of epithelial corpus cancer includes four potential routes of metastasis: contiguous extension, hematogenous dissemination, lymphatic embolization, and exfoliation with intraperitoneal spread. The associated recurrences for each of these diverse routes of spread would presuppose different adjuvant treatment strategies. In addition, determination of such disease-based therapies is predicated on the cataloging of specific pathologic or molecular factors that identify patients at high risk for harboring occult disease disseminated via one or more of these routes.[22] The following discussion will address the risk factors associated with hematogenous, lymphatic, intraperitoneal, and vaginal spread of endometrial carcinoma.

To facilitate the correlation of risk factors with specific patterns of recurrence, the outcomes of 612 consecutive patients with endometrial carcinoma managed surgically at Mayo Clinic Rochester were assessed. Inclusion criteria required hysterectomy with removal of existing adnexal structures and absence of a diagnosis of other malignancies within 5 years prior to or after the detection of endometrial cancer. All surgical procedures were the responsibility of a gynecologic oncologist. Intraoperative frozen section was available on all surgical specimens. Hence, lymphadenectomy was usually performed when the surgeon considered the patient to be at risk for lymph node metastasis based on grade and/or depth of myometrial invasion. Postoperative adjuvant radiotherapy and occasionally hormonal or cytotoxic therapies were administered based on standard clinicopathologic prognostic indicators considered appropriate at the time treatment was initiated.

After a mean follow-up interval exceeding 6 years, 142 (23%) recurrences were documented. Information regarding the sites of failure was available in 131 cases. Clinical and pathologic characteristics evaluated for the entire population included age, stage, grade, myometrial penetration, cervical stromal invasion, body mass index, adnexal involvement, primary tumor diameter, associated hyperplasia, LVI, histologic subtype, lymph node metastases, positive peritoneal cytology, and adjuvant therapy when applicable. Logistic regression analysis and the Cox proportional hazards model were used to determine which variables were independently associated with each route of spread.

Hematogenous dissemination was defined as an initial distant failure within the lung, liver, or other sites outside of the abdominal cavity or the lymphatic system.[23] Failures via hematogenous dissemination were detected in 60 patients: 46 lung (3 associated with liver and 1 associated with bone), 9 liver, and 5 other single sites. Regression analysis identified myometrial invasion >50% as the only independent risk factor for hematogenous dissemination (Table 10.4).[23] Patients with myometrial

invasion ≤50% were associated with a 5% risk of failure at sites accessed via the hematogenous route, compared with a 23% risk if the depth of myometrial penetration was >50%.[23] For stage I (node-negative) patients, only 2% of patients with myometrial invasion <66% developed failure via hematogenous spread, compared with 29% when myometrial invasion was ≥66%.[24] As noted in Table 10.4, failures were correlated with the administration of adjuvant radiotherapy and with stage IV disease. The former presumably reflects the tendency to recommend postoperative adjuvant radiotherapy for traditional risk factors, one of which was deep myometrial invasion. The latter observation is consistent, recognizing that stage IV disease includes patients who originally had macroscopic disease in tissues/organs accessible from the pelvis through the vascular system. These findings suggest that adjuvant systemic therapy should be considered for patients at risk for occult hematogenous dissemination of disease based on the depth of myometrial invasion.

Initial sites of failure within lymph node-bearing regions were detected in 44 of the 131 patients (34%) with known sites of recurrent disease.[25] Lymphatic failure was defined as recurrent disease appearing on the pelvic sidewall, adjacent to the aorta or vena cava, or in other node-bearing regions. The median time to documented lymphatic failure was 12 months. Regression analysis identified LVI, cervical stromal invasion and lymph node metastasis as independent risk factors when all lymph node-bearing sites were included in the model (Table 10.5). As noted in Table 10.5, cervical stromal invasion and lymph node metastasis were the only independent risk factors for pelvic sidewall failure. In the absence of either of these two factors, lymphatic failures in the pelvis approached zero. These observations strongly reinforce the suggestions by other

Table 10.4 Logistic regression for predicting hematogenous dissemination

Characteristic	Odds ratio	p-value	95% confidence interval
Myometrial invasion >50%	6.00	0.003	1.80–19.94
Radiotherapy	3.47	0.06	0.95–12.68
Stage IV disease	3.50	0.16	0.60–20.36

Modified from Mariani et al. Gynecol Oncol 2007;80:233–8[23] with permission from Elsevier.

Table 10.5 Failure frequency in various lymphatic sites according to risk status

Lymphatic site(s)	Failure rate at 5 years (%)	p-value
All sites:		
Low risk[a]	0.4	<0.001
High risk[b]	31	
Pelvic sidewall:		
Low risk[a]	0	<0.001
High risk[c]	26	
Para-aortic area:		
Low risk[a]	1	<0.001
High risk[d]	33	

[a]Low risk: none of the corresponding high-risk factors.
[b]High risk: lymphovascular invasion and/or cervical stromal invasion and/or lymph node metastases.
[c]High risk: cervical stromal invasion and/or lymph node metastases.
[d]High risk: only lymph node metastases.
Modified from Mariani et al. Gynecol Oncol 2002;84:437–42[25] with permission from Elsevier.

investigators[2,4,26–28] that, following systematic lymphadenectomy, stage I (node-negative) patients are at extremely low risk for pelvic sidewall recurrence and can forego external-beam radiotherapy. Furthermore, the only independent predictor of lymphatic failure in the para-aortic area was the detection of tumor in the lymph nodes; 33% of patients with documented pelvic and/or para-aortic node metastases subsequently failed in the para-aortic area, compared with 1% when the node-bearing areas were declared negative. In addition, we have recently shown that 47% of patients with positive pelvic nodes will have para-aortic nodal involvement at the time of dissection or subsequent recurrence in the para-aortic area or both.[29] These observations should guide recommendations for and the extent of adjuvant radiotherapy in both definitively staged and inadequately staged patients. If external-beam radiotherapy is selected as adjuvant therapy to

decrease pelvic sidewall recurrence in non-staged patients, the above observations would suggest that the para-aortic area should routinely be included in the field of treatment.

Our recommendation to use external radiotherapy after lymphadenectomy in patients with positive lymph nodes is supported by retrospective data demonstrating a synergism of systematic lymph node dissection and external radiotherapy in preventing lymphatic recurrences.[30] Moreover, a high rate of pelvic recurrence in patients with advanced disease treated with systemic chemotherapy and not receiving adjuvant external-beam radiotherapy has been shown previously.[31]

Peritoneal failures were witnessed in 37 of the 131 patients (28%) with known initial sites of recurrence.[32] Peritoneal failures were defined as disease recurring in the upper abdomen or involving the pelvic peritoneum or both. Simultaneous extraabdominal sites of failure were also detected in 16 of the 37 patients (43%) with peritoneal failure. When analyzing the entire population, logistic regression identified cervical stromal invasion, nonendometrioid histology, and stage IV disease as independent risk factors. In fact, 59% of stage IV patients experienced peritoneal failures, undoubtedly a function of the presence of recognized intraabdominal disease at the time of surgical management in the majority of patients. When excluding stage IV patients, peritoneal failures were observed in 2% of the 545 stage I–III patients. Regression analysis identified non-endometrioid histology, cervical stromal invasion, positive peritoneal cytology, and lymph node metastases as independent risk factors for peritoneal failures. As noted in Table 10.6, when two or more of these factors were present, 26% of the patients experienced relapses within the abdominal cavity. Treatment strategies must also recognize that a very significant percentage

Table 10.6 Peritoneal failures in stage I–III patients according to risk status

No. of positive risk factors[a]	Patients (n)	Peritoneal failure rate (%)
0	406	<1
1	101	4
≥2	38	26

[a]Cervical stromal invasion, positive peritoneal cytology, lymph node metastases, and nonendometrioid histologic subtype.
Modified from Mariani et al. Gynecol Oncol 2003;89:236–42[32] with permission from Elsevier.

of patients with abdominal relapse (43% in this study) will also experience concomitant extraabdominal failures.[32] Hence, patients with stage IV disease, or stage I–III with two or more of the identified untoward factors, should be considered candidates for systemic adjuvant therapy.

Considering the 508 patients with stage I disease who did not receive adjuvant radiotherapy, we identified histologic grade 3 and presence of LVI as the strongest predictors of vaginal recurrence. When neither variable was present, 2% of patients experienced vaginal relapse at 5 years, compared with 11% when either risk factor was present (p <0.001) (Table 10.7).

Table 10.7 Vaginal recurrence rates according to risk factors in 508 patients with stage I endometrial cancer who did not receive adjuvant radiotherapy

Risk factor[a]	Patients[b] (n)	5-year failure rate (%)
None	448	2
Either one	57	11
Both	2	—[c]

[a]Histologic grade 3, or lymphovascular invasion, or both.
[b]Neither histologic grade nor information about lymphovascular invasion was available for 1 patient.
[c]Of the 2 patients, 1 had vaginal relapse 63 months after primary surgery.
Reprinted from Mariani A et al. Gynecol Oncol 2005;97: 820–7.[33]

Depth of myometrial invasion was not a significant predictor of vaginal recurrence.[33]

Predictors of different patterns of tumor dissemination in endometrial cancer are summarized in Table 10.8. Using these risk factors, subgroups of patients were subsequently identified with predictable regional or distant patterns of recurrence that might potentially benefit from disease-based adjuvant therapies.[22]

From 1984 to 1996, at Mayo Clinic Rochester, 1109 patients with endometrial cancer were managed surgically. Based on data from their medical records, 915 patients with epithelial endometrial cancer met the following inclusion criteria: (i) treatment included hysterectomy and removal of existing adnexal structures and (ii) no other malignancy was diagnosed within 5 years before or after the diagnosis of endometrial cancer (except for carcinoma in situ or skin cancer other than melanoma).

Five-year recurrence rates are stratified by different sites of recurrence and risk factors and listed in Table 10.9. Considering the overall population of 915 patients, 190 (21%) had identifiable relapse of disease. The site of recurrence was unknown in 14 patients. Excluding these 14 patients, we observed 84 (9%) hematogenous recurrences, 57 (6%) lymphatic recurrences, 57 (6%) peritoneal recurrences, and 41 (5%) vaginal recurrences (Figure 10.1). More precisely, 32 of the 176 (18%) patients whose site of recurrence was known had isolated recurrence in the vagina, 37 (21%) had an isolated hematogenous relapse, 28 (16%) had an isolated lymphatic relapse, and 31 (18%) had an isolated peritoneal relapse. However, 22 patients (12.5%) had concomitant hematogenous and lymphatic recurrence, 19 (11%) had concomitant hematogenous and peritoneal recurrence, 1 (0.5%) had concomitant lymphatic and peritoneal recurrence, and 6 (3%) had concomitant recurrence in all three sites. Of all the

Table 10.8 Risk factors for hematogenous, lymphatic, and peritoneal recurrences[22–25,32,33]

Route of recurrence	Risk factors
Hematogenous:	
All stages of disease	Myometrial invasion >50%
Stage I disease, negative lymph nodes	Myometrial invasion ≥66%
Lymphatic: pelvic/para-aortic lymph nodes	Cervical stromal invasion, lymph node metastases
Peritoneal spread	Stage IV disease
	Stage II–III disease, ≥ 2 of the following variables cervical stromal invasion, positive peritoneal cytology, lymph node metastases, or type II histology (nonendometrioid subtypes)
Vaginal spread: stage I	Grade 3, lymphovascular invasion

Modified from Mariani et al. Gynecol Oncol 2004;95:120–6[22] with permission from Elsevier.

Table 10.9 Rates of recurrence at 5 years according to the different risk categories (*n* = 915)

Risk category	Recurrence rate at 5 years (%)
Hematogenous:	
All stages:	
Myometrial invasion ≤50%	4
Myometrial invasion >50%	28
Stage I (negative lymph nodes)	
Myometrial invasion <66%	2
Myometrial invasion ≥66%	34
Lymphatic:	
No risk factors	2
Cervical stromal invasion and/or positive lymph nodes	31
Peritoneal:	
Stage IV disease	63
Stage II–III disease ≥2 risk factors[a]	21
Stage I–III disease ≤1 risk factor[a]	1
Overall[b]	
Not at risk[c]	2
At risk[c]	46

[a]Cervical stromal invasion, nonendometrioid histologic subtype, positive lymph nodes, positive peritoneal cytology.
[b]Excluding vaginal recurrences.
[c]For at least one risk factor of the 3 categories of recurrence (i.e. hematogenous, lymphatic, or peritoneal).
Reprinted from Mariani et al. Gynecol Oncol 2004;95:120–6[22] with permission from Elsevier.

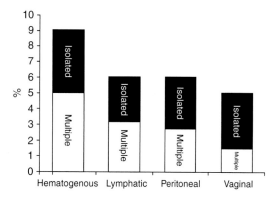

Figure 10.1 Percentage of patients with different sites of recurrence. Overall, 190 (21%) patients had recurrence: 9% hematogenous recurrences, 6% lymphatic recurrences, 6% peritoneal recurrences, and 5% vaginal recurrences. Approximately half of the patients in each category had multiple sites of relapse. Reprinted from Mariani et al. Gynecol Oncol 2004;95:120–6[22] with permission from Elsevier.

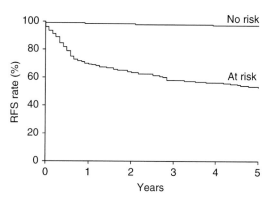

Figure 10.3 Recurrence-free survival (RFS) according to risk classification. Patients at risk for any site of recurrence (35% of the population) had a 54% 5-year RFS rate (excluding isolated vaginal recurrences) versus 98% for patients not at risk ($p < 0.001$). Reprinted from Mariani et al. Gynecol Oncol 2004;95:120–6[22] with permission from Elsevier.

recurrences, 48 (27%) had multiple sites of primary relapse (Figure 10.2).[22]

Considering the above 915 patients with endometrial cancer, the risk of recurrence at 5 years was 46% in patients with at least one

of the risk factors listed in Table 10.8 (excluding vaginal failure), and 2% in patients with no risk factors (Figure 10.3 and Table 10.9). Approximately one-third (36%) of the 915 patients have at least one of the above risk factors and are considered at risk of recurrence. However, 89% of recurrences are found within this limited group of patients.[22]

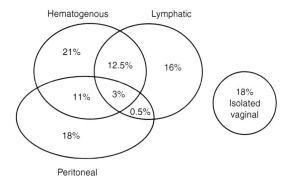

Figure 10.2 Of all recurrences, 48% had a hematogenous component (21% isolated hematogenous recurrences), 32% had a lymphatic component (16% isolated lymphatic recurrences), 32% had a peritoneal component (18% isolated peritoneal recurrences), and 18% were isolated vaginal recurrences. Approximately 27% of recurrences had multiple components of recurrence. Reprinted from Mariani et al. Gynecol Oncol 2004;95:120–6[22] with permission from Elsevier.

IDENTIFICATION OF PREDICTORS OF DIFFERENT PATTERNS OF TUMOR DISSEMINATION AFTER INADEQUATE SURGICAL STAGING

Systematic surgical staging is an important step in the management of endometrial cancer.[2] Gynecologic cancer patients managed by a gynecologic oncologist are more likely to be definitively staged surgically than patients managed by an obstetrician–gynecologist or a general surgeon.[34] Moreover, for the treatment of endometrial cancer, a lymphadenectomy is less likely to be performed in primary care hospitals than in referral centers.[35] However, most patients with endometrial cancer in the USA are treated surgically by physicians managing a very limited number (<5) of such cases annually.[36] Typically, these physicians lack detailed knowledge of the natural history of the disease and of the indications for adjuvant treatment, and lack the intraoperative expertise to perform pelvic and para-aortic lymphadenectomy and cytoreduction as indicated. Consequently, many patients receive therapy that is substandard for optimal outcomes.

Inadequate staging of endometrial cancer patients greatly compromises our ability to make appropriate recommendations for adjuvant therapy. However, referral institutions are frequently faced with the problem of making appropriate treatment decisions for patients with endometrial cancer who are referred after inadequate surgery performed elsewhere. Frequently, the only information available in these patients is the status of the tumor in the uterus and the accompanying adnexae.

In patients who have not been adequately staged, information derived from uterine and adnexal histology may assist in determining the modality and extent of postoperative therapy or the need for definitive restaging in endometrioid endometrial cancer patients. We have recently identified risk factors for pelvic and para-aortic lymph node invasion and for abdominal dissemination in patients with endometrioid disease and without adequate surgical staging.[37] Tumor diameter >2 cm, histologic grade 3, cervical stromal invasion, deep myometrial invasion, and LVI were the strongest predictors of pelvic and para-aortic dissemination, whereas adnexal metastases, and LVI predicted peritoneal spread of disease. Knowledge of the above risk factors may assist the physician in predicting the rate of lymphatic and peritoneal dissemination after incomplete surgical treatment. In fact, from 17% to >30% of patients with tumor diameter >2 cm and at least one of the above-mentioned risk factors had pelvic or para-aortic dissemination (or both), compared with 3% or less in the other remaining patients. Similarly, >40% of patients with either LVI or adnexal invasion had abdominal spread of tumor, compared with 6% of the others.[37]

PRACTICAL SUGGESTIONS FOR SURGICAL AND POSTOPERATIVE TREATMENT OF ENDOMETRIAL CANCER

After identifying a subgroup of patients who are likely not to benefit from full surgical staging[11] (see also the section on surgical treatment earlier in this chapter), guidelines were designed for the surgical treatment of endometrial cancer at the Mayo Clinic Rochester, based on our retrospective data and the current literature (Table 10.10).

As a general rule, for patients who are referred after inadequate surgical staging, risk factors for hematogenous (Tables 10.8 and 10.9), lymphatic, or abdominal dissemination can be used for practical recommendations for postoperative treatment or restaging (Figure 10.4).

With regard to postoperative treatment in patients with adequate surgical staging, in general, we suggest using chemotherapy in the presence of risk factors for hematogenous recurrence, and radiotherapy for patients with risk factors for lymphatic recurrences in the pelvic and para-aortic areas (Tables 10.8 and 10.9). With regard to the prevention of abdominal recurrences (Tables 10.8 and 10.9), we suggest the use of chemotherapy based on the results of the GOG 122 study[38] and on our finding of extra-abdominal dissemination in 43% of patients with abdominal recurrences.[32] Patients at risk of vaginal recurrence will receive vaginal brachytherapy (Tables 10.8 and 10.9).

Table 10.10 Surgical guidelines for the treatment of endometrial cancer at the Mayo Clinic Rochester (2004–06)

Treatment: Hysterectomy, bilateral salpingo-oophorectomy, peritoneal cytology, bilateral pelvic and para-aortic lymphadenectomy (up to renal vessels)

1. Can omit lymphadenectomy if:
   (A) All of the following: no myometrial invasion, endometrioid, no evidence of tumor outside the corpus (independently of grade or tumor diameter)
   (B) All of the following: endometrioid, grade 1 or 2, 0% < myometrial invasion <50%, tumor diameter ≤2 cm, no evidence of tumor outside the corpus

2. If nonendometrioid (serous, clear cells), add complete omentectomy, appendectomy, peritoneal biopsies (11 pairs: cul-de-sac, bladder peritoneum, right diaphragm, right/left colic gutters, right/left pelvic sidewall, small-/large-bowel serosa and mesentery, any suspicious area)

Reprinted from Mariani et al. Gynecol Oncol 2004;95:120–6[22] with permission from Elsevier.

The following are the current care pathways that are in effect at the Mayo Clinic Rochester for patients with early-stage endometrioid endometrial cancer. The treatment of patients with advanced or nonendometrioid endometrial tumors is described in detail in chapters 11, 14, and 15.

Patients with endometrioid tumors limited to the uterus in general do not need any therapy if negative nodes have been documented (Figure 10.5). In fact, it has been demonstrated that stage I patients with negative lymph nodes who have been treated without adjuvant external radiotherapy present a risk of recurrence at the pelvic sidewall of <1% (Table 10.11).[2] The inability of external radiotherapy to improve survival in endometrial cancer patients with tumors confined to the uterus has been shown by prospective randomized studies,[20] even in cases without any surgical staging.[19,21,39]

However, in the presence of grade 3 disease or LVI (or both), owing to the 12% risk of

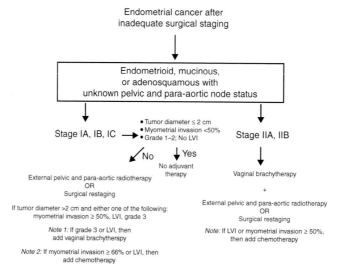

Figure 10.4 Postoperative treatment of incompletely staged early endometrioid endometrial cancer. Note that, in comparison with Figure 10.5, patients are generally recommended more aggressive treatment due to the absence of appropriate surgical staging. LVI, lymphovascular invasion.

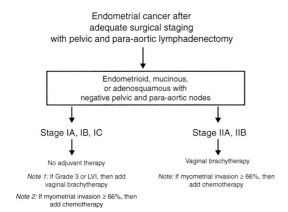

Figure 10.5 Postoperative treatment of adequately staged early endometrioid endometrial cancer. Note that, in comparison with Figure 10.4, patients are generally recommended less aggressive treatment due to the information given by appropriate surgical staging. LVI, lymphovascular invasion.

vaginal recurrence at 5 years (Figure 10.6), vaginal brachytherapy will be indicated (Figure 10.5). In fact, the effectiveness of vaginal brachytherapy in preventing vaginal recurrence has been demonstrated.[33] In our series, deep myometrial invasion (stage IC) per se is not a risk factor for vaginal recurrence, and is probably a surrogate marker for LVI or grade 3.[33]

Considering patients with stage IC endometrioid tumor with myometrial invasion ≥ 66% and negative nodes, we observed a 34% risk of distant failure at 5 years in our series (Table 10.9)[22] and a 10–16% risk in the literature.[3,40,41] For this reason, we advocate systemic therapy in this subgroup of patients (Figure 10.5).

Patients with stage II endometrioid tumor and documented negative lymph nodes who have not been treated with external radiotherapy

Table 10.11 Recurrence after lymphadenectomy in moderate- and high-risk node-negative endometrial cancer patients not receiving whole-pelvic radiotherapy

Ref	Patients (n)	Mean no. of lymph nodes	Postop BT[a]	Mean follow-up (months)	No. of recurrences	Site of recurrences
26	22	28	Yes	34	1	1 lung
						3 liver (+1 abdominal)
4	115	24	Yes	39	6	3 lung (+1 periurethral + 1 scapular)
27	105	—[b]	No	43	8	4 vagina[c]
						4 lung
						2 abdomen
28	63[d]	33	Yes	96	5[e]	1 clitoris
						1 lung
						1 unknown
Total	305				20 (6.6%)	15 distant (4.9%)
						4 vaginal[c] (1.3%)
						1 unknown (0.3%)

[a]Postoperative vaginal brachytherapy.
[b]Systematic pelvic and right aortic node dissection.
[c]All salvaged to date with radiotherapy.
[d]Personal communication with authors.
[e]Three of 5 serous papillary or clear cell.
Modified from Podratz et al. Gynecol Oncol 1998;70:163–4[2] with permission from Elsevier.

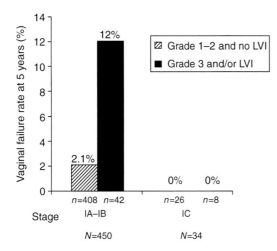

Figure 10.6 Vaginal relapse in stage I endometrioid endometrial cancer by risk group. Only patients who did not receive adjuvant radiotherapy were considered. The histogram shows the percentage of patients who had vaginal relapse according to substage (IA–IB vs IC), presence of lymphovascular invasion (LVI), and histologic grade (1–2 vs 3). Note that only patients with endometrioid tumor were considered. For three patients, no information was available about the depth of myometrial invasion or histologic grade; also, no information was available about the administration of adjuvant radiotherapy to two patients. Reprinted from Mariani et al. Gynecol Oncol 2005, 97: 820–7[33] with permission from Elsevier.

have a 1.5% risk of pelvic sidewall failure and a 1.5% risk of vaginal failure if 75% of them are managed with vaginal brachytherapy (Table 10.12). For this reason, we do not advocate the use of external radiotherapy, but we believe that patients with cervical invasion can possibly benefit from vaginal brachytherapy (Figure 10.5).

Considering four series including 66 stage II patients with endometrioid histology and negative nodes, no distant recurrences were noted.[40,42–44] In three other series of patients who had lymph node dissection, distant recurrences were reported in 2–12% of cases (Table 10.13).[45–47] One series documents an extremely high (27%) distant recurrence rate (14% rate of para-aortic recurrences). However, this study included patients with non-endometrioid tumors and those with incomplete surgical staging or only 'lymph node sampling'.[48]

In Table 10.13, distant recurrences in patients with stage II (negative nodes) endometrioid endometrial cancer are summarized. The overall rate of distant recurrences is 6%, with approximately one-third of patients being treated with external pelvic radiotherapy. Histologic grade, LVI, and depth of myometrial

Table 10.12 Local recurrences in stage II endometrioid endometrial cancer (negative nodes) and no postoperative external radiotherapy or chemotherapy

Ref	Patients (n)	Follow-up (months)	Vaginal brachytherapy	Local recurrences
45	26	60	5 (19%)	1 pelvic sidewall
47	15	74	6 (40%)	1 pelvic sidewall + 1 vaginal
48	8	40	8 (100%)	0
49	22	53	22 (100%)	0
42	15	40	12 (80%)	0
40	21	65	21 (100%)	1 vaginal
43	10	28	10 (100%)	0
44	15	36	15 (100%)	0
Total	132		99 (75%)	2 vaginal (1.5%)
				2 pelvic sidewall (1.5%)

Table 10.13 Distant recurrences in patients with stage II (negative nodes) endometrioid endometrial cancer

Ref	Patients (n)	Follow-up (months)	Median no. of lymph nodes dissected[a]	ERT/BT/both[b]	Distant recurrences[c]
45	48	60	26	22/5/0	6 (12.5%)[d]
47	48[e]	74	12 p	13/6/20	1 (2%)[f]
			3 pa		
46	42[g]	56	NA	—[h]	5 (12%)[i]
42	20	40	8 p	0/12/5	0
			0 pa		
40	21	65	>12	0/21/0	0
43	10	28	28 p	0/10/0	0
			12.5 pa		
44	15	36	23	0/15/0	0
Total	204			35 (22%)/69 (43%)/25 (15%)	12 (6%)
				Total radiotherapy 129 (80%)[j]	

[a]Pelvic (p), para-aortic (pa), or both. NA, not available.
[b]ERT, pelvic external radiotherapy; BT, brachytherapy.
[c]Outside vagina/pelvis.
[d]5 hematogenous (lung, liver, bone, brain); 1 carcinomatosis.
[e]6 patients had nonendometrioid tumor.
[f]Liver and lung, adenosquamous histologic subtype.
[g]8 patients had nonendometrioid histologic subtype.
[h]86% of the overall population of 63 patients (including also those with inadequate surgical staging) had external pelvic radiotherapy, or vaginal brachytherapy, or both.
[i]2 abdomen, 3 hematogenous (lung and bone).
[j]Excluding the 42 patients[46] with information not available.

invasion can be used to identify patients at risk of distant extrapelvic dissemination who may potentially benefit from adjuvant systemic chemotherapy.[45,46,48] In one series,[46] 16% of patients with invasion of the outer third of the myometrium had hematogenous dissemination of the disease.

Similarly to patients with stage I tumor (negative nodes), we elected to use the depth of myometrial invasion as a risk factor for distant hematogenous dissemination also in those patients with adequate surgical staging, negative nodes and cervical involvement (Figure 10.5). However, the role of adjuvant systemic chemotherapy in appropriately staged endometrioid stage II endometrial cancer remains uncertain.

In summary, there is an exigent need for a paradigm shift in the management of endometrial cancer. The continuing debate as to whether to perform lymphadenectomy versus radiotherapy is indicative of a modality-based approach to treating this disease as opposed to disease-based care pathways. Based on the above data, 25% of women with endometrial cancer at this referral center are not candidates for lymph node dissection. The remaining 75% are managed with a systematic lymph node dissection up to the renal vessels (Table 10.10).[11] Given that the GOG 99 study (with lymph node sampling)[20] and the PORTEC study (without assessment of lymph nodes)[21] have similar pelvic failure rates in the absence of radiotherapy,[39] lymph node sampling appears to be equivalent to the omission of nodal assessment. Furthermore, patients with pelvic or para–aortic nodal involvement, or those at risk for such in the absence of a formal node dissection, would appear to benefit not only from pelvic but also from extended-field radiotherapy to the para-aortic area. Our data suggested a 47% rate of either involvement or subsequent failure in the para-aortic area with positive pelvic nodes.[29] Patients at risk for intraperitoneal or hematogenous dissemination may derive benefit from traditional algorithms that include systemic therapy. Considering that 36% of all patients in our population were at risk for failure (accounting for 89% of all failures) via one of the four routes of spread

and that 46% of these patients subsequently failed despite presumed state-of-the-art management, there is an urgent requirement for gynecologic oncologists to develop quality-improvement care pathways for this disease.[22] Assuming that 39 080 new endometrial cancer cases will be diagnosed in 2007, and based on the above assumptions, 14 069 patients (36%) would be at high risk for failure and 6472 (46% of patients at risk) would be anticipated to fail. This approaches the estimated 7400 deaths predicted to occur from corpus cancer during 2007.[1] The traditional modality-based approach to treatment must be replaced with a disease-based paradigm with innovative care pathways.

REFERENCES

1. American Cancer Society. Cancer Facts and Figures 2007. http://www.cancer.org/docroot/stt/stt_0.asp.

2. Podratz KC, Mariani A, Webb MJ. Staging and therapeutic value of lymphadenectomy in endometrial cancer. Gynecol Oncol 1998; 70:163–4.

3. Morrow CP, Bundy BN, Kurman RJ, et al. Relationship between surgical–pathological risk factors and outcome in clinical stage I and II carcinoma of the endometrium: a Gynecologic Oncology Group study. Gynecol Oncol 1991;40:55–65.

4. Orr JW, Holimon JL, Orr PF. Stage I corpus cancer: Is teletherapy necessary? Am J Obstet Gynecol 1997;176:777–88.

5. Schink JC, Rademaker AW, Miller DS, Lurain JR. Tumor size in endometrial cancer. Cancer 1991;67:2791–4.

6. Creasman WT, Morrow CP, Bundy BN, et al. Surgical pathologic spread patterns of endometrial cancer. A Gynecologic Oncology Group Study. Cancer 1987;60(Suppl): 2035–41.

7. Lampe B, Kurzl R, Hantschmann P. Prognostic factors that predict pelvic lymph node metastasis from endometrial carcinoma. Cancer 1994;74:2502–8.

8. Burghardt E, Pickel H. Local spread and lymph node involvement in cervical cancer. Obstet Gynecol 1978;52:138–45.

9. Elledge RM, McGuire WL, Osborne CK. Prognostic factors in breast cancer. Semin Oncol 1992;19:244–53.

10. Kamura T, Yahata H, Shigematsu T, et al. Predicting pelvic lymph node metastasis in endometrial carcinoma. Gynecol Oncol 1999;72:387–91.

11. Mariani A, Webb MJ, Keeney GL, et al. Low-risk corpus cancer: Is lymphadenectomy or radiotherapy necessary? Am J Obstet Gynecol 2000;182:1506–19.

12. Grignon DJ, Hammond EH. College of American Pathologists Conference XXVI on Clinical Relevance of Prognostic Markers in Solid Tumors. Report of the Prostate Cancer Working Group. Arch Pathol Lab Med 1995;119:1122–6.

13. Burke HB, Henson DE. Criteria for prognostic factors and for an enhanced prognostic system. Cancer 1993;72:3131–5.

14. Inoue Y, Obata K, Abe K, et al. The prognostic significance of vascular invasion by endometrial carcinoma. Cancer 1996;78:1447–51.

15. Wilson TO, Podratz KC, Gaffey TA, et al. Evaluation of unfavorable histologic subtypes in endometrial adenocarcinoma. Am J Obstet Gynecol 1990;162:418–23.

16. Fielding LP, Fenoglio-Preiser CM, Freedman LS. The future of prognostic factors in outcome prediction for patients with cancer. Cancer 1992;70:2367–77.

17. Podczaski E, Kaminski P, Gurski K. Detection and patterns of treatment failure in 300 consecutive cases of 'early' endometrial cancer after primary surgery. Gynecol Oncol 1992;47:323–7.

18. Maggino T, Romagnolo C, Bandoni F, et al. An analysis of approaches to the management of endometrial cancer in North America: a CTF study. Gynecol Oncol 1998;68:274–9.

19. Aalders J, Abeler V, Kolstad P, Onsrud M. Postoperative external irradiation and prognostic parameters in stage I endometrial carcinoma: clinical and histopathologic study of 540 patients. Obstet Gynecol 1980;56:419–27.

20. Keys HM, Roberts AJ, Brunetto VL, et al. A phase III trial of surgery with or without adjunctive external pelvic radiation therapy in intermediate risk endometrial adenocarcinoma: a Gynecologic Oncology Group study. Gynecol Oncol 2004;92:744–51.

21. Creutzberg CL, van Putten WL, Koper PC, et al. Surgery and postoperative radiotherapy versus surgery alone for patients with stage-1 endometrial carcinoma: multicentre randomized trial. Lancet 2000;355:1404–11.

22. Mariani A, Dowdy SC, Keeney GL, et al. High-risk endometrial cancer subgroups: candidates for target-based adjuvant therapy. Gynecol Oncol 2004;95:120–6.

23. Mariani A, Webb MJ, Keeney GL, et al. Hematogenous dissemination in corpus cancer. Gynecol Oncol 2001;80:233–8.

24. Mariani A, Webb MJ, Keeney GL, et al. Surgical stage I endometrial cancer: predictors of distant failure and death. Gynecol Oncol 2002;87:274–80.

25. Mariani A, Webb MJ, Keeney GL, et al. Predictors of lymphatic failure in endometrial cancer. Gynecol Oncol 2002;84:437–42.

26. Fanning J, Nanavati PJ, Hilgers RD. Surgical staging and high dose rate brachytherapy for endometrial cancer: limiting external radiotherapy to node-positive tumors. Obstet Gynecol 1996;87:1041–4.

27. Larson DM, Broste SK, Krawisz BR. Surgery without radiotherapy for primary treatment of endometrial cancer. Obstet Gynecol 1998;91:355–9.

28. Mohan DS, Samuels MA, Selim MA, et al. Long-term outcomes of therapeutic pelvic lymphadenectomy for stage I endometrial adenocarcinoma. Gynecol Oncol 1998;70:165–71.

29. Mariani A, Keeney GL, Aletti G, et al. Endometrial carcinoma: Paraaortic dissemination. Gynecol Oncol 2004;92:833–8.

30. Mariani A, Dowdy SC, Cliby WA, et al. Efficacy of systematic lymphadenectomy and adjuvant radiotherapy in node-positive endometrial cancer patients. Gynecol Oncol 2006;101:200–8.

31. Mundt AJ, McBride R, Rotmensch J, et al. Significant pelvic recurrence in high-risk pathologic stage I–IV endometrial carcinoma patients after adjuvant chemotherapy alone: implications for adjuvant radiation therapy. Int J Radiat Oncol Biol Phys 2001;50:1145–53.

32. Mariani A, Webb MJ, Keeney GL, et al. Endometrial cancer: predictors of peritoneal failure. Gynecol Oncol 2003;89:236–42.

33. Mariani A, Dowdy SC, Keeney GL, et al. Predictors of vaginal relapse in stage I endometrial cancer. Gynecol Oncol 2005;97:820–7.

34. Orr Jr JW, Roland PY, Leichter D, Orr PF. Endometrial cancer: is surgical staging necessary? Curr Opin Oncol 2001;13:408–12.

35. Munstedt K, von Georgi R, Misselwitz B, et al. Centralizing surgery for gynecologic oncology: a strategy assuring better quality treatment? Gynecol Oncol 2003;89:4–8.

36. Corn BW, Dunton CJ, Carlson JA, et al. National trends in the surgical staging of corpus cancer: a pattern-of-practice survey. Obstet Gynecol 1997;90:628–31.

37. Mariani A, Cliby WA, Gostout BS, et al. Histologic risk factors for lymphatic or intraperitoneal dissemination in inadequately staged endometrioid endometrial cancer. Presented at the 37th Annual Meeting of the Society of Gynecologic Oncologists, Palm Springs, March 2006.

38. Randall ME, Filiaci VL, Muss H, et al. Randomized phase III trial of whole-abdominal irradiation versus doxorubicin and cisplatin chemotherapy in advanced endometrial carcinoma: a Gynecologic Oncology Group study. J Clin Oncol 2006;24:36–44.

39. Creutzberg CL. GOG-99: ending the controversy regarding pelvic radiotherapy for endometrial carcinoma? Gynecol Oncol 2004;92:740–3.

40. Horowitz NS, Peters WA III, Smith MR, et al. Adjuvant high dose rate vaginal brachytherapy as treatment of stage I and II endometrial carcinoma. Obstet Gynecol 2002;99:235–40.

41. DiSaia PJ, Creasman WT, Boronow RC, Blessing JA. Risk factors and recurrent patterns in stage I endometrial cancer. Am J Obstet Gynecol 1985;151:1009–15.

42. Rittenberg PV, Lotocki RJ, Heywood MS, Krepart GV. Stage II endometrial carcinoma: limiting post-operative radiotherapy to the vaginal vault in node-negative tumors. Gynecol Oncol 2005;98:434–8.

43. Lo KW, Cheung TH, Yu MY, et al. The value of pelvic and para-aortic lymphadenectomy in endometrial cancer to avoid unnecessary radiotherapy. Int J Gynecol Cancer 2003;13:863–9.

44. Ng TY, Nicklin JL, Perrin LC, et al. Postoperative vaginal vault brachytherapy for node-negative stage II (occult) endometrial carcinoma. Gynecol Oncol 2001;81:193–5.

45. Ayhan A, Taskiran C, Celik C, Yuce K. The long-term survival of women with surgical stage II endometrioid type endometrial cancer. Gynecol Oncol 2004;93:9–13.

46. Feltmate CM, Duska LR, Chang Y, et al. Predictors of recurrence in surgical stage II endometrial adenocarcinoma. Gynecol Oncol 1999;73:407–11.

47. Eltabbakh GH, Moore AD. Survival of women with surgical stage II endometrial cancer. Gynecol Oncol 1999;74:80–5.

48. Calvin DP, Connell PP, Rotmensch J, et al. Surgery and postoperative radiation therapy in stage II endometrial carcinoma. Am J Clin Oncol 1999;22:338–43.

49. Fanning J. Long-term survival of intermediate risk endometrial cancer (stage IG3, IC, II) treated with full lymphadenectomy and brachytherapy without teletherapy. Gynecol Oncol 2001;82:371–4.

Molecular prognostic and predictive factors in advanced endometrial cancer: implications for therapy

11

Grainger S Lanneau and D Scott McMeekin

INTRODUCTION

Endometrial cancer is the most common gynecologic cancer. Nearly 80% of the estimated 40 000 patients per year diagnosed with endometrial cancer present with disease confined to the uterus, and have an excellent prognosis.[1] Despite this, advanced and recurrent disease account for an estimated 7400 deaths per year, making endometrial cancer the eighth leading cause of cancer death in woman. In 2001, the US National Cancer Institute (NCI) convened an expert panel to develop a national 5-year plan for research priorities in gynecologic cancers. The resulting report, Priorities of the Gynecologic Cancer Progress Review Group (PRG),[2] specified that understanding tumor biology was the central key toward controlling gynecologic cancers. For endometrial cancer, one of the top research priorities defined by the PRG was to identify prognostic and predictive markers for treatment efficacy and toxicity. As we enter a molecular age of cancer therapy, specific factors that distinguish those at risk for recurrence and death, and factors that predict response to therapies, must be defined.

CLINICAL–PATHOLOGIC FACTORS

Our current understanding of prognostic factors is largely related to clinical variables (age, race, and performance status) and pathologic factors identified following surgery. The extent of extrauterine disease, as reflected in the surgical staging of endometrial cancer, is the most important prognostic factor. For example, patients with surgical stage I disease have a 5-year survival rate of 87%, whereas the 5-year survival rates for patients with nodal metastases (stage IIIC) or abdominal or distant disease spread (stage IVB) are 32% and 5%, respectively.[3] Tumor-specific factors such as grade, cell type, depth of myometrial invasion, presence of lymphovascular space involvement (LVSI), and volume of residual disease have been associated with prognosis in several studies. The Gynecologic Oncology Group (GOG) has demonstrated relationships between tumor characteristics (grade and depth of myometrial invasion) and extrauterine spread in a large prospective study of patients with disease clinically confined to the uterus.[4] In the absence of pathologic risk factors, negative LVSI, cytology/adnexal spread, lymph nodes, or gross disease outside the uterus, the GOG found that the risk of recurrence was only 8%.[5] Depending on the number of risk factors present, recurrence rates with one, two, and three positive factors were 20%, 40%, and 63%, respectively. For patients with advanced or recurrent cancers treated with chemotherapy, the GOG has found poorer performance status, treatment of recurrent disease (compared with advanced disease), non-white race, and clear cell and papillary serous histologic types to be independent predictors of poorer survival.[6] The prognostic information derived from clinical and pathologic information has withstood the test of time and has proven itself to be clinically useful and relevant. Molecular markers that act as surrogates for tumor grade or histologic type will have limited utility.

TYPE I AND II ENDOMETRIAL CANCERS: A MODEL FOR DISCUSSION

One of the paradigms for bridging the gap between clinical–pathologic prognostic factors and molecular ones can be seen in the relatively simple, yet attractive classification system of endometrial cancers suggested by Bokhman[7] (Table 11.1). Endometrial cancers are thought to broadly arise from one of two different pathways: estrogen-dependent or estrogen-independent. Based on the clinical and histologic features, endometrial cancers have been divided into type I and type II tumors. Type I tumors are more common (85%), tend to be found in younger women, and develop via a precursor lesion of atypical hyperplasia. These tumors are associated with a predisposing history of hyperestrogenism. They tend to be well differentiated and have minimal myometrial invasion, and as a result typically have a favorable outcome. Type II tumors account for a small percentage of endometrial carcinomas, occur in an older population, and frequently develop in the face of an atrophic endometrium. About half of all relapses occur in this group. Papillary serous (PS), clear cell, and perhaps grade 3 tumors fit into the type II category. Despite the broad generalizations of the two categories,

Table 11.1 Comparison between type I and type II endometrial cancers

	Type I	*Type II*
Clinical features[7]		
Risk factors	Unopposed estrogen	Age
Race	White>Black	White=Black
Differentiation	Well differentiated	Poorly differentiated
Histology	Endometrioid	Nonendometrioid
Stage	I/II	III/IV
Prognosis	Favorable	Not favorable
Molecular features[8]		
Ploidy	Diploid	Aneuploid
KRAS overexpression	Yes	Yes
HER2/neu (ERBB2) overexpression	No	Yes
TP53 overexpression	No	Yes
PTEN mutations	Yes	No
Microsatellite instability	Yes	No

Reprinted from Kufe DW, Pollock RE, Weichselbaum RR, eds. Cancer Medicine, 6th edn. Hamilton, Ontario: BC Decker, 2003.

translational science data lends support for a separation into these groups at a molecular level. For example, mutations of *TP53* are common in uterine papillary serous carcinoma (UPSC), and rare in type I tumors. In type I tumors, *PTEN* mutations are common, but are rare with UPSC. Global gene expression profiles by have also been shown to differ between type I and II tumors.[9]

Environmental factors play an important role in endometrial carcinoma, and its increasing frequency has been attributed to dietary and hormonal factors as well as an aging population. Carcinogenesis in endometrial cancer is preceded by successive stages of initiation, promotion, and progression. Each step involves morphologic, biochemical, and cytologic changes that result from various cellular gene interactions. Molecular-based evidence suggests that carcinogenesis of the endometrium evolves through several different pathways. Tumors arise by the accumulation of inherited and somatic alterations in genes important for growth, regulation, angiogenesis, invasion, and metastasis. A variety of specific genetic alterations have been described in endometrial cancer, and their understanding will be the key to better diagnostics and treatment (Table 11.2).[10,11] As most patients with endometrial cancer have early-stage disease, much of the information about prognostic and predictive factors have come from study in patients with early-stage disease. Less is known specifically about patients with advanced-stage disease.

HORMONE RECEPTOR STATUS

Just as molecular markers may be associated with prognosis, molecular findings may also predict whether or not particular tumors are more or less likely to respond to a particular therapy.

Despite the development of several targeted biologic agents for treatment of cancer, it has been challenging to define which targets are relevant. Clinical trials have shown that the mere presence of a target does not guarantee that tumor growth can be inhibited by inhibition of the target. Hormonal status was amongst the first biologic markers to be predictive of response in the treatment of endometrial cancer. As early as 1951, Kelley observed that endometrial cancers were sensitive to progesterone. The GOG has completed several studies evaluating the role of hormonal therapy in patients with advanced and recurrent disease. In one study with 331 women, the response rate to 150 mg/day medroxyprogesterone acetate (MPA) was 18%, and in another study, using megestrol acetate (MA) at 800 mg/day, the response rate was 24%.[12,13] A subsequent study compared MPA at 200 or 1000 mg/day in 299 patients. The response rate to low-dose therapy was 25%, versus 15% with the higher-dose regimen.[14] The duration of response ranged from 2.5 to 3.2 months.

The presence of estrogen and progestin receptors in tumors has been thought to be associated with a greater likelihood of response to hormonal agents. For example, in the GOG trial comparing high- and low-dose MPA, for all patients, the response rate for progestin receptor (PR)-negative tumors was 8%, versus 37% when PR was positive ($p < 0.001$). Likewise, when primary tumors were estrogen receptor (ER)-negative, the response rate was 7%, versus 26% when tumors were ER-positive ($p < 0.005$). Tumor grade appears to be a surrogate for receptor status and response, with 37% grade 1, 23% grade 2, and 9% grade 3 tumors having a response to MPA (Table 11.3). The extent to which receptor status is prognostic is uncertain. Kadar et al[15] showed that in early-stage disease, increasing concentrations of

Table 11.2 Genetic changes associated with endometrial cancer

Gene	Function	Mechanism	Frequency[a]
KRAS	Oncogene	• Mutation	10–30%
HER2/neu (ERBB2)	Oncogene	• Amplification	10–20%
TP53	Tumor suppressor	• Mutation	• Mutation 10–20%
		• Deletion	• Deletion 30%
		• Other	• Overexpression 20–30%
CDKN1A (p21$^{Wafl/Cip1}$)	Tumor suppressor	• Via p53	• Loss of expression 15–40%
		• Other mechanisms	
PTEN/MMAC1	Tumor suppressor	• Mutation (germline, somatic)	• Germline in Cowden's disease
		• Deletions	• Sporodic forms:
		• Methylation	deletion/mutation 30–50%
			methylation 20%
			loss of expression 10–15%
MLH1	DNA repair	• Mutation	• Germline mutation
		• Methylation	frequent in HNPCC families
			• Methylation 71–92% of sporadic
			tumors showing MSI
			• Loss of expression 10–15%
MSH2	DNA repair	• Mutation	• Germline mutation in
		• Methylation	HNPCC families
			• Methylation infrequent in
			sporadic forms
			• Loss of expression 15–20%
MSH6	DNA repair	• Mutation	• Germline mutation in
			HNPCC families
			• Loss of expression 10–15%
CDKN2A (p16^{INK4A}, p14^{ARF})	Tumor suppressor	• Mutation	• Mutation, deletion,
		• Deletion	methylation 2–6%
		• Methylation	• Loss of expression 20–70%

[a]HNPCC, hereditary nonpolyposis colorectal cancer; MSI, microsatellite instability.
Adapted from Salvesen HB, Akslen LA. APMIS 2002;110:673–89.[11]

ER and PR were associated with survival, with PR being an independent predictor for survival in a multivariate analysis. It is unknown if ER/PR status is an independent predictor of survival in patients with advanced or recurrent disease, however.

A more sophisticated understanding of hormonal status is evolving. For example, PR downregulation has been noted with chronic exposure to progestins, and this may explain the short duration of response noted in clinical trials.

It has been observed that estrogens (including tamoxifen) increase PR concentrations, and it has been hypothesized that estrogenic stimulation in combination with progestins may counterbalance PR downregulation. The GOG conducted two phase II studies in patients with advanced or recurrent endometrial cancer which added tamoxifen to progestin therapy.[16,17] In one trial, 27% of patients had a response with the sequential use of MA for 3 weeks, followed by 3 weeks

Table 11.3 Relationship between grade of tumor and response to progestins

Ref	Treatment[a]	Grade	n	Response rate (%)
18	Various progestins	1	10	40
		2	71	15
		3	73	2
13	MA 800 mg/d	1	14	37 (grade 1–2)
		2	17	—
		3	27	8
14	MPA 200 mg/d vs	1	59	37
	1000 mg/d	2	113	23
		3	127	9
16	Tam 40 mg/d + alternating	1	15	Overall 33
	wkly MP 200 mg/d	2	17	
		3	27	
17	MA 160 mg/d × 3 wks	1	16	38
	alternating with Tam	2	17	24
	40 mg/d × 3 wks	3	22	22

[a]MA, megestrol acetate; MPA, medroxyprogesterone acetate; Tam, tamoxifen.

of tamoxifen. In the second, a 33% response rate was observed when alternating weekly cycles of MPA were added to daily tamoxifen treatment.

In the setting of recurrent disease, most data on tumor ER/PR status have been determined from the primary tumor (Figure 11.1). Whether or not receptors are present at the same concentrations or remain functional in primary versus recurrent disease, or at metastatic sites, is unknown. In the GOG studies, response to progestins was not shown to be different in patients with advanced versus recurrent disease or based on site of recurrence. In one study using alternating tamoxifen and MA, the response rate for extrapelvic disease was 31%, compared with 14% in patients with disease limited to the pelvis, however.[17]

PRs have been separated into two major isoforms: PRA and PRB. These isoforms are differentially expressed and have different functions.[19] In endometrial cancers, PRA may induce cell senescence and PRB a secretory phenotype.

In vitro experiments suggest that PRB may be more important for growth inhibition. In poorly differentiated tumors, PRB is more commonly lost. In one series, patients with PRB-negative tumors had poorer survival than those positive for PRB.[20] Whether or not a

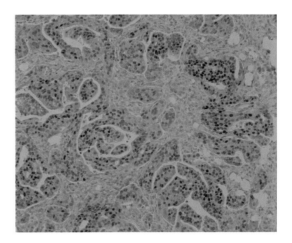

Figure 11.1 ER immunohistochemical staining of an endometrioid tumor. Photo provided by Dr Rosemary Zuna, University of Oklahoma, Oklahoma City, OK.

particular progestin isoform will be more or less likely associated with response to hormonal manipulation remains to be seen.

DNA MISMATCH REPAIR

The human genome is punctuated with repetitive nucleotides sequences or 'microsatellites'. These repetitive di-, tri-, and tetranucleotides are frequently located between genes and have been classified as 'junk DNA'. The highly polymorphic microsatellite DNA is composed of repetitive 2–6 base-pairs of variable size, with an estimated 35 000–100 000 copies in the human genome.[21] Cancers may arise through multiple frameshift mutations in microsatellite sequences throughout the genome. These mutations result from defects in replication error repair of repeated sequences. On a molecular basis, alterations of DNA mismatch repair affect 20% of endometrial cancers, predominantly in type I tumors. Germline mutations of one of the mismatch repair genes *MSH2*, *MLH1*, or *MSH6* are associated with hereditary endometrial cancers, whereas promoter hypermethylation of *MLH1* appears to be associated with sporadic cancers. These changes are thought to be the earliest genetic event in endometrial carcinogenesis. Mutated or inactivated mismatch repair genes lead to accumulations of single base-pair mismatches, as well as insertions or deletions in tandem repeats. Genomic instability and accumulation of subsequent mutations in cancer-related genes such as *PTEN* or *KRAS* may result from microsatellite instability.

Studies have also noted dual pathways that demonstrate microsatellite stability and instability (MSI) in endometrial carcinomas. Germline mutations of mismatch repair genes occur in patients with hereditary nonpolyposis colorectal cancer (HNPCC).[22] Endometrial cancer is the most common extracolonic neoplasia associated with women affected by HNPCC, and MSI has been demonstrated in both familial and sporadic forms. These carcinomas are clinically related to type I tumors, since they occur at a younger age, and are histologically mucinous or endometrioid.[23] In one large series, 94% of tumors with MSI were of endometrioid type, compared with 23% that were nonendometrioid ($p = 0.001$).[24] Tumors with MSI display a high background of genetic instability, tend to be diploid, occur via the p53-independent pathway, and involve loss of *MLH1* expression. A second pathway thought to be related to sporadic cases of endometrial cancer is hypermethylation of the *MLH1* promoter, which causes gene inactivation through a 'second hit' in cells already carrying a gene mutation or deletion.[25] Tumors with hypermethylation of the *MLH1* promoter occur via a distinct pathway of endometrial carcinogenesis separate from aneuploidy or p53 disturbances.[26,27] Black et al[24] compared 93 endometrial cancers with MSI to 380 tumors without MSI. While patients with MSI-positive tumors had a trend toward more advanced cancers and deeper myometrial invasion, disease-free and disease-specific survival were poorer with MSI-negative tumors. Response to a particular therapy does not seem to be related to MSI status.

PTEN

PTEN (phosphatase and tensin homolog deleted on chromosome 10) is the most frequently altered gene in endometrial carcinoma. *PTEN* mutations are thought to be an early event in endometrial carcinogenesis, with 30–50% of endometrial cancers having a mutation.[28] *PTEN* has been mapped to chromosome 10q23, and is thought to function as a tumor suppressor gene. It is involved in focal adhesion, regulation, cellular migration, and tumor cell proliferation.[29] It is expressed most highly in an estrogen-rich environment. Progestins affect *PTEN* expression and promote involution of *PTEN*-mutated endometrial cells in various histopathologic settings.[30] Patients with *PTEN*-related endometrial cancers typically have type I tumors, have nonmetastatic disease, and are felt to have a more favorable prognosis.[31] In a study of 98 patients, the prognostic significance of *PTEN* expression (suggesting active *PTEN*) was assessed in patients with node-positive endometrial cancer.[32] The survival rate was significantly higher for *PTEN*-expressing tumors (48-month survival rate 63% for *PTEN*-positive vs 30% for *PTEN*-negative). The survival difference was most pronounced when chemotherapy was used, with the 48-month survival rates for *PTEN*-positive and *PTEN*-negative tumors being 80% and 30%, respectively. Expression of *PTEN* was an independent predictor of survival. These data suggest that *PTEN* expression is a favorable prognostic factor, and may also be predictive of response.

An important component of the *PTEN* pathway is the mammalian target of rapamycin (mTOR). Loss of PTEN protein function leads to activation of Akt, which leads to upregulation of mTOR. mTOR regulates the production of proteins critical for cell growth and division via activation of S6 ribosomal protein kinase1 and inhibition of the eIF4E inhibitor 4E-BP1. mTOR inhibits the turnover of cyclin D1, and stimulates the elimination of the cyclin-dependent kinase (cdk) inhibitor p27^{Kip1}.[29] Therefore, mTOR controls processes required for cell growth and division. In a variety of cancer cell lines, inhibition of mTOR by rapamycin and rapamycin analogs induces a phenotype similar to that induced by nutrient starvation, with G_1 arrest, reduction in cell size, and downregulation of protein synthesis.

Slomovitz et al[33] performed immunohistochemical staining of endometrial cancers from 95 patients, and found phosphorylated mTOR (p-mTOR) to be expressed in 53% of cancers. Primary endometrioid and PS tumors and recurrent tumors stained for p-mTOR similarly. Based on in vitro and early clinical data, mTOR inhibitors are being studied in patients with persistent or recurrent endometrial cancer. Recent data suggest that mTOR inhibitors such as rapamycin are able to restore tamoxifen response in tamoxifen-resistant MCF-7 breast cancer cells.[34] Demonstration of expression of mTOR in advanced endometrial cancers has not been an eligibility criteria in ongoing clinical trials with mTOR inhibitors. As such, it is not known if mTOR expression is sufficient for response. Currently, the use of mTOR as a prognostic indicator is premature.

TP53

Mutations in the *TP53* tumor suppressor gene (encoding the p53 protein) have been suggested to be among the most common genetic change in cancers. p53 enables cells to repair themselves after DNA damage and acts as a check on cell proliferation during stressful events. Ultimately, *TP53* acts as a tumor suppressor gene essential for cell cycle arrest and programmed cell death.[35] In endometrial cancer, *TP53* mutations are relatively uncommon, being found in only 10–20% of cancers. *TP53* mutation is more commonly observed in PS histologic types, is thought to be a late event in type I endometrial cancers, and is rarely found in endometrial hyperplasia.

Several studies have suggested that *TP53* mutation is a prognostic factor associated with aggressive histologic subtypes and poor prognosis.[36–38] Mutated *TP53* is thought to lead to accumulation of a more stable p53 protein, which frequently can be observed to accumulate and be observed with immunohistochemical (IHC) staining of tumors (commonly referred to as 'overexpression') (Figure 11.2). There is debate as to how closely IHC staining of p53 protein reflects actual mutations at a DNA level. In a study evaluating 44 patients with and 44 patients without recurrence, overexpression by IHC was significantly associated with recurrent endometrial carcinoma in stage I disease (odds ratio 3.8; 95% confidence interval (CI) 1.5–9.8), independently of tumor grade and myometrial invasion.[38] It is uncertain as to the predictive effect of p53 overexpression on different treatments in endometrial cancer. In one series of 59 patients with endometrioid tumors, *TP53* mutation was associated with poorer survival, but radiation improved survival in the group with *TP53* mutations, suggesting a possible predictive role.[39]

HER2/neu (ERBB2)

HER2/neu (also known as *ERBB2*) is a proto-oncogene that encodes the transmembrane growth factor receptor p185^{ErbB-2}, which is a

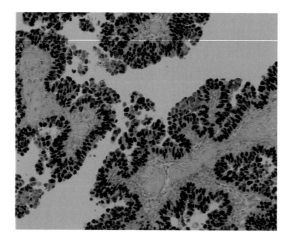

Figure 11.2 p53 immunohistochemical staining of a serous tumor. Photo provided by Dr Rosemary Zuna, University of Oklahoma, Oklahoma City, OK.

receptor tyrosine kinase structurally similar to the epidermal growth factor receptor (EGFR).[40] Abnormal expression of *HER2* is commonly observed in a variety of primary tumors, suggesting that its overexpression may contribute to tumorigenesis. *HER2* overexpression has been identified in 25–30% of breast cancers, 10–30% of ovarian carcinomas, and 10–15% of endometrial cancers.[41,42] In endometrial cancer, one study found that overexpression was identified in 27% of patients with metastatic disease, compared with 4% of those with disease limited to the uterus.[43] An inverse relationship between *HER2* and PR expression was also noted. The GOG evaluated 273 patients with advanced or recurrent disease participating in a phase III chemotherapy trial, and found that 15% of patients had gene amplification.[44]

Trastuzumab (Herceptin) is a monoclonal antibody that targets the receptor p185^{ErbB-2}. Like PRs as a predictor of response for progestational agents, *HER2* is required for activity of trastuzumab. In breast cancer, as a single agent, trastuzumab produced a modest response rate of 15%, with higher responses noted when it was used in combination with chemotherapy in those heavily pretreated and with metastatic disease. The GOG has presented preliminary results of a phase II study with trastuzumab in patients with advanced or recurrent endometrial cancer, and observed no objective responses in 23 patients.[45] Of note, using eligibility criteria that required tumors to have two- to threefold overexpression by IHC (Herceptest) or gene amplification by fluorescence in situ hybridization (FISH), only 7 of 23 were FISH-positive. In many, but not all, cases, *HER2* overexpression is due to gene amplification. It has been shown that response to trastuzumab is particularly related to amplification of the *HER2* gene, rather than overexpression demonstrated by IHC staining of tumors. Given this finding, and the initial low response rate seen with trastuzumab, the GOG has modified eligibility of the phase II trial to now include only those patients with amplification of *HER2* as seen with FISH.

Patients with PS histology may have a greater frequency of *HER2* overexpression.[46] Slomovitz et al[47] evaluated 68 patients with PS tumors for *HER2* overexpression and amplification. In multivariate analysis, lymph node status and *HER2* overexpression by IHC were the only factors associated with decreased overall survival (p <0.05). Gene amplification of *HER2* was rare. In another study evaluating 483 patients with tissue microarrays, *HER2* amplification was seen in 29% of serous, 15% of grade 3, 3% of grade 2, and 1% of grade 1 endometrioid cancers.[48] By multivariate analysis *HER2* overexpression (by IHC) in the presence of *HER2* amplification (by FISH) correlated with poorer survival, with a hazard ratio of 2.3 (95% CI 1.25–5.32). *HER2* appears to be an important prognostic factor in a small population of endometrial cancer patients.

GENE EXPRESSION PROFILES

While individual molecular changes that relate to prognosis have been identified, broad surveys of patterns of overall gene expression have been suggested to have utility in defining different patient populations.[49] For example, gene expression profiling using cDNA microarray technology has shown different patterns of gene expression between normal and malignant endometrium, type I and type II endometrial cancers, and serous, endometrioid, and clear cell histologies from ovarian and endometrial cancers.[8,50,51] Array technology has also been used to define prognosis in breast, ovarian,

and endometrial cancers. In one study of 75 patients with early-stage endometrial cancer, risk of recurrence could be predicted based on a gene expression-based risk score.[52] No single gene or signature gene list correlated with recurrence; however, a risk score could be created based on genes most associated with recurrence. The high-risk pattern was independent of other well-known clinicopathologic risk factors. This study was weakened by a lack of uniform surgical staging. This makes the relevance of genetic/molecular markers compared with standard surgical prognostic factors more difficult to interpret. Gene expression arrays have also been predictive of response in breast and ovarian cancers. For example, Hartman et al[53] identified a 14-gene predictive model that had a 95% positive predictive value for early relapse after paclitaxel/platinum chemotherapy in patients with ovarian cancer. Similar data to predict response to chemotherapy have yet to be developed for endometrial cancers.

ANGIOGENESIS

In 2004, Hurwitz et al[54] showed a significant increase in progression-free survival and survival in previously untreated metastatic colorectal cancer patients who were treated with a vascular endothelial growth factor (VEGF) antibody, bevacizumab, plus chemotherapy, as compared with chemotherapy plus placebo. These findings provided clinical proof of the utility of antiangiogenic therapy in cancer treatments. VEGF is a potent regulator of angiogenesis, and sustained VEGF production by tumor and surrounding stroma is thought to be crucial in establishing the angiogenic process. In endometrial cancer, tumor microvessel density (MVD) counts have been used as a surrogate measure for angiogenic activity. Increased MVD counts have been shown in hyperplastic and malignant endometrium compared with normal controls, and correlate with increasing stage.[55] Salvesen et al[56] showed that the 5-year survival rate was 57% versus 90% in patients with higher versus lower MVD, and that MVD was an independent predictor of survival in a multivariate analysis.

IHC detection of cytoplasmic VEGF within tumors has been associated with prognosis in some, but not all, studies.[57,58] In one study of 228 patients, there was a correlation between VEGF expression and LVSI, nodal metastases, depth of myometrial invasion, and disease-free survival.[58] Patients with cancer have been shown to have significantly higher levels of serum VEGF than normal subjects. The measurement of circulating VEGF levels is a more feasible approach in the situation of recurrent or persistent endometrial cancer, where cancer tissue is not always available. Several studies using enzyme-linked immunosorbent assay (ELISA) of serum demonstrated significantly higher levels of circulating VEGF in endometrial cancer patients in comparison with healthy controls.[59] In one series of 53 patients, higher VEGF levels were associated with recurrence.[60] It has also been hypothesized that measuring VEGF levels in serum and plasma might reflect the efficacy of antiangiogenic therapies. In one study of 72 patients with endometrial cancer, circulating VEGF levels were associated with tumor stage, which decreased significantly after treatment, and then increased at clinical relapse.[61]

Data are mixed with regard to the prognostic and predictive roles of VEGF. For example, VEGF expression did not correlate with the incidence of metastases, recurrence, and survival in one study of 47 patients.[57] The reason for the discrepancies between studies may lie in the varying expression pattern of VEGF in early- versus late-stage endometrial cancer. VEGF is highly expressed in early-stage and well-differentiated uterine endometrial cancers, but is expressed at lower levels with advancement of clinical stage and dedifferentiation. In colorectal cancer, neither MVD nor VEGF expression proved to be predictive of response to bevacizumab, and the addition of the antibody to chemotherapy improved survival regardless of the expression of VEGF.[62]

CONCLUSIONS

A variety of clinical prognostic factors providing information to predict risk of recurrence or death exist in endometrial cancer. As our understanding of molecular and genetic changes of endometrial cancer continues to develop, any information about tumor biology must be balanced by what information is readily available from clinical–pathologic data. To date, mutations in *TP53*, *PTEN*, and *HER2* have shown prognostic significance in several studies. The extent to which prognostic information is independent of stage, grade, and histologic type remains to be seen. The extent of disease spread as reflected in the surgical stage remains the strongest predictor of survival in endometrial carcinoma. Better prognostic information is important, but predictive information as to how a tumor will or will not respond to potential therapies is most desired. Data derived from cDNA microarrays in combination with other high-throughput technologies will hopefully lead to better diagnostics and future treatments. The most well-developed predictive factor is hormone receptor status. For evolving targeted therapies, the presence of a marker may not be sufficient to see clinical activity. Surrogate measures for activity should be developed.

REFERENCES

1. American Cancer society. Cancer Facts and Figures 2007. http.//www.cancer.org/docroot/stt/stt_0. asp.

2. Priorities of the Gynecologic Cancer Progress Review Group. National Cancer Institute. http://planning.cancer.gov.pdfprgreports/gynreport.pdf, November 2001.

3. Creasman W, Odicino F, Maisonneuve P, et al. Carcinoma of the corpus uteri. J Epidem Biostat 1998;3:35–61.

4. Creasman WT, Morrow CP, Bundy BN, et al. Surgical pathologic spread patterns of endometrial cancer. Cancer 1987;60:2035–41.

5. Morrow CP, Bundy BN, Kurman RJ, et al. Relationship between surgical–pathological risk factors and outcome in clinical stage I and II carcinoma of the endometrium: a Gynecologic Oncology Group study. Gynecol Oncol 1991;40:55–65.

6. McMeekin DS, Filiaci VL, Thigpen T, et al. Importance of histology in advanced and recurrent endometrial cancer patients participating in 1st-line chemotherapy trials: a Gynecologic Oncology Group trial. Gynecol Oncol 2005;96:940–1 (Abst 69).

7. Bokhman JV. Two pathogenetic types of endometrial carcinoma. Gynecol Oncol 1983;15:10–17.

8. Berchuck A, Maxwell GL, Risinger JL. Genetic alterations in endometrial cancer. Hung J Gynecol Oncol 1997;2:153–7.

9. Cao QJ, Belbin T, Socci N, et al. Distinctive gene expression profiles by cDNA microarrays in endometrioid and serous carcinomas of the endometrium. Int J Gynecol Pathol 2004;23:321–9.

10. Berchuck A, Boyd J. Molecular basis of endometrial cancer. Cancer 1995;76:2034–40.

11. Salvesen HB, Akslen LA. Molecular pathogenesis and prognostic factors in endometrial cancer. APMIS 2002;110:673–89.

12. Thigpen T, Blessing J, DiSaia P. Oral medroxyprogesterone acetate in advanced or recurrent endometrial cancer: results of therapy and correlation with estrogen and progesterone levels: the Gynecologic Oncology Group experience. In: Baulier E, Iacobelli S, McGuire W, eds. Endocrinology and Malignancy. Carnforth, UK: Parthenon, 1986:446–54.

13. Lentz S, Brady M, Major F, et al. High-dose megestrol acetate in advanced or recurrent endometrial carcinoma: a Gynecologic Oncology Group study. J Clin Oncol 1996;14:357–61.

14. Thigpen T, Brady M, Alvarez R, et al. Oral medroxyprogesterone acetate in the treatment of advanced or recurrent endometrial carcinoma: a dose response study by the Gynecologic Oncology Group. J Clin Oncol 1999;17:1736–44.

15. Kadar N, Malfetano J, Homesley H. Steroid receptor concentrations in endometrial carcinoma: effect on survival in surgically staged patients. Gynecol Oncol 1993;50:281–6.

16. Whitney C, Brunetto V, Zaino R, et al. Phase II study of medroxyprogesterone acetate plus tamoxifen in advanced endometrial carcinoma: a Gynecologic Oncology Group study. Gynecol Oncol 2004;92:4–9.

17. Fiorica J, Brunetto V, Hanjani P, et al. Phase II trial of alternating courses of megestrol acetate and tamoxifen in advanced endometrial carcinoma: a Gynecologic Oncology Group study. Gynecol Oncol 2004;92:10–14.

18. Podratz K, O'Brien P, Malkasian G, et al. Effects of progestational agents in treatment of endometrial carcinoma. Obstet Gynecol 1985;66:106–10.

19. Leslie K, Stein MP, Kumar N, et al. Progesterone receptor isoform identification and subcellular localization in endometrial cancer. Gynecol Oncol 2005;96:32–41.

20. Miyamoto T, Watanabe J, Hata H, et al. Significance of progesterone receptor A and B expressions in endometrial adenocarcinoma. J Steroid Biochem Mol Biol 2004;92:111–18.

21. Jacks T, Weinberg A. Cell cycle control and its watchman. Nature 1996;381:643–4.

22. Lynch HT, de la Chapelle A. Hereditary colorectal cancer. N Engl J Med 2003;348:919–32.

23. Parc YR, Halling K, Burgart L, et al. Microsatellite instability and *hMLH1/hMLH2* expression in young endometrial carcinoma patients: association with family and histopathology. Int J Cancer 2000;86:60–6.

24. Black D, Soslow R, Levine D, et al. Clinicopathologic significance of defective DNA mismatch repair in endometrial cancer. J Clin Oncol 2006;24:1745–53.

25. Jones PA, Laird PW. Cancer epigenetics comes to age. Nat Genet 1999;21:163–7.

26. MacDonald ND, Salvesen HB, Ryan A, et al. Frequency and prognostic impact of microsatellite instability in a large population based study of endometrial carcinomas. Cancer Res 2000;60:1750–2.

27. Salvesen HB, MacDonald N, Ryan A, et al. Methylation of *hMLH1* in a population-based series of endometrial carcinomas. Clin Cancer Res 2000;6:3607–13.

28. Tashiro H, Blazes MS Wu R, et al. Mutation in *PTEN* are frequent in endometrial carcinomas but rare in other gynecologic malignancies. Cancer Res 1997;57:3935–40.

29. Sansal I, Sellers W. The biology and clinical relevance of the *PTEN* tumor suppressor pathway. J Clin Oncol 2004;22:2954–63.

30. Zheng W, Baker HE, Mutter GL. Involution of *PTEN*-null endometrial glands with progestin therapy. Gynecol Oncol 2004;92:1008–13.

31. Salvesen HB, Stefansson I, Kretzschmar EI, et al. Significance of *PTEN* alterations in endometrial carcinoma: a population-based study of mutations, promoter methylation and PTEN protein expression. Int J Oncol 2004;25:1615–23.

32. Kanamori Y, Kigawa J, Itamochi H, et al. *PTEN* expression is associated with prognosis for patients with advanced endometrial carcinoma undergoing postoperative chemotherapy. Int J Cancer 2002; 100:686–9.

33. Slomovitz BM, Wu W, Broaddus R, et al. mTOR inhibition is a rational target for the treatment of endometrial cancer. J Clin Oncol 2004;22:14S (Abst 5076).

34. Treeck O, Wackwitz B, Haus U, Ortmann O. Effect of a combined treatment with mTOR inhibitor RAD001 and tamoxifen in vitro on growth and apoptosis of human cancer cells. Gynecol Oncol 2006;102:292–9.

35. Levine AJ. p53, the cellular gatekeeper for growth and division. Cell 1997;88:323–31.

36. Pisani AL, Barbuta Da, Chen D, et al. Her-2/neu, p53, and DNA analysis as prognosticators for survival in endometrial carcinoma. Obstet Gynecol 1995;85:729–34.

37. Moll UM, Chalas E, Auguste M, et al. Uterine papillary serous carcinoma evolves via a p53 driven pathway. Hum Pathol 1996;27: 1295–1300.

38. Pijnenborg J, van de Broek L, Dam de Veen G, et al. *TP53* overexpression in recurrent endometrial carcinoma. Gynecol Oncol 2006;100:397–404.

39. Saffari B, Bernstein L, Hong DC, et al. Association of *p53* mutations and codon 72 single nucleotide polymorphism with lower overall survival and responsiveness to adjuvant radiotherapy in endometrioid endometrial carcinomas. Int J Gynecol Cancer 2005;15:952–63.

40. Akiyama T, Sudo C Ogawara H, et al. The product of the human c-erb-2 gene: a 185 kilodalton glycoprotein with tyrosine kinase activity. Science 1986;232:1644–6.

41. Slamon DJ, Godolphin W, Jones LA, et al. Studies of the Her-2/*neu* proto-oncogene in human breast and ovarian carcinoma. Science 1989;244:707–12.

42. Berchuck A, Kamel A, Whitaker R, et al. Overexpression of Her-2/*neu* is associated with poor survival in advanced epithelial ovarian cancer. Cancer Res 1990;50: 4087–91.

43. Bigsby RM, Li AX, Bomolaski J, et al. Immunohistochemical study of Her-2/*neu*, epidermal growth factor receptor and steroid receptor expression in normal and malignant endometrium. Obstet Gynecol 1992;79: 95–100.

44. Grushko TA, Ridderstrale K, Olopade OI, et al. Identification of Her-2/*NEU* oncogene amplification by fluorescence in situ hybridization in endometrial carcinoma from patients included in GOG trial 177. Proc Am Soc Clin Oncol 2003;22:Abst 1880.

45. Fleming GF, Sill MA, Thigpen JT, et al. Phase II evaluation of trastuzumab in patients with advanced or recurrent endometrial carcinoma: a report on GOG 181B. Proc Am Soc Clin Oncol 2003,22:Abst 1821.

46. Santin A, Bellone S, Van Stedum S, et al. Determination of HER2/*neu* status in uterine serous papillary carcinoma: comparative analysis of immunohistochemistry and fluorescence in situ hybridization. Gynecol Oncol 2005;98:24–30.

47. Slomovitz B, Broaddus RR, Burke TW, et al. Her-2/*neu* overexpression and amplification in uterine papillary serous carcinoma. J Clin Oncol 2004;22:3126–32.

48. Morrison C, Zanagnolo V, Ramirez N, et al. HER-2 is an independent prognostic factor in endometrial cancer: association with outcome in a large cohort of surgically staged patients. J Clin Oncol 2006;24:2376–85.

49. Quackenbush J. Microarray analysis and tumor classification. N Engl J Med 2006;354: 2463–72.

50. Mutter G, Baak J, Fitzgerald J, et al. Global expression changes of constitutive and hormonally regulated genes during endometrial neoplastic transformation. Gynecol Oncol 2001;83:177–85.

51. Zorn K, Bonome T, Gangi L, et al. Gene expression profiles of serous, endometrioid, and clear cell subtypes of ovarian and endometrioid cancer. Clin Cancer Res 2005;11:6422–30.

52. Ferguson S, Olshen A, Viale A, et al. Stratification of intermediate-risk endometrial cancer patients into groups at high risk and low risk for recurrence based on tumor gene expression profiles. Clin Cancer Res 2005;11:2252–7.

53. Hartman L, Lu K, Linette G, et al. Gene expression profiles predict early relapse in ovarian cancer after platinum–paclitaxel chemotherapy. Clin Cancer Res 2005; 11:2149–55.

54. Hurwitz H, Fehrenbacher L, Novotny W, et al. Bevacizumab plus irinotecan, fluorouracil, leucovorin for metastatic colorectal cancer. N Engl J Med 2004;350:2335–42.

55. Abulafia O, Triest WE, Sherer DM, et al. Angiogenesis in endometrial hyperplasia and stage I endometrial carcinoma. Obstet Gynecol 1995;86:479–85.

56. Salvesen HB, Iversen OE, Akslen LA. Independent prognostic importance of microvessel density in endometrial cancer. Br J Cancer 1998;77:1140–4.

57. Fine BA, Valente PT, Feinstein GI, et al. VEGF, flt-1, and KDR/flk-1 as prognostic indicators in endometrial carcinoma. Gynecol Oncol 2000;76:33–9.

58. Hirai M, Nakagawara A, Oosaki T, et al. Expression of vascular endothelial growth factors (VEGF-A/VEGF-1 and VEGF-C/VEGF-2) in postmenopausal uterine endometrial carcinoma. Gynecol Oncol 2001; 80:181–8.

59. Peng XP, Li JD, Li MD, et al. Clinical significance of vascular endothelial growth factor in sera of patients with gynaecological malignant tumors. Aizheng 2002;21:181–5.

60. Chen C, Cheng WF, Lee CN, et al. Cytosol vascular endothelial growth factor in endometrial

carcinoma: correlation with disease-free survival. Gynecol Oncol 2001;80:207–12.

61. Bai X, Mi R. Expression of basic fibroblastic growth factor and microvessel density in endometrial carcinoma. Zhonghua Fu Chan Ke Za Zhi 2000;35:348–51.

62. Jubb A, Hurwitz H, Bai W, et al. Impact of vascular endothelial growth factor A expression, thrombospondin-2 expression, and microvessel density on the treatment effect of bevacizumab in metastatic colorectal cancer. J Clin Oncol 2006;24:217–27.

Endometrial cancer associated with defective DNA mismatch repair   12

Karen H Lu and Russell R Broaddus

INTRODUCTION

Defective DNA mismatch repair is one of the most common and well-characterized genetic defects detected in endometrial cancer, occurring in approximately 20–25% of all cases.[1] Defective DNA mismatch repair in endometrial cancer can be either inherited or acquired (sporadic). For women with inherited defective DNA mismatch repair, known as Lynch syndrome, the onset of endometrial cancer is usually at a younger age. This chapter describes the clinicopathologic significance of both acquired and inherited defective DNA mismatch repair in endometrial cancer. While there are fewer direct clinical implications for endometrial cancer patients with acquired defective DNA mismatch repair, there are significant clinical implications for patients with Lynch syndrome. This chapter also discusses the clinical management of women with Lynch syndrome.

HOW IS DEFECTIVE DNA MISMATCH REPAIR IDENTIFIED?

DNA mismatch repair proteins fix mistakes that commonly occur during DNA replication. This system of DNA mismatch repair was initially described in prokaryotes, and it was

subsequently found to be highly conserved across species. In humans, a defective DNA mismatch repair system was found to the underlying cause of Lynch syndrome (hereditary nonpolyposis colorectal cancer, HNPCC), an inherited cancer susceptibility syndrome characterized by early-onset colon cancer and endometrial cancer. Prior to the identification of the genes, the diagnosis of Lynch syndrome was based on clinical criteria, called the Amsterdam criteria (Table 12.1).[2] The specific genes responsible for Lynch syndrome are *MLH1, MSH2, MSH6,* and *PMS2.* Germline mutations in *MLH1* and *MSH2* account for >90% of cases of Lynch syndrome. Individuals with Lynch syndrome have inherited one allele of a mismatch repair gene that is nonfunctional due to mutation. Subsequent somatic loss of function of the corresponding normal allele results in defective DNA mismatch repair. This molecular defect is manifested clinically by a substantially increased risk of colon and endometrial cancer, as well as increased risks of ovarian, small bowel, stomach, renal pelvis, and ureteral cancers. In Lynch syndrome, the gene mutation is inherited in an autosomal dominant fashion, and each child has a 50% risk of inheriting the mutation. However, not all individuals who have germline Lynch syndrome

Table 12.1 Amsterdam II criteria

Patient must meet *all* of the following:
- Three or more relatives with a histologically verified HNPCC-associated cancer (or cancer of the endometrium, small bowel, ureter, or renal pelvis), one of whom is a first-degree relative of the other two; FAP should be excluded
- HNPCC-associated cancer involving at least two generations
- One or more HNPCC-associated cancer cases diagnosed before the age of 50 years

HNPCC, hereditary nonpolyposis colorectal cancer; FAP, familial adenomatous polyposis.
Reprinted from Vasen HF et al. Dis Colon Rectum 1991; 34:424–5.[2]

mutations will have cancer (incomplete penetrance). Other unidentified genetic and environmental factors likely play a role. Overall, Lynch syndrome accounts for <5% of colon cancers and <5% of endometrial cancers. However, identification of these individuals is crucial for two key reasons. First, individuals with germline Lynch syndrome mutations are at very high risk for developing second cancers. Second, identification of the specific genetic defect in an individual with a colon or endometrial cancer allows their relatives to undergo predictive genetic testing. By identifying women with endometrial cancer with Lynch syndrome, clinicians can have a significant impact on the patient and her family.

DNA mismatch repair defects can also be acquired, rather than inherited. In sporadic colon and endometrial adenocarcinomas, loss of MLH1 protein expression occurs due to an epigenetic modification, methylation of the *MLH1* gene promoter.[3] Such methylation is a common mechanism of downregulating gene expression, and is not passed on to children.

From a clinical standpoint, mismatch repair can be identified in human tumors. In addition, molecular tools can help distinguish acquired mismatch repair (sporadic cancer) from inherited mismatch repair (Lynch syndrome). A polymerase chain reaction (PCR)-based assay termed microsatellite instability analysis identifies those tumors with defective mismatch repair. Microsatellites are regions of the DNA in which there are single, di-, tri-, or quadranucleotide repeats (e.g. CACACA). A microsatellite instability (MSI) assay compares an individual's tumor DNA with normal DNA. When a different number of nucleotides are found in these repeat sequences in tumor compared with normal tissue, this is indicative of an abnormally functioning DNA mismatch repair system. Six different microsatellite regions of DNA are examined, as defined by the NIH consensus panel. These include BAT25, BAT26, BAT40, D5S346, D2S123, and D17S250.[4] By convention, if allelic shift is detected in one of the six microsatellites, the tumor is designated as microsatellite instability–low (MSI-L). The clinical significance, if any, of MSI-L tumors is not currently known. If a tumor has allelic shift in two or more of the six microsatellites, the tumor is designated as microsatellite instability–high (MSI-H). This analysis can be performed on formalin-fixed paraffin imbedded tissue. An example of this analysis is shown in Figure 12.1.

Another method for examining tumors for defective DNA mismatch repair is to perform immunohistochemistry for each of the DNA mismatch repair proteins. Loss of immunohistochemical expression of any of these proteins indicates lack of the protein in the tumor. An example of immunohistochemistry is shown in Figure 12.2. Immunohistochemistry is readily available in most clinical pathology laboratories, whereas MSI analysis is a PCR-based

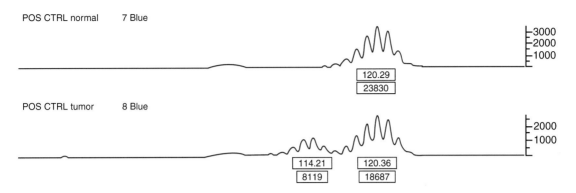

POS CTRL normal   7 Blue

120.29
23830

POS CTRL tumor   8 Blue

114.21
8119

120.36
18687

Figure 12.1 Chromatogram of BAT26 microsatellite instability analysis. DNA was extracted from formalin-fixed, paraffin-embedded sections of an endometrial carcinoma. DNA from microscopically confirmed normal ovary was used as normal tissue control. Allelic shift is present when the tumor DNA has more peaks on the chromatogram compared with the normal DNA. In this case, the tumor DNA has at least four more peaks than the normal DNA. Thus, for BAT26, there is allelic shift. Allelic shift in at least two of the six markers analyzed is indicative of MSI-H.

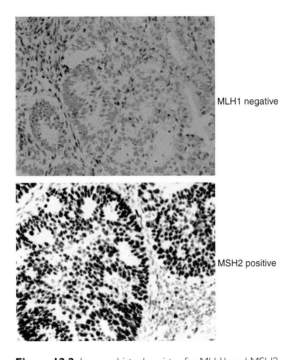

MLH1 negative

MSH2 positive

Figure 12.2 Immunohistochemistry for MLH1 and MSH2. Immunohistochemistry was performed using formalin-fixed, paraffin-embedded sections of an endometrial carcinoma. Tumor cell nuclei are strongly positive for MSH2 (dark brown staining). However, tumor cell nuclei do not stain for MLH1. Note that adjacent stromal cells do stain positive for MLH1. Adjacent stromal cells, inflammatory cells, and normal endometrium can serve as useful internal positive controls for immunohistochemical analysis.

assay that may only be available in larger laboratories.

Clinically, in a patient who is suspected of having Lynch syndrome (young age of onset of colon or endometrial cancer or a strong family history of colon or endometrial cancer), immunohistochemistry and MSI analysis can be performed on the tumor tissue first. If microsatellite instability is present and there is loss of immunohistochemical expression of one of the DNA mismatch repair proteins, directed germline testing using a peripheral blood sample with full sequencing of the appropriate gene can be performed. Such germline testing is important, as it can identify the exact mutation in the affected DNA mismatch repair gene. Knowledge of this exact mutation is a necessary tool for identifying other mutation carriers in a family. If a family member is found to have such a mutation, intensified cancer screening can be initiated.

ACQUIRED DEFECTIVE DNA MISMATCH REPAIR

When a tumor is MSI-H and has loss of immunohistochemical expression of MLH1, epigenetic silencing by hypermethylation of the promoter of *MLH1* may be the cause. The presence of hypermethylation of the *MLH1* promoter is a strong indicator that the patient has sporadic, not acquired, DNA mismatch repair. A number of studies have found that microsatellite instability occurs in approximately 20% of all endometrial cancers.[1] When specific histologies are examined, acquired defective DNA mismatch repair secondary to *MLH1* methylation occurs primarily in endometrioid endometrial cancers; *MLH1* methylation is uncommon in nonendometrioid tumors. Overall, for women with endometrial cancer associated with sporadic, acquired defective DNA mismatch repair, the age of diagnosis is the same as for women without defective DNA mismatch repair.

There is an abundance of literature examining microsatellite instability in colon cancer. Interestingly, MSI-H colon cancer is associated with an improved clinical outcome, compared with microsatellite-stable colon cancers.[5] In addition, MSI-H colon cancers tend to be unresponsive to 5-fluorouracil (5-FU)-based chemotherapy regimens, the primary chemotherapy for colon cancer.[1,6–14] A number of studies have examined the clinical significance of MSI-H endometrial cancer. In one of the largest studies, Black et al[1] examined 473 patients with endometrial cancer. Of these patients, 93 (20%) were MSI-H. Compared with the microsatellite-stable tumors, MSI-H tumors were predominantly endometrioid (94% vs 23%), had a higher proportion with myometrial invasion, and were of more advanced stage. Overall, the patients with MSI-H tumors had

a better disease-free survival and disease-specific survival.

INHERITED DEFECTIVE DNA MISMATCH REPAIR AND RISK OF ENDOMETRIAL CANCER

Individuals with Lynch syndrome have inherited one allele in a mismatch repair gene that is nonfunctional. Loss of the corresponding allele results in defective mismatch repair. This molecular defect is manifested clinically by a substantially increased risk of colon and endometrial cancer. The estimates of endometrial cancer risks for individuals with a germline *MLH1* and *MSH2* mutation are 40–60% (Figure 12.3).[15,16] In fact, for mutation-positive women, these two studies found that the risk of endometrial cancer is higher than the risk of colon cancer. Aarnio et al[15] reported a 60% lifetime risk for endometrial cancer in women with Lynch/HNPCC, as compared with a 54% lifetime risk for colon cancer. Dunlop et al[16] reported a 42% risk of endometrial cancer and a 30% risk of colon cancer in mutation-positive women. Vasen et al[17] examined cancer risks in *MLH1* mutation

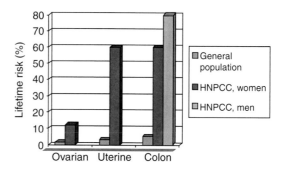

Figure 12.3 Lifetime risk for colon, endometrial, and ovarian cancer in men and women with Lynch syndrome (hereditary nonpolyposis colorectal cancer, HNPCC) compared with the general population risk.

carriers separately from *MSH2* mutation carriers. They reported a 35–40% risk of endometrial cancer in women with *MSH2* mutations and a 25% risk in women with *MLH1* mutations. They also reported that the risk of developing colon cancer in women with either *MLH1* or *MSH2* germline mutations was 50–60%. Green et al[18] examined a large *MSH2* kindred in Newfoundland and found that, for women, the cumulative risk by age 70 of endometrial cancer was 79% and the cumulative risk of colon cancer was 64%. Data from all of these studies were obtained from Lynch/HNPCC families that had documented *MLH1* and *MSH2* germline mutations. The reported risks of endometrial cancer in these studies are higher than the previously reported risk of 20%, which was based on families that fulfilled Amsterdam criteria but had not undergone genetic testing.[19] Clearly, women with Lynch/HNPCC have a significant risk for endometrial cancer, and that risk may, in fact, exceed their colon cancer risk.

Wijnen et al[20] reported an excess of endometrial cancers in female carriers of *MSH6* germline mutations. Truncating *MSH6* mutations were identified in 10 of 214 Lynch/HNPCC kindreds in which an *MLH1* or *MSH2* mutation had not been identified. Wijnen et al[20] reported that the frequency of endometrial cancer and hyperplasia was 73% in their cohort of female *MSH6* mutation carriers, compared with 29% in *MSH2* mutation carriers and 31% in *MLH1* mutation carriers. Hendriks et al[21] examined a large number of individuals from 20 families with *MSH6* mutations. They reported that women with *MSH6* mutations had a 71% cumulative risk of endometrial cancer by age 70, which was substantially higher than their risk for colon cancer. In addition, they found that the mean age of endometrial cancer in these women was 55 years, with a sharp increase in risk after age 50.

Ovarian cancer in Lynch/HNPCC has been poorly described and is not well understood. The risk of ovarian cancer in women with a Lynch/HNPCC mutation has been reported to be 12%.[15] Vasen et al[17] reported that the risk of ovarian cancer with an *MSH2* mutation was approximately 10%, while the risk with an *MLH1* mutation was lower at 3%. Green et al[18] reported a 36% risk of ovarian cancer in a large kindred with an *MSH2* mutation. Other cancer risks for individuals with Lynch syndrome include cancers of the small bowel, stomach, ureter, renal pelvis, and brain. Similar to ovarian cancer, very little is known about these tumors in Lynch/HNPCC.

Identifying individuals with Lynch syndrome

Identifying individuals with Lynch syndrome has important clinical implications. First, patients with Lynch syndrome have a substantial risk of developing a second primary cancer. Second, identifying the specific gene mutation in a woman with endometrial cancer and Lynch syndrome allows her family members to undergo predictive genetic testing. Historically, gastrointestinal surgeons, medical oncologists, and gastroenterologists have identified individuals as being at risk for Lynch syndrome. The gynecologic community has played a less significant role in identifying such individuals. Therefore, published criteria that are used to assist clinicians in identifying individuals with Lynch syndrome are primarily focused on colon cancer. The revised Bethesda criteria include criteria relating to family history, age of onset of cancer, synchronous and metachronous cancers, and specific histopathologic features of colon cancer (Table 12.2).[4] In contrast,

Table 12.2 The Revised Bethesda Guidelines for testing colorectal tumors for microsatellite instability (MSI)

Tumors from individuals should be tested for MSI in the following situations:

1. Colorectal cancer diagnosed in a patient who is less than 50 years of age
2. Presence of synchronous, metachronous colorectal, or other HNPCC-associated tumors,[a] regardless of age
3. Colorectal cancer with the MSI-H[b] histology[c] diagnosed in a patient who is less than 60 years of age[d]
4. Colorectal cancer diagnosed in one or more first-degree relatives with an HNPCC-related tumor, with one of the cancers being diagnosed under age 50 years
5. Colorectal cancer diagnosed in two or more first- or second-degree relatives with HNPCC-related tumors, regardless of age

---

[a]Hereditary nonpolyposis colorectal cancer (HNPCC)-related tumors include colorectal, endometrial, stomach, ovarian, pancreas, ureter and renal pelvis, biliary tract, and brain (usually glioblastoma as seen in Turcot syndrome) tumors, sebaceous gland adenomas and keratoacanthomas in Muir–Torre syndrome, and carcinoma of the small bowel.
[b]MSI-H (microsatellite instability–high) in tumors refers to changes in two or more of the five National Cancer Institute-recommended panels of microsatellite markers.
[c]Presence of tumor-infiltrating lymphocytes, Crohn-like lymphocytic reaction, mucinous/signet-ring differentiation, or medullary growth pattern.
[d]There was no consensus among the Workshop participants on whether to include the age criteria in guideline 3; participants voted to keep less than 60 years of age in the guidelines.
Reprinted from Umar A et al. J Natl Cancer Inst 2004;96:261–8.[4]

there have been no well-defined guidelines for identifying individuals with endometrial cancer as potentially having Lynch syndrome.

We have examined a large series of women from Lynch syndrome families who had both a colorectal and an endometrial or ovarian cancer in their lifetime.[22] Of the 117 women, 16 had a colorectal cancer and an endometrial/ovarian cancer diagnosed simultaneously. Of the remaining 101 women, 52 (51%) had an endometrial or ovarian cancer diagnosed first. Forty-nine (49%) women had a colorectal cancer diagnosed first. By identifying that an endometrial cancer patient has Lynch syndrome, clinicians may institute screening for colon cancer and prevent the development of a potentially lethal second cancer. Developing criteria to assist gynecologists and gynecologic oncologists in identifying which women with endometrial cancer may have Lynch syndrome is crucial. The revised Bethesda criteria focuses specifically on individuals with colon cancer.[4]

A more multidisciplinary set of guidelines that would provide all clinicians with simple criteria for screening would be useful for the early identification of women with Lynch syndrome.

A study by Berends et al[23] examined a cohort of women under age 50 with endometrial cancer, and determined the prevalence of germline mutations in *MLH1*, *MSH2*, or *MSH6*. Among 63 women tested, they identified 5 individuals with germline mutations (8%). In those women with endometrial cancer who were less than 50 years of age and had a first-degree relative with a Lynch syndrome-associated cancer, the prevalence of a mismatch repair gene mutation was 23%. Berends et al recommended that women with endometrial cancer under age 50 with a first-degree relative with colon or other Lynch syndrome-associated cancer should be considered for Lynch syndrome genetic testing.

Individuals with synchronous or metachronous colon and endometrial tumors are likely to have Lynch syndrome. In a study by Millar et al,[24] 18% (7 of 40) women with synchronous or metachronous colon and endometrial cancers had a germline *MLH1* or *MSH2* mutation. Individuals with synchronous endometrial and ovarian cancers have been identified in Lynch syndrome families. However, synchronous endometrial and ovarian cancers occur in about 10% of all ovarian cancers and 5% of all endometrial cancers, and are not likely to be an accurate indicator of Lynch syndrome.[25] Clearly, more work needs to be done to assist the gynecologist or gynecologic oncologist in identifying those individuals with Lynch syndrome.

Endometrial cancer phenotype in Lynch/HNPCC

As discussed previously, sporadic MSI-H endometrial cancer due to *MLH1* methylation (acquired or nonhereditary cancer) is associated almost exclusively with endometrioid tumors, higher International Federation of Gynecology and Obstetrics (FIGO) grade, and advanced stage.[23,26–29] Do MSI-H tumors due to inherited DNA mismatch repair deficiency have the same phenotype? We examined a series of endometrial cancers from women with documented Lynch syndrome germline mutations.[30] Our study demonstrated that Lynch syndrome-associated endometrial cancer, while sharing the common molecular abnormality of MSI, actually includes a broader spectrum of tumor histotypes, including endometrioid adenocarcinoma, papillary serous carcinoma, clear cell carcinoma, and malignant mixed müllerian tumor. In fact, the endometrial tumor spectrum for Lynch syndrome more closely mirrored that of the general population than that for *MLH1* methylation: 78% were stage I, 10% were stage 2, and 12% were stage III or IV. Myometrial invasion

of >50% of the uterine wall occurred in 26% of cases. Only 44% of the endometrioid tumors were grade 1, with the majority being grade 2 or 3. In all, nearly 25% of all cancers had pathologic features (deep myometrial invasion >50% myometrial wall thickness; cervix involvement; lymph node or adnexal metastasis; i.e. stage IC–IV) that would necessitate adjuvant therapy following hysterectomy.

A few other studies have described the clinicopathologic features of Lynch syndrome-associated endometrial cancer. Vasen et al[26] identified 125 women with endometrial cancer from families fulfilling the Amsterdam criteria from seven countries. At the time of the study, genetic testing was not available. The median age of diagnosis of endometrial cancer in their cohort was 48 years, with a range 27–72 years. Information on presenting symptoms, histology, and grade of tumor were not reported. Interestingly, 61% of 125 cases had a second primary cancer (usually colon cancer) either before or after the diagnosis of endometrial cancer. Vasen at al[26] reported excellent survival, with only 12% dying of their endometrial cancer. A study by Boks et al[31] also examined survival of endometrial cancer patients with Lynch syndrome. They compared 50 patients with endometrial cancer and Lynch syndrome (based on either germline test results or the revised Amsterdam criteria) with 100 age- and stage-matched women with sporadic endometrial cancer. The overall 5-year cumulative survival rates were similar: 88% for women with Lynch syndrome and 82% for women with sporadic endometrial cancer. In the cohort of women with Lynch syndrome, the majority (78%) had early-stage disease and 92% had endometrioid histology. Among the 22% of women with Lynch syndrome and advanced-stage disease, it was unclear whether prognosis was improved compared with that of a sporadic population with advanced-stage disease. In Lynch syndrome-associated colon cancer, overall survival appears to be more favorable compared with that for sporadic colon cancer.[32] Additional studies will be needed to determine if this holds true for Lynch/HNPCC-associated endometrial cancer. Comparing outcomes in advanced-stage patients may be important, as prognosis for early-stage endometrial cancer is highly favorable.

Typical endometrioid endometrial cancer develops through a stepwise pathway from normal endometrium, to complex hyperplasia with atypia, to carcinoma. It is unclear whether Lynch/HNPCC-associated endometrial cancer follows this pattern. In one study by Berends et al,[33] two patients with known mutations had endometrial hyperplasia without concurrent endometrial cancer and three patients had endometrial hyperplasia with concurrent endometrial cancer. Berends et al[33] demonstrated loss of the appropriate protein by immunohistochemistry in the hyperplasias and the cancers, suggesting that the mismatch repair defect may occur early in endometrial carcinogenesis. Zhou et al[34] examined PTEN mutations, an early and frequent event in sporadic endometrial cancer, in Lynch/HNPCC-associated tumors. They examined 41 endometrial cancers from mutation-positive Lynch/HNPCC families, and found that 68% demonstrated weak or absent staining for PTEN protein by immunohistochemisty. Of 20 cases, 18 had somatic PTEN mutations, involving the 6(A) tracts in exon 7 or 8. Zhou et al[34] concluded that PTEN mutations are critical in the pathogenesis of both sporadic and Lynch/HNPCC-associated endometrial cancer. Additional studies of the histologic and molecular phenotype of endometrial cancer in women with Lynch syndrome/HNPCC are necessary to better define the differences between sporadic endometrial

cancer and endometrial cancer arising in Lynch syndrome/HNPCC.

Clinical management

Screening and prevention

There have to date been limited studies evaluating screening for endometrial cancer in women with Lynch syndrome. Nevertheless, clinical guidelines have been established that recommend screening for endometrial cancer beginning at age 25–35 years.[35] Modalities for endometrial cancer screening include transvaginal ultrasound and an office endometrial sampling.

The use of transvaginal ultrasound to evaluate the thickness of the endometrial stripe as a screening tool for Lynch syndrome is not likely to be beneficial. Screening for endometrial cancer is primarily focused on the premenopausal age group. In this population, the thickness of the endometrial stripe changes with the menstrual cycle, and is unlikely to be a sensitive or specific test for endometrial cancer. Two studies have reported their experience with ultrasound as a screening modality for endometrial cancer. Dove-Edwin et al[36] examined the outcome of endometrial cancer surveillance by ultrasound in 269 women with Lynch syndrome. Women who were screened included those who were mutation-positive, those who had Lynch syndrome based on Amsterdam criteria, and those who did not fulfill the Amsterdam criteria but had a family history suggestive of Lynch syndrome. No cancers were detected in 522 ultrasounds. However, two interval cases of endometrial cancer occurred. One patient had a normal surveillance ultrasound 2 years prior to developing postmenopausal bleeding. The second patient had a normal surveillance ultrasound 6 months prior to a diagnosis of a stage I endometrial cancer. Dove-Edwin et al[36] concluded that ultrasound may not be an effective method to detect early endometrial cancer. In a study by Rijcken et al,[37] 41 women with Lynch syndrome were enrolled in a screening program, in which 179 transvaginal ultrasounds were performed. Of those, 17 were defined to be abnormal based on thickness or irregularity of lining. Of these 17 patients, 14 had a follow-up endometrial biopsy that was within normal limits. One patient had an endometrium thickened to 27 mm on ultrasound, and a biopsy revealed complex atypical hyperplasia. Two additional patients had ultrasounds with an irregular endometrium, and both had focal complex atypical hyperplasia on biopsy. However, ultrasound failed to identify one patient who developed endometrial cancer. She had a normal transvaginal ultrasound and developed vaginal bleeding 8 months later. At the time of diagnosis, she had a stage IB, grade 2 endometrioid adenocarcinoma.

The endometrial pipelle biopsy is an office procedure that provides adequate tissue for pathologic diagnosis and is a reasonable screening modality. Studies performed in women presenting with abnormal vaginal bleeding have shown that the sensitivity of an office endometrial pipelle is equivalent to a dilatation and curettage (D&C) performed in the operating room.[38] Our current recommendations for our patients who are known mutation carriers include an annual office endometrial biopsy. We also include an annual transvaginal ultrasound in order to evaluate the ovaries. Annual CA-125 testing can be included as part of the screening program, but false positives in the premenopausal age range are common.

The oral contraceptive pill (OCP) has been shown to decrease the risk of endometrial cancer by 50% in women at the general population risk.[39] In addition, the OCP has also been shown to substantially decrease the risk of ovarian cancer. We are currently conducting a chemoprevention study in women with Lynch syndrome using the OCP or medroxyprogesterone acetate (Depo-Provera). While the endpoint for this study will not be reduction in incidence of disease, we will examine the effect of these agents on surrogate molecular biomarkers in the endometrium.

Prophylactic surgery

We have examined the efficacy of prophylactic hysterectomy in a large number of women with documented germline mutations associated with Lynch syndrome.[40] Sixty-one women underwent prophylactic hysterectomy and were matched with 210 women who did not undergo hysterectomy. None of the women who underwent prophylactic hysterectomy developed endometrial cancer, whereas 69 women in the control group (33%) did. No other studies of prophylactic gynecologic surgery had previously been published for women with Lynch syndrome. These findings helped provide substantive data supporting this prevention strategy for women with Lynch syndrome, and, importantly, provided a basis for consensus groups to make clinical recommendations. The Cancer Genetics Studies Consortium had stated in their 1997 Guidelines[35] that there was insufficient data either for or against prophylactic hysterectomy for the prevention of endometrial cancer. Based on our study, their most recent published guidelines[41] state 'Evidence supports the efficacy of prophylactic hysterectomy and oophorectomy.' Women with Lynch syndrome should be counseled that prophylactic hysterectomy and bilateral salpingo-oophorectomy is a reasonable management option to consider. When childbearing is complete, a laparoscopically assisted vaginal hysterectomy and bilateral salpingo-oophorectomy or a total abdominal hysterectomy bilateral salpingo-oophorectomy (TAH–BSO) can be performed. For women with Lynch syndrome undergoing colon surgery, concurrent prophylactic TAH–BSO can be considered.

For those gynecologists or gynecologic oncologists performing prophylactic hysterectomy and bilateral salpingo-oophorectomy in women who are known mutation carriers, consideration of finding an occult endometrial or ovarian cancer should be given. We reported a case of an asymptomatic, 48-year-old woman who was a known *MSH2* mutation carrier and who underwent a prophylactic vaginal hysterectomy and bilateral salpingo-oophorectomy. At the time of final pathologic review, she was found to have a grade 2 endometrial cancer with involvement of the endocervical glands and 5/12 mm invasion of the uterine wall. Because the endometrial cancer was not identified at the time of surgery, no staging was performed. The patient therefore underwent restaging performed via laparotomy.[29] We recommend that in women who are known mutation carriers undergoing prophylactic hysterectomy, a preoperative endometrial biopsy be performed. In addition, we recommend that the uterus be examined intraoperatively by a pathologist for occult disease.

CONCLUSIONS

Defective DNA mismatch repair occurs in approximately 20–25% of all cases of endometrial cancer. The majority of these cases are noninherited or acquired, and result from hypermethylation, or 'silencing' of the *MLH1* promoter. For women with inherited defective DNA mismatch repair, known as Lynch syndrome, the onset of endometrial cancer is usually at a younger age and the risk of developing a second cancer is high. Gynecologic oncologists and gynecologists play a key role in identifying these individuals. In addition to asking about family history of endometrial and colon cancer, tumor studies including microsatellite instability testing and immunohistochemistry can assist in differentiating acquired from inherited defective DNA mismatch repair. While studies have shown a preponderance of endometrioid cancers associated with acquired MSI, inherited MSI endometrial cancers have a broader spectrum of disease.

REFERENCES

1. Black D, Soslow RA, Levine DA, et al. Clinicopathologic significance of defective DNA mismatch repair in endometrial carcinoma. J Clin Oncol 2006;24:1745–53.

2. Vasen HF, Mecklin JP, Khan PM, Lynch HT, et al. The International Collaborative Group on Hereditary Non-Polyposis Colorectal Cancer (ICG-HNPCC). Dis Colon Rectum 1991;34:424–5.

3. Gurin CC, Federici MG, Kang L, et al. Causes and consequences of microsatellite instability in endometrial carcinoma. Cancer Res 1999; 59:462–6.

4. Umar A, Boland CR, Terdiman JP, et al. Revised Bethesda Guidelines for hereditary nonpolyposis colorectal cancer (Lynch syndrome) and microsatellite instability. J Natl Cancer Inst 2004;96:261–8.

5. Gryfe R, Kim H, Hsieh ET, et al. Tumor microsatellite instability and clinical outcome in young patients with colorectal cancer. N Engl J Med 2000;342:69–77.

6. Caduff RF, Johnston CM, Svoboda-Newman SM, et al. Clinical and pathological significance of microsatellite instability in sporadic endometrial carcinoma. Am J Pathol 1996; 148:1671–8.

7. Fiumicino S, Ercoli A, Ferrandine G, et al. Microsatellite instability is an independent indicator of recurrence in sporadic stage I–II endometrial adenocarcinoma. J Clin Oncol 2001;19:1008–14.

8. Maxwell GL, Risinger JI, Alvarez A, et al. Favorable survival associated with microsatellite instability in endometrioid endometrial cancers. Obstet Gynecol 2001;97:417–22.

9. Wong YF, Ip TY, Chung TK, et al. Clinical and pathologic significance of microsatellite instability in endometrial cancer. Int J Gynecol Cancer 1999;9:406–10.

10. Tibiletti MG, Furlan D, Taborelli M, et al. Microsatellite instability in endometrial cancer: relation to histological subtypes. Gynecol Oncol 1999;73:247–52.

11. MacDonald ND, Salvesen HB, Ryan A, et al. Frequency and prognostic impact of microsatellite instability in a large population-based study of endometrial carcinomas. Cancer Res 2000;60:1750–2.

12. Baldinu P, Cossu A, Manca A, et al. Microsatellite instability and mutation analysis of candidate genes in unselected sardinian patients with endometrial carcinoma. Cancer 2002;94:3157–68.

13. Basil JB, Goodfellow PJ, Rader JS, et al. Clinical significance of microsatellite instability in endometrial carcinoma. Cancer 2000; 89:1758–64.

14. Catasus L, Machin P, Matias-Guiu X, et al. Microsatellite instability in endometrial carcinomas: clinicopathologic correlations in a series of 42 cases. Hum Pathol 1998;29: 1160–4.

15. Aarnio M, Sankila R, Pukkala E, et al. Cancer risk in mutation carriers of DNA-mismatch-repair genes. Int J Cancer 1999;81:214–18.

16. Dunlop MG, Farrington SM, Carothers AD, et al. Cancer risk associated with germline DNA mismatch repair gene mutations. Hum Mol Genet 1997;6:105–10.

17. Vasen HF, Stormorken A, Menko FH, et al. *MSH2* mutation carriers are at higher risk of cancer than *MLH1* mutation carriers: a study of hereditary nonpolyposis colorectal cancer families. J Clin Oncol 2001;19:4074–80.

18. Green J, O'Driscoll M, Barnes A, et al. Impact of gender and parent of origin on the phenotypic expression of hereditary nonpolyposis colorectal cancer in a large Newfoundland kindred with a common *MSH2* mutation. Dis Colon Rectum 2002;45:1223–32.

19. Watson P, Vasen HF, Mecklin JP, et al. The risk of endometrial cancer in hereditary nonpolyposis colorectal cancer. Am J Med 1994;96:516–20.

20. Wijnen J, de Leeuw W, Vasen H, et al. Familial endometrial cancer in female carriers of *MSH6* germline mutations. Nat Genet 1999; 23:142–4.

21. Hendriks YM, Wagner A, Morreau H, et al. Cancer risk in hereditary nonpolyposis colorectal cancer due to *MSH6* mutations: impact on counseling and surveillance. Gastroenterology 2004;127:17–25.

22. Lu K, Dinh M, Kohlmann W, et al. Gynecological malignancy as a 'sentinel cancer' for women with HNPCC. Gynecol Oncol 2004;92:421.

23. Berends MJ, Wu Y, Sijmons RH, et al. Toward new strategies to select young endometrial cancer patients for mismatch repair gene mutation analysis. J Clin Oncol 2003;21: 4364–70.

24. Millar AL, Pal T, Madlensky L, et al. Mismatch repair gene defects contribute to the genetic basis of double primary cancers of the colorectum and endometrium. Hum Mol Genet 1999;8:823–9.

25. Soliman PT, Slomovitz BM, Broaddus RR, et al. Synchronous primary cancers of the

endometrium and ovary: a single institution review of 84 cases. Gynecol Oncol 2004;94: 456–62.

26. Vasen HF, Watson P, Mecklin JP, et al. The epidemiology of endometrial cancer in hereditary nonpolyposis colorectal cancer. Anticancer Res 1994;14:1675–8.

27. Smith RA, Cokkinides V, Eyre HJ. American Cancer Society guidelines for the early detection of cancer, 2006. CA Cancer J Clin 2006; 56:11–25; quiz 49–50.

28. NCCN Clinical Practice Guidelines in Oncology: Genetic Familial High-Risk Assessment: Breast and Ovarian. Rockledge, PA: National Comprehensive Cancer Network, 2006.

29. Chung L, Broaddus R, Crozier M, et al. Unexpected endometrial cancer at prophylactic hysterectomy in a woman with hereditary nonpolyposis colon cancer. Obstet Gynecol 2003;102:1152–5.

30. Broaddus RR, Lynch HT, Chen LM, et al. Pathologic features of endometrial carcinoma associated with HNPCC: a comparison with sporadic endometrial carcinoma. Cancer 2006;106:87–94.

31. Boks DE, Trujillo AP, Vooqd AC, et al. Survival analysis of endometrial carcinoma associated with hereditary nonpolyposis colorectal cancer. Int J Cancer 2002;102:198–200.

32. Watson P, Lin KM, Rodriguez-Bigas MA, et al. Colorectal carcinoma survival among hereditary nonpolyposis colorectal carcinoma family members. Cancer 1998;83:259–66.

33. Berends MJ, Hollema H, Wu Y, et al. MLH1 and MSH2 protein expression as a pre-screening marker in hereditary and non-hereditary endometrial hyperplasia and cancer. Int J Cancer 2001;92:398–403.

34. Zhou XP, Kuismanen S, Nystrom-Lahti M, et al. Distinct *PTEN* mutational spectra in hereditary non-polyposis colon cancer syndrome-related endometrial carcinomas compared to sporadic microsatellite unstable tumors. Hum Mol Genet 2002;11:445–50.

35. Burke W, Peterson G, Lynch P, et al. Recommendations for follow-up care of individuals with an inherited predisposition to cancer. I. Hereditary nonpolyposis colon cancer. Cancer Genetics Studies Consortium. JAMA 1997;277:915–19.

36. Dove-Edwin I, Boks D, Goff S, et al. The outcome of endometrial carcinoma surveillance by ultrasound scan in women at risk of hereditary nonpolyposis colorectal carcinoma and familial colorectal carcinoma. Cancer 2002; 94:1708–12.

37. Rijcken FE, Mourits MJ, Kleibeuker JH, et al. Gynecologic screening in hereditary nonpolyposis colorectal cancer. Gynecol Oncol 2003;91:74–80.

38. Dijkhuizen FP, Mol BW, Brolmann HA, et al. The accuracy of endometrial sampling in the diagnosis of patients with endometrial carcinoma and hyperplasia: a meta-analysis. Cancer 2000;89:1765–72.

39. Combination oral contraceptive use and the risk of endometrial cancer. The Cancer and Steroid Hormone Study of the Centers for Disease Control and the National Institute of Child Health and Human Development. JAMA 1987;257:796–800.

40. Schmeler KM, Lynch HT, Chen LM, et al. Prophylactic surgery to reduce the risk of gynecologic cancers in the Lynch syndrome. N Engl J Med 2006;354:261–9.

41. Chen S, Wang W, Lee S, et al. Prediction of germline mutations and cancer risk in the Lynch syndrome. JAMA 2006;296:1479–87.

Molecular profiling in endometrial cancer: current research and implications for the future

13

Michael A Bidus, John I Risinger, and G Larry Maxwell

INTRODUCTION

According to the American Cancer Society (ACS), an estimated 39 080 new cases of uterine cancer will be diagnosed in 2007 making this the fourth most common cancer in women.[1] In addition to the significant effects on the patients and their families, endometrial cancer places a significant burden on the healthcare system. Specifically, the Agency for Healthcare and Quality Research estimated that over $770M, was spent on the inpatient management of patients with endometrial cancer in 2004.[2] An improved understanding of the molecular etiology of endometrial cancer offers to facilitate development of future chemopreventive agents and improved therapeutics for patients with more advanced forms of this disease. Development of molecularly based therapies will ultimately provide a more targeted approach toward decreasing the morbidity and mortality associated with this disease as well as the significant monetary affects on the American healthcare system. In addition, novel molecular diagnostic techniques provide opportunities for prediction of prognosis that could direct more targeted surgery and adjuvant therapies.

TARGETED MOLECULAR PROFILING

Epidemiologic and clinical studies of endometrial cancer have suggested that there are two distinct types of endometrial cancer. Type I endometrial cancers, which account for approximately 75% of endometrial cancer cases, are usually endometrioid in histology, are well differentiated, and present with early-stage disease. These tumors are frequently associated with a history of unopposed estrogen exposure or other hyperestrogenic risk factors such as obesity. Patients with type I endometrial cancer typically have a favorable prognosis with appropriate therapy. In contrast, type II endometrial cancers are more often moderately to poorly differentiated and nonendometrioid in histology. These tumors are usually metastatic at presentation, and are more likely to recur despite aggressive surgical and medical management (Table 13.1).[3] However, not all cancers can be neatly characterized as either pure type I or II lesions, and endometrial cancers can also be viewed as a continuous spectrum with respect to etiology and clinical behavior. Nonetheless, as the genetic events involved in the development of endometrial cancer have been elucidated,

Table 13.1 Clinical phenotypes of endometrial cancer

	Type I	*Type II*
Race	Caucasian > African–American	Caucasian = African–American
Grade	Well differentiated	Poorly differentiated
Histology	Endometrioid	Nonendometrioid
Stage	I/II	III/IV
Prognosis	Favorable	Unfavorable
Precursor	Atypical hyperplasia	Endometrial intraepithelial carcinoma

it has been found that specific alterations are frequently seen in either type I or II cases.

The majority of genetic alterations characteristic of endometrioid (typically type I) and nonendometrioid (typically type II) endometrial cancers were discovered via more conventional candidate gene-based approaches (namely, allelotyping, functional chromosomal transfer analysis, comparative genomic hybridization, conventional cytogenetic data, etc.) used to focus on specific genes and/or regions of chromosomes that might be involved in endometrial carcinogenesis. This approach has been very successful in identifying critical target genes, and suggests that distinct molecular alterations may be characteristic of endometrioid versus nonendometrioid endometrial cancers (Table 13.2). In summary, endometrioid cancers display an increased incidence of alterations in the *PTEN* tumor suppressor gene and activating mutations within the *CTNNB1* and *KRAS2* genes,[4,5] as well as defects in mismatch repair that result in microsatellite instability.[6–8] Nonendometrioid cancers rarely, if ever, contain *PTEN* mutations or microsatellite instability,[9] but are more likely to be characterized by *TP53* mutation, and widespread aneuploidy.[10–12] Although these changes have been described in some endometrial cancers, our group has found that many endometrial cancers do not contain these molecular alterations. In an examination of 87 cancers, we found that the majority of cases did not contain alteration at any of these loci, even when many were advanced-stage.[13] These findings suggest that other molecular pathways and mechanisms of gene inactivation remain unrecognized when a mutational analysis is undertaken. In the

Table 13.2 Endometrial cancer: molecular profiles of histologic types

	Endometrioid	*Nonendometrioid*
Ploidy	Near-diploid	Aneuploid
HER2/*neu* (*ERBB2*) overexpression	Infrequent	Frequent
TP53 mutation	Infrequent	Frequent
KRAS2 activating mutation	Frequent	Infrequent
PTEN mutation	Frequent	Infrequent
Microsatellite instability	Frequent	Infrequent
CTNNB1 mutation	Frequent	Infrequent

absence of ubiquitous gene mutation, we and others have subsequently evaluated the role of epigenetic mechanisms in endometrial cancer. Promoter hypermethylation or hypomethylation events that involve important growth-regulatory pathways (i.e. cell cycle control, apoptosis, cell adhesion/invasion, DNA repair, etc.) have been implicated in carcinogenesis of the endometrium.[14,15]

Although a targeted analysis of gene mutations and promoter methylation has provided useful information regarding molecular alterations associated with endometrial cancer, it must be acknowledged that a survey approach is extremely limited and biased based on the loci examined. We have subsequently pursued microarray methods of gene expression analysis in an effort to describe more comprehensively the molecular profile of endometrial cancers. This chapter will focus on commonly used high-throughput genomic analysis techniques and their application in the field of cancer biology with a specific emphasis on endometrial cancer.

TISSUE PREPARATION

Tissue specimens used in molecular profiling experiments (particularly in the setting of high-throughput techniques) should be obtained from tissue repositories and other laboratories that collect tissues using International Society for Biological and Environmental Repositories (IBESR) best practice guidelines.[16] Timely freezing of harvested tissue specimens is essential for maintaining the integrity of gene expression measured using microarray.[17] Procurement and processing of specimens for storage within 60 minutes using a standardized protocol is a 'best practice' consistent with IBESR guidelines and will facilitate more accurate high-throughput analysis.[16]

Laser capture microscopy

Solid tumors can often be architecturally heterogeneous when visualized microscopically as a result of invasive interdigitation of cancerous cells into a normal tissue interface. Inclusion of normal cells in a tumor specimen that is processed using gene expression analysis can potentially mask the unique expression profile of the cancer cell population. Although many investigative groups have minimized the ratio of normal to cancer cells by dissecting the specimen grossly using sterile razor blades and needles, the development of laser capture microscopy (LCM) has facilitated more rapid and reliable isolation of pure cell populations for study.[18]

LCM is initially used to examine histologic samples placed on the stage of the microscope. The cells of interest can be identified through direct visualization of morphology or through immunohistochemical staining. A laser is used to 'microdissect' or outline the specific cell populations, which are then removed in a manner that is unique depending on the chosen LCM platform. The Pixcell II–Arcturus system uses a low-power infrared laser to melt a thermoplastic film contained in a cap placed over the surface of the cells of interest. When the cap is lifted, the microdissected specimen remains attached to the cap and is preserved for further evaluation.[19] A second system, PALM LCM, has an ultraviolet laser projecting from underneath the membrane-coated (i.e. polyethylene glycol) slide containing the overlying tissue specimen. During the microdissection, the laser is used to cut through the membrane and tissue in a perimeter around the cells of interest. Once this is complete, the focal point of the laser changes to facilitate catapulting of the tissue specimen of interest into an overlying cap containing buffer.[20] Finally, the Leica system is an LCM that uses an ultraviolet laser to cut a specimen placed into a membrane (no glass), and once the particular area has been completely circumscribed, the specimen falls into a tube by gravity.[21] All three systems are practical and efficient for isolation of specific populations of cells that are free of contaminants and provide samples that are acceptable for use in molecular analysis.

LCM has the advantages of preserving cellular morphology, tissue architecture, and molecular composition of DNA, RNA, or protein, and can be used on cytology samples, archival specimens, or fresh/frozen tissue samples. Comparisons of LCM-prepared versus grossly dissected frozen tissue samples in breast cancer research have shown that microdissection can enhance the sensitivity of evaluating target gene transcript expression levels.[22] Microarray studies involving endometrial cancer have used macrodissected material that is characterized by a minimum cancer-to-normal cell background ratio of $\geq 50\%$. The use of microdissected versus macrodissected material is an area of controversy. Opponents of the use of microdissected material would caution that the inclusion of stroma may result in contamination of the specimen, potentially masking detection of differentially expressed genes by epithelial cells or alternatively introducing transcripts that are characteristic of stromal expression. Advocates of the use of macrodissected material would prefer having sampling of the entire molecular milieu since epithelial–stromal interactions may be important in the neoplastic processes. DNA or RNA should be extracted using standard procedures. As a quality control measure, investigators should both quantify the amount of extracted DNA or RNA and check the integrity of the isolated molecular component, which can be performed in batch using chip-based techniques (e.g. Agilent Pico-Chip).

PROCESSING OF DNA MICROARRAYS: cDNA AND OLIGONUCLEOTIDE ARRAYS

The microarray chip or slide consists of a template upon which the genes of an organism are represented by single-stranded cDNA or oligonucleotide probes that are precisely arranged using an automated robotic spotting process. This potentially results in the representation of >40 000 transcripts, including the estimated 30 000 known genes in the human genome, on a single chip.

Using this technique, RNA is extracted from a tissue specimen and, through reverse transcription, cDNA or cRNA is made that is fluorescently labeled. Binding of the labeled cDNA or cRNA to the microarray chip probes provides a measure of the relative transcript expression of representative genes. Although hybridization has been used for decades to detect and quantify nucleic acids, the miniaturization of the process has facilitated the review of gene expression on a genomic scale.

The use of an oligonucleotide platform such as Affymetrix involves the synthesis of biotin-labeled cRNA that is used to hybridize to oligomers on the microarray chip. Approximately 11–16 probes are selected among all possible 25-mers to represent each transcript. For each probe designed to be perfectly complementary to a target sequence, a partner probe is generated that is identical except for a single base mismatch in its center. These probe pairs, called the perfect match probe (PM) and the mismatch probe (MM), allow subtraction of signals caused by nonspecific hybridization. The difference in hybridization signals between the partners, as well as

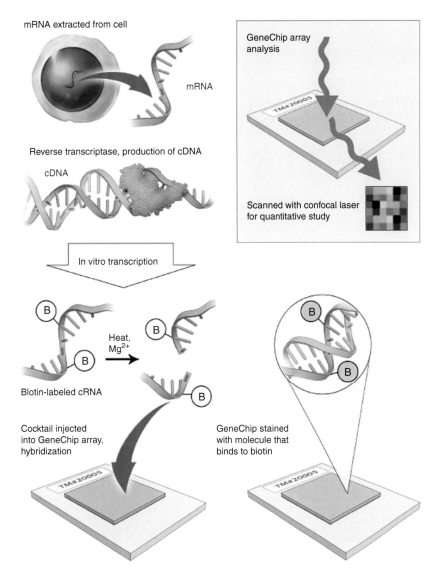

Figure 13.1 Oligonucleotide array. RNA is extracted from the dissected tissue specimen, and reverse transcription and in vitro transcription is used to create biotin-labeled cRNA representative of each case. Hybridization of the cRNA with the oligomers on the microarray is performed and the chip is scanned to quantitate binding.

their intensity ratios, serve as indicators of specific transcript abundance (Figure 13.1).[23]

Microarray experiments using a cDNA chip require both a tissue specimen cRNA and a 'universal standard' cRNA, each of which is labeled with either cytochrome 3 (green) or cytochrome 5 (red). The 'universal standard' represents RNA from multiple tissue types that is pooled and is available from several commercial suppliers (including Stratagene and Clontech), with minimal batch-to-batch variability according to the manufacturers. Following hybridization of the mixture containing both the labeled specimen and universal standard cRNAs with the microchip containing cDNA probes, the microarray scanner determines whether known probes on the microchip bind to either or both of the cytochromes. Determination of the ratio of expression of the two cytochromes facilitates an estimation of target expression in the specimen (Figure 13.2).[23]

There are advantages to each approach. Oligonucleotides, by virtue of their small size in terms of numbers of base pairs, are shorter than the probes used in cDNA arrays and are therefore more specific. Multiple oligonucleotides can be used to represent an entire gene sequence as well as potential alterations,

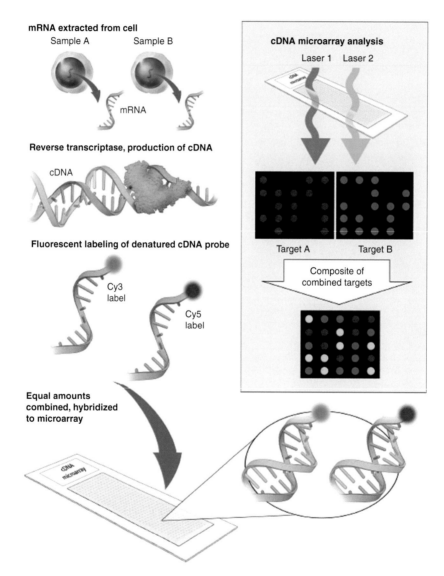

Figure 13.2 cDNA microarray. For each case, RNA is extracted from the dissected tissue specimen and a control. Reverse transcription is used to create either (cytochrome 3) Cy3-labeled or Cy5-labeled cDNA for the cases in the study versus control groups. Hybridization of the cDNA with the primers on the microarray is performed and the chip is scanned to quantitate binding.

facilitating the detection of single-nucleotide polymorphisms in addition to gene mutations, insertions, or deletions. Unfortunately, oligonucleotides are oriented in one direction (either sense or antisense), requiring labeling of the sample RNA to reflect 3′ or 5′ orientation. In comparison, cDNA microarrays have longer probes, allowing for high sensitivity for gene detection. cDNA microarrays are also more versatile in that the probes are double-stranded, allowing for the hybridization of either sense or antisense RNA. Disadvantages of cDNA microarrays include reduced specificity, and the possibility of cross-hybridization due to multiple repeat sequences or homologs present across different genes.

Current protocols for the fluorescent labeling of RNA require large quantities of RNA, which can pose a challenge to investigators. Degradation that occurs during the microdissection of tissue specimens can pose time constraints that limit the amount of material that can be collected. Even when using equipment fitted with robotic microscope stage instrumentation, investigators may be required to dissect material from multiple slides. An alternative for utilizing limited material in array analysis is to use the polymerase chain reaction (PCR) to amplify total cDNA before labeling. Although this technique may bias expression results, it may also serve to facilitate discovery of genes that are expressed at low abundance yet are differentially expressed between groups.[24,25]

Another controversial issue associated with microarray analysis of cancer involves the selection of the optimal control. Many of the microarray experiments to date involving endometrial cancer have focused on comparison between two groups of cancers that are phenotypically different, obviating the need for identification of a suitable control. Comparison of endometrial cancers with a 'normal' endometrial specimen is more challenging. Should only epithelial cells or a combination of epithelium and stroma be used? Should postmenopausal or perimenopausal endometrium be used? Does endometrial cancer arise from these differentiated cells or does it derive from a yet to be clarified precursor stem cell? Investigations evaluating multiple controls are forthcoming. Investigations comparing ovarian cancer with normal ovarian tissue have shown that the normal control that is selected can strongly influence the genes that are identified as differentially expressed.[26] Although alterations in epithelial–stromal interactions may be important in identifying differentially expressed genes that distinguish cancers, it is also possible that the additional stroma may impede detection of subtle yet important changes in epithelial gene expression that can be a signature for a particular cancer. In the assessment of whole-ovary (WO) samples, ovarian surface epithelium (OSE) brushings, OSE exposed to short-term culture, and immortalized cell lines, the majority of differentially expressed genes were unique to each cancer compared with normal specimens, with none of the genes being present on all five gene lists of differentially expressed transcripts.[26] We expect a similar challenge to be associated with the microarray analysis of endometrial cancer versus normal endometrium. However, these quality control experiments are necessary in the context of microarray studies involving endometrial cancer so that investigative groups can select the more appropriate control in approaching a specific research objective.

ANALYSIS OF MICROARRAY DATA

Interpretation of statistical tests assumes that the data have equal variances and are collected from normal populations. Invariably, some degree of systematic variation in the microarray data can exist due to potential sources such as scanner-introduced bias, irregularities in hybridization, differing intensities of dye incorporation, and unequal quantities of starting RNA. Log transformation and permutation tests can improve normality, facilitate identification of outliers, and assist in the interpretation of the raw expression data.[27] Once the data have been normalized, the expression data can be analyzed using several approaches, including class discovery, class comparison, and class prediction.[28]

Class discovery

Class discovery is a powerful analytical tool that can assist the researcher in identifying classes of disease distinguished by unique molecular profiles. Clustering and other methods of unsupervised analysis can be used to organize multivariate data into groups based on similarities in gene expression. Cases within a cluster are more closely related to one another than to a case in a different cluster. Hierarchical methods are used to successively merge clusters (using dendrograms to display relatedness) so that at each level of the hierarchy, clusters within the same group are more similar to each other than to those in another group.[28]

The applications of class discovery in endometrial cancer microarray experiments have been demonstrated in an analysis by Ferguson et al[29] involving 39 endometrial cancer patients, 10 of whom had a history of recent tamoxifen use and 29 of whom did not. A supervised class comparison analysis was performed, but failed to identify a statistically significant difference in gene expression between the two groups. However, when unsupervised hierarchical cluster analysis (class discovery analysis) was performed on all 39 cases independently

of tamoxifen exposure, two highly distinct classes of tumors were noted, characterized by distinctly different gene expression profiles. These two groups were similar in age, parity, histologic type, and stage of disease, but differed significantly in tumor grade. One group was composed primarily of grade I tumors, while the other group consisted primarily of grade II and III tumors.[29] Based on clinical studies, tumor grade has long been known to be a sensitive indicator of disease spread. This study provided strong molecular evidence that tumor grade may define biologically distinct tumors.

Class comparison

Class comparison analysis is designed to detect or describe differences between two known groups, such as type I and type II endometrial carcinoma. Principal component analysis and multidimensional scaling are unsupervised methods of analysis. This type of analysis enables the overall genomic expression pattern of a sample to be expressed as a point in a three-dimensional figure and facilitates identification of clustering of samples according to similar global gene expression profiles (Figure 13.3). The disadvantage of this visualization tool is that information can be lost in the reduction of thousands of dimensions of information into a three-dimensional figure, and therefore this form of unsupervised analysis may not always project the separation of clusters in significantly different groups.[28]

Binary comparison is a supervised method of class comparison analysis that identifies genes that are differentially expressed between two groups using standard statistical tests such as the Wilcoxon rank-sum test, ANOVA, or *t*-test. Heat maps are typically used to display differentially expressed genes detected in the comparative analysis of groups (Figure 13.4), with

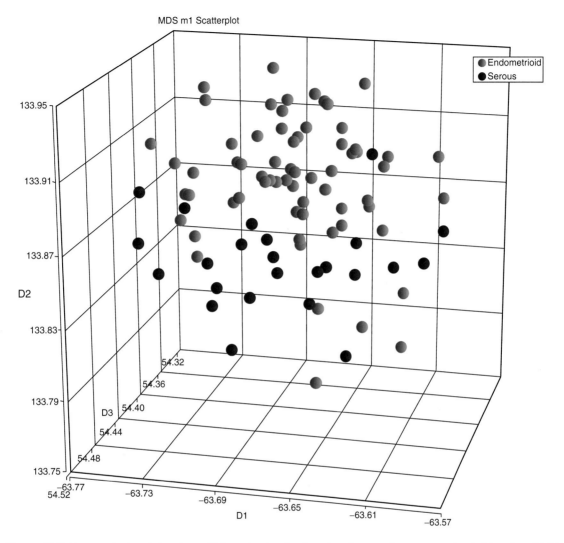

Figure 13.3 Unsupervised analysis using multidimensional scaling based on the overall gene expression in 66 endometrioid (green) and 24 papillary serous (blue) carcinomas.

red typically used to represent upregulation and green to depict downregulation of genes.

Binary comparison according to tumor phenotype

Molecular differences between endometrial cancer and normal endometrium

Identification of genes differentially expressed in a comparison of endometrial cancer and normal endometrium offers the opportunity to identify targets for chemoprevention strategies. Mutter et al[30] used microarray technology to analyze global gene expression profiles in tissue samples from 4 patients with cycling normal endometrium and 10 patients with endometrioid adenocarcinoma of the endometrium. Binary comparison analysis in conjunction with complex statistical analysis techniques was used to demonstrate that 50 genes could discriminate

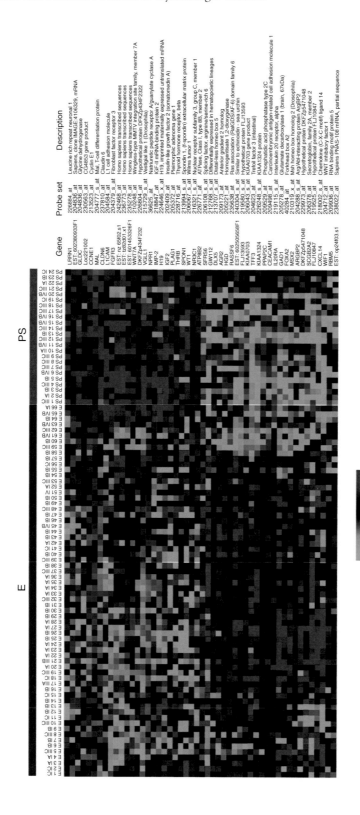

Figure 13.4 Supervised analysis identifying genes that are differentially expressed when comparing global gene expression between 66 endometrioid carcinomas and 24 papillary serous carcinomas. The 25 most upregulated and 25 most downregulated genes at p <0.001 are illustrated. Each sample in the heat map is labeled with histology, stage of disease and coded tumor number. The heat map was color-coded using red for upregulation from normal endometrium and green for downregulation.

between normal and malignant endometrium. In addition, after analyzing the gene expression profiles from the normal endometrium and accounting for genes differentially expressed in the proliferative versus secretory phases of the menstrual cycle, this analysis demonstrated that the gene expression profiles of adenocarcinoma cases more closely resembled the expression profiles of the proliferative-phase normal endometrium samples.[30] While these results are interesting in that the majority of endometrial carcinomas arise in a background of proliferative endometrium, these results should be interpreted with caution. The carcinoma patients in this study were all postmenopausal, while the normal endometrial samples were obtained from premenopausal normally cycling women. The hormonal milieu present in the endometrium from these two groups is arguably vastly different, and therefore it is expected that the gene expression profiles between these two groups would likewise be different.

Molecular differences between different histologic groups

The clinical outcome of patients with endometrial cancer can often be determined to some extent by whether they have an endometrioid (typically type I) or nonendometrioid (typically type II) tumor.[3] Although mutation and expression analysis of targeted genes has demonstrated that there appear to be unique molecular profiles associated with different histologic subtypes of endometrial cancer, microarray techniques facilitate analysis of gene expression on a more comprehensive level. Our group initially used cDNA microarrays to evaluate the gene expression profiles of 19 endometrioid cancers, 13 papillary serous endometrial cancers, 3 clear cell carcinomas, and 7 normal endometria.[31] Multidimensional scaling analysis

showed distinct clustering of genes between each of the histologic subtypes, and unsupervised analysis of the microarray results revealed 191 genes that were differentially expressed by a factor of two within the histologic groups. Twenty-four of these genes could distinguish between endometrioid and serous subtypes. Real-time PCR confirmed that folate-binding protein was overexpressed in papillary serous endometrial cancers (up to 60-fold) compared with normal endometrium, suggesting that this gene should be further evaluated as a potential biomarker associated with this histologic subtype.[31] Similar small studies of endometrial cancer have been performed by other investigational groups using cDNA microarrays, and have confirmed these conclusions.[32,33]

More recently, our group performed a more extensive analysis of global gene expression in 119 uterine cancers using oligonucleotide arrays.[34] In this analysis, we choose to also include mixed müllerian tumors of the uterus, since these sarcomas share some features characteristic of both papillary serous tumors (i.e. poor prognosis) and endometrioid carcinomas (i.e. association with obesity and tamoxifen exposure). Unsupervised and supervised analysis of global gene expression in 66 endometrioid, 24 papillary serous, and 29 endometrial carcinosarcomas confirmed that distinct patterns of gene expression characterize each of these histologic subtypes of uterine cancer. Two-sample t-tests comparing endometrioid and papillary serous, endometrioid and mixed müllerian tumor, and papillary serous and mixed müllerian tumor pairs identified 1055, 5212, and 1208 differentially expressed genes, respectively, at $p < 0.001$. In addition, we found that when we performed supervised analysis on a subset of papillary serous and endometrioid cancers that were matched for stage and grade, we obtained a much shorter list of differentially expressed genes.[34] These findings suggested that although the global gene expression patterns for these histologic subtypes are distinct, they also share genetic alterations that are common to both types. Other investigators have shown further that both endometrioid and papillary serous subtypes of carcinoma have unique gene expression profiles when originating in the endometrium versus the ovary, despite clinical features that more advanced forms of these histologic subtypes share irrespective of the primary site of origin.[35]

Node prediction

Although the majority of endometrial cancers are confined to the uterus at the time of diagnosis, approximately 15% have occult extrauterine spread.[36] Unfortunately, contemporary radiologic and laboratory testing are suboptimal at accurate identification of patients likely to have node metastasis. Development of an accurate diagnostic test would enhance patient care by identifying patients at high risk for nodal metastasis who should be referred to a gynecologic oncologist versus those at low risk who could be managed by the general obstetrician/gynecologist. One potential application of gene expression profiling is in the prediction of nodal metastasis in the preoperative patient with endometrial cancer. Bidus et al[37] evaluated the expression profiles of 41 patients with endometrioid endometrial cancer. Of these 41 patients, 12 had positive lymph nodes. Supervised analysis of the expression profiles revealed 450 genes that were differentially expressed between the node-positive and node-negative groups. Overexpressed genes in the lymph node-positive group included *CDC2* and *MAD2L1*, both of which are cell cycle checkpoint genes.[37] This study

showed that it was possible to demonstrate expression profiles associated with lymphatic spread of tumor. Such results offer promise that, one day, gene expression profiles of preoperative tissue biopsies may reliably predict the presence or absence of lymphatic spread, thereby impacting the clinical decisions regarding the performance of lymph node sampling in endometrial carcinoma.

Risk of recurrence

'Intermediate-risk' patients with stage IB, IC, or II (occult) endometrial cancer have an approximately 15% risk of recurrence, and multiple studies have evaluated the options of adjuvant therapy to maximize disease-free survival.[38,39] Tests that are more accurate than staging classification at prediction of recurrence would prove invaluable in selection of patients for adjuvant therapies in order to minimize treatment-related patient morbidity and optimize survival. Ferguson et al[40] used binary comparison analysis of DNA microarray data to demonstrate that endometrial carcinoma patients who are thought to be at intermediate risk for recurrence can be segregated into a group at low risk for recurrence and another group at high risk based upon global gene expression profiling. In this study, tissue samples from 13 recurrent endometrial cancer patients and 62 disease-free patients, all originally classified as at intermediate risk for recurrence based upon traditional histologic and pathologic criteria, underwent global gene expression profiling using oligonucleotide microarray analysis. Binary comparison analysis was used to select differentially expressed genes in the high-risk group relative to the low-risk group to create a risk score. This score, a linear combination of the individual gene expression values weighted by the regression coefficients of the genes in the model, was then shown to be associated with a statistically significant increased risk of recurrence when the entire cohort was analyzed.[40] While the stratification of patients into low- and high-risk groups based upon risk score did not correlate perfectly with recurrence, this study demonstrates how binary comparison analysis can be applied to molecular research and translated into clinically meaningful applications and results.

Binary comparison according to tumor genotype

Gene expression profiling is useful not only to identify distinct profiles of histologically different tumors, but also to investigate differences in histologically similar but genetically dissimilar tumors as a method of explaining differences in outcomes. Previous evidence has suggested that microsatellite instability (MSI) is a favorable prognostic factor in endometrioid endometrial cancer,[41,42] and this clinical behavior may be explained by a unique global gene expression pattern. Risinger et al[43] explored this phenomenon in patients with early-stage endometrioid endometrial cancers that were histologically similar but had different MSI phenotypes. Using DNA microarrays to test the hypothesis that MSI tumors have a unique genetic profile, they performed gene expression analysis on 16 microsatellite-stable cancers and 12 MSI cancers. They found that 109 gene transcripts differed by at least twofold between the two groups. Moreover, the gene encoding for the SFRP1 protein was frequently downregulated and associated with promoter hypermethylation in the MSI group compared with the microsatellite-stable group, demonstrating that MSI tumors are genetically different from microsatellite-stable tumors, even though they are histologically identical. This genetic difference is a possible explanation

for the difference in outcome associated with MSI.[43]

Class prediction

Unlike class comparison, where one is trying to describe differences between two groups, or class discovery, where one is attempting to identify subgroups, class prediction analysis involves predicting which class or group a sample will belong to based upon its global gene expression profile. In this case, unknown samples are placed into a preexisting classification based upon the gene expression profile of the sample. The gene expression profile of the class must be known and be sufficiently accurate in terms of predictability to be used as a model. Several class prediction methods that are commonly used include support vector machine, linear discriminant analysis, nearest centroid classifier, and compound covariate. Prediction can be performed by leaving one sample out at a time for cross-validation and using all other samples for classification. Alternatively, development of a prediction model based on a training set and subsequent testing of the model on a validation set is an even more optimal approach to class prediction.[28] Although there have been no reports of class prediction of clinical endpoints in endometrial cancer to date, our group is currently undertaking validation of a model aimed at prediction of nodal metastasis in endometrial cancer.

VALIDATION OF GENE EXPRESSION

Gene expression data from microarray experiments ideally should be validated using an alternative laboratory-based method. Commonly used techniques include real-time PCR, in situ hybridization, northern blot, and immunohistochemistry. In a poll of investigators using tissue microarrays produced by the US National Cancer Institute (NCI), users reported that changes in gene expression correlated with differences in protein expression <50% of the time.[25] These discrepancies can be related to the specificity and sensitivity of the antibody probe as well as post-translational processes affecting the expression of protein relative to the mRNA transcript.

Tissue microarrays

Because gene expression arrays do not always correlate with protein expression, immunohistochemistry is commonly used for validation of gene expression at the protein level in tissue. The development of tissue microarray (TMA) technology has revolutionized the analysis of global gene expression by utilizing high-throughput techniques on multiple tissue specimens simultaneously. A TMA is created by obtaining 0.6–2.0 mm core biopsies from each donor tissue block and transferring these core tissue samples to a predrilled recipient paraffin block. Each of the donor cores is arranged in rows and columns sequentially with 0.8 mm spacing. Once all of the core samples have been placed in the TMA array block, 5 μm sections are cut from the TMA block and transferred to glass slides for processing using immunohistochemistry or other in situ procedures (i.e. FISH or mRNA in situ hybridization) (Figure 13.5). Using this spacing arrangement, tissue specimens from several hundred patients can be represented in one slide instead of hundreds of slides. Quality control of the cases on each array can be enhanced by having multiple duplicate, triplicate, or quadruplicate tissue specimens from each representative case, accounting for histologic variations in the spectrum of pathology changes. Approximately 300 slides

typically can be generated from a single TMA assay block. In addition, each donor block can provide multiple core tissue specimens that can be used to create hundreds of TMAs, each of which can provide hundreds of slides for molecular analysis, thereby giving a process that utilizes the donor tissue specimens in a much more tissue-preserving fashion. The entire process may be performed manually or in an automated fashion using robotics. Data analysis of TMA can be accomplished through manual reading of the TMA by the pathologist, or through automated image capture and analysis techniques, which provide an opportunity to further enhance the standardization and timeliness of the technique.[44,45]

Recently our group has used TMA to validate overexpression and amplification of a known oncogene that was detected during array analysis of endometrial cancers. An exploratory analysis by our group of 10 papillary serous carcinomas and 10 normal endometrial specimens using a comparative genomic hybridization (CGH) array detected significant DNA copy changes at 91 of 287 cytolocations evaluated (unpublished work). In this study, we noted that 50% of the cancers showed gains at cytolocation 17q11.2, which encodes HER2/neu. A subsequent oligonucleotide microarray comparison of 24 papillary serous carcinomas and 10 normal endometrial specimens revealed that HER2 was overexpressed by at least twofold at $p < 0.001$ (unpublished work). In a review of previous studies of HER2 overexpression in endometrial cancer, we acknowledged that the low rates of overexpression may have been the result of a preponderance of endometrioid cancers comprising the sample set undergoing analysis.[46,47] Recent clinical data was also conflicting regarding the incidence (18–62%) of HER2 overexpression in patients with papillary serous subtypes of

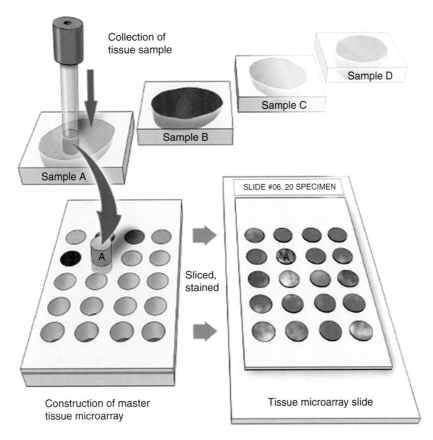

Figure 13.5 Tissue microarray. Core biopsies are created from multiple donor blocks and sequentially transferred to a recipient block that has been predrilled with rows and columns of holes for the transferred tissue cores. Once construction of the tissue microarray block is complete, slides can be cut containing representative specimens from the donor cases.

endometrial cancer.[48–50] A TMA comprising endometrial cancers from 483 patients was subsequently used to further evaluate this controversy. In this analysis, both HER2 overexpression and amplification correlated with survival, which was shorter in patients who overexpressed (median 5.2 years) and/or showed amplification of HER2 (median 3.5 years) compared with those who did not (median 13 years). Pure papillary serous endometrial carcinomas showed the highest frequency of both overexpression (43%) and amplification (29%). In addition, mixed epithelial cancers with serous differentiation showed a lower rate of both overexpression (26%) and amplification (7%). These findings suggested that previous reports involving uterine papillary serous carcinomas may have had lower rates for overexpression resulting from inclusion of these mixed epithelial subtypes of cancer. Our data also suggested that therapies that target HER2 may have a role in the treatment of papillary serous endometrial carcinomas that are pure in histologic composition (Figure 13.6).[51] The use of TMA proved to be invaluable in providing a large group of well-annotated specimens with which to validate our array findings.

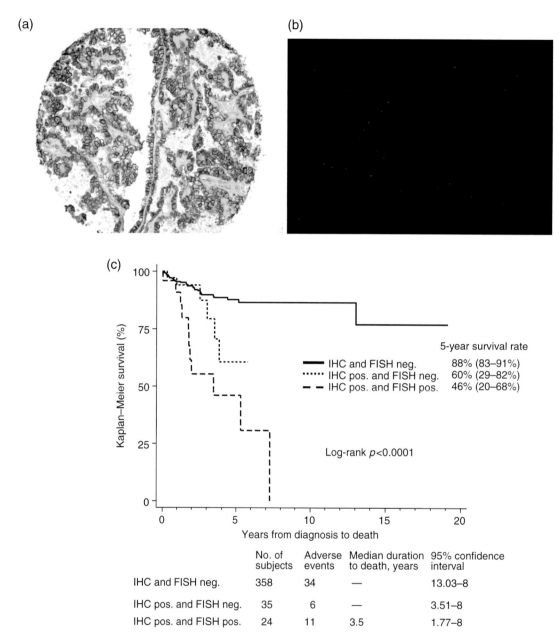

Figure 13.6 The utility of tissue microarray in confirming gene expression. (a) Positive (3 out of 3 scoring system) immunohistochemistry (IHC) with strong membranous staining in >10% cells of a serous carcinoma. (b) Corresponding fluorescence in situ hybridization (FISH) demonstrating a high level of HER2/*neu* amplification. (c) Kaplan–Meier survival curve for 396 patients with endometrial cancer represented on tissue microarray.

FUTURE DIRECTIONS

In this chapter, we have reviewed the common techniques involved with high-throughput genomic analysis in an attempt to clarify the benefits, advantages, and disadvantages of these molecular biologic technologies. In addition, we have discussed recent studies utilizing microarray techniques in the study of endometrial carcinoma. It is expected that these techniques will lead directly to improvements in diagnosis, prognosis, and treatment as we learn more about the biology of endometrial carcinoma.

REFERENCES

1. Jemal A, Siegel R, Ward E. Cancer statistics. CA Cancer J Clin 2007;57:43–66.

2. http://www.ahrq.gov/

3. Deligdisch L, Holinka CF. Endometrial carcinoma: two diseases? Cancer Detect Prev 1987;10:237–46.

4. Kong D, Suzuki A, Zou TT, Sakurada A, et al. *PTEN1* is frequently mutated in primary endometrial carcinomas. Nat Genet 1997;17:143–4.

5. Risinger JI, Hayes AK, Berchuck A, Barrett JC. *PTEN/MMAC1* mutations in endometrial cancers. Cancer Res 1997;57:4736–8.

6. Risinger JI, Hayes K, Maxwell GL, Barrett C, Berchuck A. *PTEN* mutation in endometrial cancers is associated with favorable clinical and pathologic characteristics. Clin Cancer Res 1998;4:3005–10.

7. Risinger JI, Berchuck A, Kohler MF, et al. Genetic instability of microsatellites in endometrial carcinoma. Cancer Res 1993;53: 5100–3.

8. Maxwell GL, Risinger JI, Alvarez AA, Barrett JC, Berchuck A. Microsatellite instability is associated with favorable survival in endometrial carcinomas. Obstet Gynecol 2001;97:417–22.

9. Black D, Soslow RA, Levine DA, et al. Clinicopathologic significance of defective DNA mismatch repair in endometrial carcinoma. J Clin Oncol 2006;24:1745–53.

10. Lukes AS, Kohler MF, Pieper CF, et al. Multivariable analysis of DNA ploidy, p53, and HER-2/*neu* as prognostic factors in endometrial cancer. Cancer 1994;73:2380–5.

11. Kohler MF, Berchuck A, Davidoff AM, et al. Overexpression and mutation of p53 in endometrial carcinoma. Cancer Res 1992;52: 1622–7.

12. Kohler MF, Carney P, Dodge R, et al. p53 overexpression in advanced-stage endometrial adenocarcinoma. Am J Obstet Gynecol 1996;175:1246–52.

13. Risinger JI, Maxwell GL, Chandramouli GVR, Berchuck A, Barrett JC. Molecular genetic profiles of serous and endometrioid endometrial cancers, genes downregulated in endometrial cancers and the role of epigenetics. In: Kuramoto H, Nishida M, eds. Cell and Molecular Biology of Endometrial Cancer. Tokyo: Springer-Verlag, 2003:245–51.

14. Herman JG, Baylin SB. Promoter-region hypermethylation and gene silencing in human cancer. Curr Top Microbiol Immunol 2000;249:35–54.

15. Risinger J, Maxwell GL, Berchuck A, Barrett C. Promoter hypermethylation as an epigenetic component in type I and type II cancers. Ann NY Acad Sci 2003;983:209–12.

16. ISBER (International Society for Biological and Environmental Repositories). Best practices for repositories I: collection, storage and retrieval of human biological materials for research. Cell Preserv Technol 2005;3:5–48.

17. Spruessel A, Steimann G, Jung M, et al. Tissue ischemia time affects gene and protein expression patterns within minutes following

surgical tumor excision. BioTechniques 2004; 36:1–8.

18. Hunt JL, Finkelstein SD. Microdissection techniques for molecular testing in surgical pathology. Arch Pathol Lab Med 2004;128: 1372–8.

19. Espina V, Milia J, Wu G, Cowherd S, Liotta LA. Laser capture microdissection. Meth Mol Biol 2006;319:213–29.

20. Nijaz Y, Sticvh M, Sagmuller B, et al. Noncontact laser microdissection and pressure catapulting: sample preparation for genomic, transcriptomic and proteomic analysis. Meth Mol Med 2005;114:1–24.

21. Kolble K. The Leica microdissection system: design and applications. J Mol Med 2000;78:B24–5.

22. Becette V, Vignaud S, Regnier C, et al. Gene transcript assay by real-time RT–PCR in epithelial breast cancer cells selected by laser microdissection. Int J Biol Markers 2004;19: 100–8.

23. Holloway AJ, van Laar RK, Tothill RW, Bowtell DDL. Options available-from start to finish for obtaining data from DNA microarrays II. Nat Genet 2002;32(Suppl): 481–9.

24. Emmert-Buck MR, Strausberg RL, Krizman DB, et al. Molecular profiling of clinical tissue specimens: feasibility and applications. Am J Pathol 2000;156:1109–15.

25. Chuaqui RF, Bonner RE, Best CJM, et al. Post-analysis follow-up and validation of microarray experiments. Nat Genet 2002;32(Suppl):509–14.

26. Zorn KK, Jazaeri AA, Awtrey CS, et al. Choice of normal ovarian control influences determination of differentially expressed genes in ovarian cancer expression profiling studies. Clin Cancer Res 2003;9:4811–18.

27. Quackenbush J. Microarray data normalization and transformation. Nat Genet 2002; 32:496–501.

28. Slonim DK. From patterns to pathways: gene expression data analysis comes of age. Nat Genet 2002;32:502–8.

29. Ferguson SE, Olshen AB, Viale A, et al. Gene expression profiling of tamoxifen-associated uterine cancers: evidence for two molecular classes of endometrial carcinoma. Gynecol Oncol 2004;92:719–25.

30. Mutter GL, Baak JP, Fitzgerald JT, et al. Global expression changes of constitutive and hormonally regulated genes during endometrial neoplastic transformation. Gynecol Oncol 2001;83:177–85.

31. Risinger J, Maxwell GL, Chandramouli GVR, et al. Microarray analysis reveals distinct gene expression profiles among different histologic types of endometrial cancer. Cancer Res 2003;63:6–11.

32. Cao QJ, Belbin T, Socci N, et al. Distinctive gene expression profiles by cDNA microarrays in endometrioid and serous carcinomas of the endometrium. Int J Gynecol Pathol 2004;23:321–9.

33. Moreno-Bueno G, Sanchez-Estevez C, Cassia R, et al. Differential gene expression profile in endometrioid and nonendometrioid endometrial carcinoma: STK15 is frequently overexpressed and amplified in nonendometrioid carcinomas. Cancer Res 2003;63: 5697–702.

34. Maxwell GL, Chandramouli GVR, Dainty L, et al. Microarray analysis of endometrial carcinomas and mixed mullerian tumors reveals distinct gene expression profiles associated with different histologic types of uterine cancer. Clin Cancer Res 2005;11:4056–66.

35. Zorn KK, Bonome T, Gangi L, et al. Gene expression profiles of serous, endometrioid, and clear cell subtypes of ovarian and endometrial cancer. Clin Cancer Res 2005;11: 6422–30.

36. Creasman WT, Morrow CP, Bundy BN, et al. Surgical pathologic spread patterns of endometrial cancer. A Gynecologic Oncology

Group study. Cancer 1987;60(8 Suppl.): 2035–41.

37. Bidus MA, Risinger JI, Chandramouli GVR, et al. Prediction of lymph node metastasis in patients with endometrioid endometrial cancer using expression microarray. Clin Cancer Res 2006;12:83–8.

38. Keys HM, Roberts JA, Brunetto VL, et al. A phase III trial of surgery with or without adjunctive external pelvic radiation therapy in intermediate risk endometrial adenocarcinoma: a Gynecologic Oncology Group study. Gynecol Oncol 2004;92:744–51.

39. Macdonald OK, Sause WT, Lee RJ, et al. Adjuvant radiotherapy and survival outcomes in early-stage endometrial cancer: a multi-institutional analysis of 608 women. Gynecol Oncol 2006;103:661–6.

40. Ferguson SE, Olshen AB, Viale A, Barakat RR, Boyd J. Stratification of intermediate-risk endometrial cancer patients into groups at high risk or low risk for recurrence based on tumor gene expression profiles. Clin Cancer Res 2005;11:2252–7.

41. Black D, Soslow RA, Levine DA, et al. Clinicopathologic significance of defective DNA mismatch repair in endometrial carcinoma. J Clin Oncol 2006;24:1745–53.

42. Maxwell GL, Risinger JI, Alvarez AA, Barrett JC, Berchuck A. Favorable survival associated with microsatellite instability in endometrioid endometrial cancers. Obstet Gynecol 2001;97:417–22.

43. Risinger JI, Maxwell GL, Chandramouli GVR, et al. Gene expression profiling of microsatellite unstable and microsatellite stable endometrial cancers indicates distinct pathways of aberrant signaling. Cancer Res 2005;65: 5031–7.

44. Giltnane JM, Rimm DL. Technology insight: identification of biomarkers with tissue microarray technology. Nat Clin Pract Oncol 2004;1:104–11.

45. Eguiluz C, Viguera E, Millan L, Perez J. Multitissue array review: a chronological description of tissue array techniques, applications and procedures. Pathol Res Pract 2006;202:561–8.

46. Berchuck A, Rodriguez G, Kinney RB, et al. Overexpression of HER-2/*neu* in endometrial cancer is associated with advanced stage disease. Am J Obstet Gynecol 1991;164:15–21.

47. Lukes AS, Kohler MF, Pieper CF, et al. Multivariable analysis of DNA ploidy, p53, and HER-2/*neu* as prognostic factors in endometrial cancer. Cancer 1994;73:2380–5.

48. Mariani A, Sebo TJ, Katzmann JA, et al. HER-2/*neu* overexpression and hormone dependency in endometrial cancer: analysis of cohort and review of literature. Anticancer Res 2005;25:2921–7.

49. Slomovitz BM, Broaddus RR, Burke TW, et al. Her-2/*neu* overexpression and amplification in uterine papillary serous carcinoma. J Clin Oncol 2004;22:3126–32.

50. Santin AD, Bellone S, Van Stedum S, et al. Determination of HER2/*neu* status in uterine serous papillary carcinoma: comparative analysis of immunohistochemistry and fluorescence in situ hybridization. Gynecol Oncol 2005; 98:24–30.

51. Morrison C, Zanagnolo V, Ramirez N, et al. HER-2 is an independent prognostic factor in endometrial cancer: association with outcome in a large cohort of surgically staged patients. J Clin Oncol 2006;24: 2376–85.

Prognostic markers of uterine papillary serous carcinoma

14

Brian M Slomovitz and Warner K Huh

INTRODUCTION

First described by Hendrickson et al[1] in 1982, uterine papillary serous carcinoma (UPSC) is an aggressive histologic subtype of endometrial cancer that has distinct clinical and pathologic characteristics and accounts for a disproportionate number of recurrences and deaths.[2] While this subtype comprises <10% of cases of endometrial cancer, it accounts >50% of recurrences and deaths due to this disease.[1] These tumors occur more frequently in the absence of hyperestrogenism and endometrial hyperplasia, and most arise from atrophic endometrium. The 5-year overall survival rate for patients with stage I UPSC is 45–70% and that for patients with stage III or IV disease is 7–37%.[3–9]

CLINICOPATHOLOGIC FEATURES

While prognostic markers for typical endometrial carcinoma (i.e. endometrioid endometrial carcinoma, EEC) are well characterized, only limited information is available that allows us to predict clinical behavior for patients with UPSC. Traditional pathologic criteria (lymphovascular space invasion (LVSI), depth of myometrial invasion, and lymph node involvement) are not predictive of metastatic disease or site of recurrence for UPSC. However, stage, lymph node status, LVSI, and depth of uterine invasion are predictors of survival. Several investigators have confirmed that depth of myometrial invasion and LVSI are significant pathologic determinants of a poor prognosis.[6,10,11] Significantly, it is not uncommon for patients with no myometrial invasion to have distant disease at the time of initial diagnosis. Up to 40% of patients with no myometrial invasion will have advanced disease at the time of surgical staging. Therefore, complete surgical evaluation, including lymph node dissection and omental biopsy, is indicated at the time of initial surgery. In addition, mixed adenocarcinomas with serous components portend a clinical course similar to that of pure UPSC. Therefore, patients with either endometrioid carcinoma or clear cell carcinoma with serous components should be treated as if they have UPSC.[6,8]

Unlike most other gynecologic tumors, patients with stage IA tumors may have unusually aggressive disease. In the study by Gehrig et al,[12] 6 had stage IA UPSC and were given adjuvant therapy, and 2 went on to have documented vaginal recurrences. In the study by Carcangiu et al[8] of 13 patients with stage IA UPSC, all except 1 received adjuvant therapy, and 2 of the 13 patients had recurrences in the abdomen 9 months after their initial diagnosis. One had received adjuvant whole-abdominal radiotherapy, and the other had received adjuvant platinum-based chemotherapy. In the large retrospective series of 129 patients from the

MD Anderson Cancer Center, 20% of patients with stage IA disease had recurrent disease.[6]

ADJUVANT THERAPY AND PROGNOSIS

Radiotherapy

The addition of adjuvant therapy to the surgical treatment of patients with early-stage UPSC is controversial. In the largest series of patients with stage I disease who were surgically staged, Huh et al[13] found that the recurrence rates and overall survival were similar between surgical stage I patients with UPSC who were managed conservatively ($n=40$) and those treated with adjuvant radiotherapy ($n=12$). The absence of pelvic sidewall failures suggested minimal or no benefit for adjuvant radiotherapy. Huh et al[13] found that 43% of patients had distant recurrent disease. They concluded that the use of adjuvant chemotherapy in these patients should be further investigated. In the accompanying editorial, Podratz and Mariani[14] state, 'It is reasonable to suggest that treatment strategies should be predicated on the anticipated pattern of recurrence', suggesting that adjuvant chemotherapy may be indicated.

Whole-abdominal radiotherapy has been shown to have poor response rates and high recurrence rates even when applied in the adjuvant setting.[15] The necessary hepatic and renal shielding may be partially responsible for poor responses. The pattern of failure for early-stage patients with UPSC following whole-abdominal radiotherapy was evaluated in a study by the Gynecologic Oncology Group (GOG 94).[16] In this trial, 62% (8 of 13) of patients with UPSC recurred in the radiated field. Only one of these recurrences was limited to the pelvis.

Chemotherapy

Adjuvant chemotherapy for patients with UPSC has been evaluated. A summary of studies reporting on patients with stage I UPSC is shown in Table 14.1. Kelly et al[17] reported an improved survival in stage I patients treated with adjuvant based therapy. In this study, patients with stage IA disease did well whether or not they received adjuvant therapy. Among the patients with stage IB and IC disease, 1 of 22 patients who received adjuvant platinum-based chemotherapy had recurrent disease, compared with 14 of 18 recurrences in those patients who did not have adjuvant chemotherapy. Kelly et al[17] concluded that platinum-based chemotherapy improved survival in patients with stage I UPSC and that patients with stage IA UPSC with no residual disease could be observed without additional therapy.

Dietrich et al[18] reported on a multi-institutional study of 29 patients with stage I UPSC treated with adjuvant chemotherapy. Twenty-one of these patients were treated with carboplatin and paclitaxel. Only one patient recurred in the vagina after three cycles of therapy. The mean follow-up for the remaining 20 patients was 41 months (range 13–138 months). The authors[18] concluded that this combination after surgery was effective.

An early study by Price et al[19] reported on cyclophosphamide, doxorubicin, and cisplatin in 14 patients with UPSC treated in the adjuvant setting. Six of these patients had stage I disease and three had stage II disease. Eleven (58%) were alive without disease with a median follow-up of 24 months. The remaining eight patients (one stage II, two stage III, and five stage III) were dead of disease, with a median survival of 14 months. In this study, three patients had a distant recurrence, three had a regional recurrence, and one had a local recurrence in

Table 14.1 Summary of stage I UPSC studies

Ref	n	FIGO stage	Follow-up (months)	Recurrence rate (%)
Observation (surgery only)				
13	40	IA (13), IB (17), IC (10)	24	17
Elit	27	IA (19), IB (7), IC (1)	42	19
17	21	IA (16), IB (4), IC (2)	—	29
Bristow	11	IA (4), IB (7)	47	9
Gallion	9	IA (9)	—	0
3	5	IA (3), IB (2)	47	0
Gehrig	6	IA (6)	24	33
Chemotherapy[a]				
13	7	IA (2), IB (3), IC (2)	50	0
Elit	6	IA (3), IB (2), IC (2)	36	66
18	29	IA (7), IB (17), IC (5)	41	5
17	32	IA (9), IB (16), IC (7)	37–57	3

[a]Paclitaxel and carboplatin.

the pelvis. One patient had recurrent disease only documented by an elevated CA–125 level.

Zanotti et al[20] treated nine patients (three stage I, one stage II, three stage III, and two stage IV) with paclitaxel- and platinum-based chemotherapy who had no evidence of disease after surgical staging. The progression-free interval in this group was 35 months (range 6–72 months) and the treatment was well tolerated. Ramondetta et al[21] treated five patients with no measurable disease with paclitaxel in the adjuvant setting. Three of these patients developed recurrent disease (at a median of 7 months) and two were disease-free at 14 and 56 months. All of these patients had advanced-stage disease.

Combined radio- and chemotherapy

Combined chemotherapy and radiotherapy may play a role in the management of patients with early-stage disease. Turner et al[22] reported the application of vaginal radiation at a high dose rate in combination with chemotherapy in surgical stage I patient. The 5-year survival rate was 94%, which is higher than in most other studies for patients with stage I disease.

Proposed collaborative trials will evaluate the role of chemotherapy combined with radiation for the adjuvant therapy of patients with stage I disease. These studies will help to determine the role of combination therapy for patients with intermediate- to high-risk disease.

MOLECULAR FACTORS

Typical EECs have four common genetic alterations: *PTEN* mutations, *KRAS* mutations, microsatellite instability (MSI), and B-catenin mutations. Although *TP53* mutations are uncommon in patients with EEC, they are commonly found in women with UPSC. While 80–90% of UPSCs show overexpression of p53 protein by immunohistochemistry (IHC), this only represents those patients with *TP53* missense mutations (Figure 14.1). Other genetic abnormalities yield aberrant functioning p53 without IHC overexpression. Most, if not all, of UPSCs have loss of *TP53* control. In addition, 78% of cases of endometrial intraepithelial carcinoma, the precursor lesion of UPSC, have mutations in *TP53*. Therefore, mutations are likely an early event in the pathogenesis of this disease. Baergen et al[23] identified a consistent *TP53* mutation in the primary and metastatic tumors in four women with UPSC or its precursor, endometrial intraepithelial carcinoma.

Aberrant expression of both transmembrane and intracellular proteins has been evaluated in these tumors. The human HER2/*neu* (*ERBB2*) gene product, also called p185[HER2] and c-ErbB-2, is a member of the epidermal growth factor receptor (EGFR) transmembrane receptor tyrosine kinase family.[24,25] Overexpression of HER2/*neu* has been found to play a role in cellular transformation, tumorigenesis, and metastasis.[26] In breast cancers, 25–30% of tumors overexpress HER2/*neu*.[27,28] Overexpression of HER2/*neu* is considered a negative prognostic factor for women with breast cancer, being associated with a shorter disease-free interval and worse overall survival.[28–31] In ovarian cancer, early data reported up to 30% overexpression of HER2/*neu*.[32] Most recently, results from the GOG found that a significantly lower percentage (11.4%, or 95 of 837) of ovarian cancers overexpressed HER2/*neu* by immuno-histochemistry.[33]

In a study by Slomovitz et al[34] of 68 patients with UPSC, there was an 18% incidence of HER2/*neu* overexpression. Gene amplification of HER2/*neu* was rare. In addition, Slomovitz et al demonstrated that HER2/*neu* overexpression was the strongest predictor of overall survival and disease-specific survival when compared with traditional pathologic features (Figure 14.2). Coronado et al[35] examined different histologic subtypes of endometrial cancer and reported that HER2/*neu* expression was more frequent in the case of advanced-stage disease, nonendometrioid subtypes, deep myometrial invasion, and high-grade histology. They did not find HER2/*neu* to be an independent prognostic factor. In 100 cases of all histologic subtypes of endometrial cancer, Lukes et al[36] found that HER2/*neu* overexpression was a predictor of recurrent or persistent disease. Berchuck et al[37] concluded

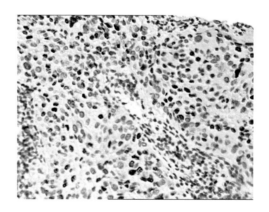

Figure 14.1 p53 immunohistochemistry.

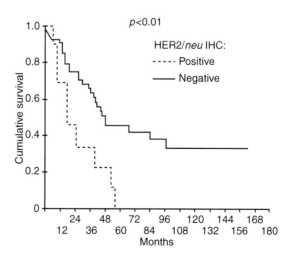

Figure 14.2 HER2/*neu* immunohistochemistry (IHC) and overall survival Kaplan–Meier curves.

that HER2/*neu* expression in all types of endometrial cancer was associated with an increased incidence of death from persistent or recurrent disease.

Other cellular proteins have been found to be overexpressed in tumors from patients with UPSC. Imatinib (Gleevec/Glivec) is a tyrosine kinase inhibitor that specifically targets Kit, Abl, and platelet-derived growth factor receptor (PDGFR). It has been shown to be an effective treatment for patients with chronic myelogenous leukemia (CML) and gastrointestinal stromal tumors (GISTs). In a study evaluating the expression of these kinases in a series of primary and recurrent UPSCs, most tumors expressed Abl and PDGFR.[38]

Expression of these kinases did not have prognostic implications.

SUMMARY

Typical predictors of high stage and poor outcome are not present in patients with UPSC. All patients with UPSC should undergo complete surgical staging, even in the absence of uterine invasion. While adjuvant therapy appears to provide a clinical benefit, even in patients with stage I disease, our current knowledge of this disease does not allow us to know which tumors will recur and which will follow a more indolent course. A better understanding of these tumors on a molecular level is needed.

REFERENCES

1. Hendrickson M, Ross J, Eifel P, Martinez A, Kempson R. Uterine papillary serous carcinoma: a highly malignant form of endometrial adenocarcinoma. Am J Surg Pathol 1982;6: 93–108.

2. Rose PG. Endometrial carcinoma. N Engl J Med 1996;335:640–9.

3. Grice J, Ek M, Greer B, et al. Uterine papillary serous carcinoma: evaluation of long-term survival in surgically staged patients. Gynecol Oncol 1998;69:69–73.

4. Bristow RE, Asrari F, Trimble EL, Montz FJ. Extended surgical staging for uterine papillary serous carcinoma: survival outcome of locoregional (stage I–III) disease. Gynecol Oncol 2001;81:279–86.

5. Bristow RE, Duska LR, Montz FJ. The role of cytoreductive surgery in the management of stage IV uterine papillary serous carcinoma. Gynecol Oncol 2001;81:92–9.

6. Slomovitz BM, Burke TW, Eifel PJ, et al. Uterine papillary serous carcinoma (UPSC): a single institution review of 129 cases. Gynecol Oncol 2003;91:463–9.

7. Piura B, Meirovitz M, Shmulman M, et al. Uterine papillary serous carcinoma: study of 19 cases. Eur J Obstet Gynecol Reprod Biol 1998;79:69–73.

8. Carcangiu ML, Chambers JT. Uterine papillary serous carcinoma: a study on 108 cases with emphasis on the prognostic significance of associated endometrioid carcinoma, absence of invasion, and concomitant ovarian carcinoma. Gynecol Oncol 1992;47:298–305.

9. Carcangiu ML, Chambers JT. Early pathologic stage clear cell carcinoma and uterine papillary serous carcinoma of the endometrium: comparison of clinicopathologic features and survival. Int J Gynecol Pathol 1995;14:30–8.

10. Goff BA, Kato D, Schmidt RA, et al. Uterine papillary serous carcinoma: patterns of metastatic spread. Gynecol Oncol 1994;54: 264–8.

11. Sherman ME, Bitterman P, Rosenshein NB, Delgado G, Kurman RJ. Uterine serous carcinoma. A morphologically diverse neoplasm with unifying clinicopathologic features. Am J Surg Pathol 1992;16:600–10.

12. Gehrig PA, Groben PA, Fowler WC Jr, Walton LA, Van Le L. Noninvasive papillary serous carcinoma of the endometrium. Obstet Gynecol 2001;97:153–7.

13. Huh WK, Powell M, Leath CA 3rd, et al. Uterine papillary serous carcinoma: comparisons of outcomes in surgical stage I patients with and without adjuvant therapy. Gynecol Oncol 2003;91:470–5.

14. Podratz KC, Mariani A. Uterine papillary serous carcinomas: the exigency for clinical trials. Gynecol Oncol 2003;91:461–2.

15. Frank AH, Tseng PC, Haffty BG, et al. Adjuvant whole-abdominal radiation therapy in uterine papillary serous carcinoma. Cancer 1991;68:1516–19.

16. Sutton G, Bundy B, Axelrod J, et al. Whole abdominal radiotherapy in stage I–II papillary serous or clear cell cancers of the uterus (a GOG study). Gynecol Oncol 2002;84:479–536 (Abst 205).

17. Kelly MG, O'Malley D M, Hui P, et al. Improved survival in surgical stage I patients with uterine papillary serous carcinoma (UPSC) treated with adjuvant platinum-based chemotherapy. Gynecol Oncol 2005;98:353–9.

18. Dietrich CS 3rd, Modesitt SC, Depriest PD, et al. The efficacy of adjuvant platinum-based chemotherapy in stage I uterine papillary serous carcinoma (UPSC). Gynecol Oncol 2005;99:557–63.

19. Price FV, Chambers SK, Carcangiu ML, et al. Intravenous cisplatin, doxorubicin, and cyclophosphamide in the treatment of uterine papillary serous carcinoma (UPSC). Gynecol Oncol 1993;51:383–9.

20. Zanotti KM, Belinson JL, Kennedy AW, Webster KD, Markman M. The use of paclitaxel and platinum-based chemotherapy in uterine papillary serous carcinoma. Gynecol Oncol 1999;74:272–7.

21. Ramondetta L, Burke TW, Levenback C, et al. Treatment of uterine papillary serous carcinoma with paclitaxel. Gynecol Oncol 2001;82:156–61.

22. Turner BC, Knisely JP, Kacinski BM, et al. Effective treatment of stage I uterine papillary serous carcinoma with high dose-rate vaginal apex radiation (^{192}Ir) and chemotherapy. Int J Radiat Oncol Biol Phys 1998;40:77–84.

23. Baergen RN, Warren CD, Isacson C, Ellenson LH. Early uterine serous carcinoma: clonal origin of extrauterine disease. Int J Gynecol Pathol 2001;20:214–19.

24. Coussens L, Yang-Feng TL, Liao YC, et al. Tyrosine kinase receptor with extensive homology to EGF receptor shares chromosomal location with *neu* oncogene. Science 1985;230:1132–19.

25. Akiyama T, Kadooka T, Ogawara H, Sakakibara S. Characterization of the epidermal growth factor receptor and the erbB oncogene product by site-specific antibodies. Arch Biochem Biophys 1986;245:531–6.

26. Chazin VR, Kaleko M, Miller AD, Slamon DJ. Transformation mediated by the human HER-2 gene independent of the epidermal growth factor receptor. Oncogene 1992;7:1859–66.

27. Slamon DJ, Clark GM, Wong SG, et al. Human breast cancer: correlation of relapse and survival with amplification of the HER-2/*neu* oncogene. Science 1987;235:177–82.

28. Slamon DJ, Godolphin W, Jones LA, et al. Studies of the HER-2/*neu* proto-oncogene in human breast and ovarian cancer. Science 1989;244:707–12.

29. Andrulis IL, Bull SB, Blackstein ME, et al. *neu*/erbB-2 amplification identifies a poor-prognosis group of women with node-negative breast cancer. Toronto Breast Cancer Study Group. J Clin Oncol 1998;16:1340–9.

30. Gusterson BA. Identification and interpretation of epidermal growth factor and c-erbB-2 overexpression. Eur J Cancer 1992;28:263–7.

31. Gusterson BA, Gelber RD, Goldhirsch A, et al. Prognostic importance of c-erbB-2 expression in breast cancer. International (Ludwig) Breast Cancer Study Group. J Clin Oncol 1992;10:1049–56.

32. Berchuck A, Kamel A, Whitaker R, et al. Overexpression of HER-2/*neu* is associated with poor survival in advanced epithelial ovarian cancer. Cancer Res 1990;50:4087–91.

33. Bookman MA, Darcy KM, Clarke-Pearson D, Boothby RA, Horowitz IR. Evaluation of monoclonal humanized anti-HER2 antibody, trastuzumab, in patients with recurrent or refractory ovarian or primary peritoneal carcinoma with overexpression of HER2: a phase II trial of the Gynecologic Oncology Group. J Clin Oncol 2003;21:283–90.

34. Slomovitz BM, Broaddus RR, Burke TW, et al. Her-2/*neu* overexpression and amplification in uterine papillary serous carcinoma. J Clin Oncol 2004;22:3126–32.

35. Coronado PJ, Vidart JA, Lopez-Asenjo JA, et al. p53 overexpression predicts endometrial carcinoma recurrence better than HER-2/*neu* overexpression. Eur J Obstet Gynecol Reprod Biol 2001;98:103–8.

36. Lukes AS, Kohler MF, Pieper CF, et al. Multivariable analysis of DNA ploidy, p53, and HER-2/*neu* as prognostic factors in endometrial cancer. Cancer 1994;73:2380–5.

37. Berchuck A, Rodriguez G, Kinney RB, et al. Overexpression of HER-2/*neu* in endometrial cancer is associated with advanced stage disease. Am J Obstet Gynecol 1991;164:15–21.

38. Slomovitz BM, Broaddus RR, Schmandt R, et al. Expression of imatinib mesylate-targeted kinases in endometrial carcinoma. Gynecol Oncol 2004;95:32–6.

Predictors of outcome in malignant mixed müllerian tumors of the uterus

15

Elizabeth D Euscher, Robin A Lacour, and Lois M Ramondetta

INTRODUCTION

Malignant mixed müllerian tumors (MMMTs) are uncommon but aggressive gynecologic malignancies that may arise in the vagina, uterine cervix, uterine corpus, ovary or fallopian tube. Of these sites, the uterine corpus is most commonly affected.[1] MMMTs are defined by the presence of an intimate admixture of carcinoma and sarcoma. The carcinomatous component may be endometrioid, serous, clear cell, or any combination of these.[2–5] The sarcomatous component is, by convention, designated either homologous (resembling a sarcoma primary in the uterus) or heterologous (resembling a sarcoma usually arising extrinsic to the uterus) (Figure 15.1). Of the heterologous elements that have been described, rhabdomyosarcoma is most commonly observed, followed by chondrosarcoma and fibrosarcoma.[2–6] It is not unusual to see a mixture of heterologous elements. In the majority of MMMTs, both tumor components are usually high-grade.[4–6]

To reflect the biphasic nature of MMMT, the current World Health Organization (WHO) classification now designates uterine MMMTs as 'mixed epithelial and mesenchymal tumors'.[7] The rarity of the disease and confusing nomenclature have resulted in limited understanding. MMMTs have historically been grouped with all other uterine sarcomas for clinical trials. In addition, much of the early work, and a few of the later studies, focused on the sarcomatous component with regard to prognosis. Early reports attempted to correlate heterologous versus homologous elements with prognosis and found a survival advantage with homologous sarcoma.[8,9] A preponderance of later studies found no such differences in survival.[4,6,10–14] With that said, it is the epithelial component, müllerian in origin, that appears to have the greatest influence on survival. Typically, recurrences of MMMTs are composed of carcinoma of endometrioid or papillary serous subtype. However, recurrences and distant metastases composed of sarcoma or mixed carcinoma and sarcoma also occur.

These tumors usually present in women over the age of 50 and peak in incidence during the seventh and eighth decades. MMMTs are more common in African-American than Caucasian patients. MMMTs are more likely than endometrial stromal sarcomas (ESS) or leiomyosarcomas (LMS) to present with postmenopausal bleeding. Abnormal bleeding usually occurs as a result of the origin of MMMTs in the endometrium, rather than in the myometrium. As a result, the presence of malignancy can usually be determined preoperatively

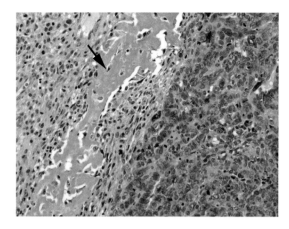

Figure 15.1 High-grade serous carcinoma (right half of image) is sharply demarcated from high-grade sarcoma with heterologous element, which in this example is osteosarcoma (osteoid marked by arrow).

Table 15.1 Survival by stage for malignant mixed müllerian tumors

Stage	5-year survival rate (%)	Ref
I	53	15
II–III	8.5	15
IV	0–16	16

with an endometrial biopsy. Patients typically present with a bulky, polypoid mass extending into, and even through, the endocervical canal. In contrast to LMS, uterine MMMTs metastasize at early stages to pelvic and para-aortic lymph nodes.

Recurrence rates for stage I and II MMMTs are 50%.[15] Distant metastases account for 50–80% of all recurrences. The most common sites of metastasis are the lung and omentum. Features associated with poor prognosis include adnexal spread, lymph node metastasis, and high grade of tumor. Unfortunately, the 5-year survival rate in patients with MMMTs is often <20% (Table 15.1).[15,16]

As stated above, the rarity of MMMTs, as well as confusing nomenclature, have precluded full understanding of the disease and of prognostic factors. Furthermore, as with all endometrial cancers, surgical staging was not incorporated into the evaluation process until 1988, and therefore full pelvic and abdominal evaluations were not always performed at the time of surgery. Many clinical–epidemiologic, surgical, and histologic–molecular factors have been evaluated in order to better understand determinants of prognosis. In spite of efforts to elucidate prognostic factors based on tumor characteristics, the most consistently demonstrated factor that best predicts prognosis is pathologic stage.[2,4,9,17–19]

EPIDEMIOLOGIC FACTORS: AGE AND RACE

A possible negative effect of increased age at the time of diagnosis has been suggested,[20] but many studies have shown no effect or an opposite effect of age.[21,22] Whether age is a predictor of poor prognosis independently or because of associated comorbidities that preclude aggressive chemotherapy, the answer is not known.[2,23] Others have shown the appearance of a trend toward more advanced disease in younger women, as well as in African-American women.[10]

PARITY AND MENOPAUSAL FACTORS

There have been some associations with later onset of menopause and lengthened overall survival.[21,24] Parity has been shown to be protective as well as an insignificant influence.[13,21]

CLINICAL FACTORS

Tumor size

In a small study ($n = 35$), the size and weight of the uterus appeared to have no association with extent of disease.[10] However, a tumor size >8 cm and a carcinoma-to-sarcoma ratio of >1 were associated with more extensive disease.

Stage at presentation and lymph node involvement

There has been some attempt to identify high-risk subgroups within early-stage MMMT (stage I and II). While some believe that the depth of myometrial invasion is predictive of stage but not necessarily a significant prognostic variable,[5,10,11,18] others have shown at least a trend toward an adverse prognosis with increased depth.[2,4,6,12,25] Higher stages usually had deeper myometrial invasion,[4] and in clinical stage I and II patients, the presence of extrauterine disease at the time of surgery correlated with the depth of myometrial invasion.[2,6] Yamada et al[26] showed that the 5-year survival rate of patients with disease confined to the uterus was significantly better compared with others (74% vs 24%; $p = 0.0013$). In this study, pathologic factors predictive of recurrence in patients with MMMT included stage and depth of invasion at presentation, as well as the presence of adnexal and serosal involvement, lymph node metastasis, and positive cytology. However, only intraperitoneal disease was associated with poor survival. In a large Gynecologic Oncology Group (GOG) trial, the presence of adnexal metastasis, positive peritoneal cytology, and cervical involvement, as well as invasion to the outer 50% of the uterine wall were identified as negative predictors of survival.[27] When evaluated by stage, the presence of adnexal spread, lymph node involvement, tumor size, lymphovascular space invasion (LVSI), depth of invasion, and positive peritoneal cytology were related to progression-free interval (PFI) in stage I and II disease by univariate analysis.[27]

Peritoneal cytology

Almost all studies evaluating the presence of positive peritoneal washings have shown this to be a significant negative prognostic factor.[12,27,28] Kanbour et al[28] reported that 20% of stage I tumors were associated with positive peritoneal cytology, and the finding is almost always predictive of fatal disease.

Effects of debulking

Clearly, evidence of disease outside the uterus is a poor prognostic factor. With that said, it appears that most studies have found significant survival benefits to surgically debulking patients presenting with uterine MMMT. Patients with minimal residual disease may have longer survival than those with gross residual disease remaining after surgical debulking.[29,30] However, this has not been seen in all studies.[2]

PATHOLOGIC EVALUATION

Histologic type and grade

More recently, attention has shifted to the carcinomatous component of MMMT and how its characteristics may influence survival. Two studies have demonstrated that a clear cell or serous component is associated with an increased likelihood of extrauterine disease.[6,13] Another author has suggested that a carcinoma-to-sarcoma ratio >1 is also associated with advanced stage.[10] Grading the sarcoma was another potential avenue in the effort to define poor prognostic factors. The early reports that sarcoma grade may adversely affect prognosis have been refuted. [4,6,11,13,31–33] Most likely, tumor grade does not impact survival, since most of these tumors are high-grade. Furthermore, the mitotic index of sarcoma has also not been useful in predicting prognosis.[34,35]

Lymphovascular space invasion

LVSI may also predict extrauterine disease and prognosis,[6,10] although this has not been a consistent finding. [2,4,5,11]

Molecular

Although immunohistochemistry and molecular pathology have been widely utilized in other areas of gynecologic pathology, their use in the context of MMMT has been relatively less studied. For the most part, immunohistochemistry has been applied in an effort to better demonstrate the biphasic nature of this tumor, as well as to demonstrate heterologous differentiation. Although antibodies to desmin and MyoD1 can support the histologic impression of the presence of rhabdomyoblasts, other antibodies to epithelial and mesenchymal antigens have been less than perfect. Often the sarcomatous areas coexpress epithelial markers, and endometrioid histotypes are frequently vimentin-positive.[5,36] Other authors have utilized antibodies to oncogene products, such as p53, in order to test whether these biphasic tumors are potentially monoclonal. Indeed, p53 can be coexpressed by both the sarcoma and the carcinoma in MMMT.[19] However, expression of p53 in MMMT does not portend an adverse prognosis. In the same study, the authors also found no link between increased Ki-67 (a marker of cellular proliferation) and a worse prognosis.[19]

In the future, there may be an increased role for the detection of oncogenes for the purpose of target-specific therapy. Some have studied HER2/neu (ERBB2) by immunohistochemistry in MMMT, with the reported percentage of tumors expressing the antigen ranging from 19% to 100%.[37,38] In the lower range of expression, the scoring system accepted for HER2/neu expression in breast carcinoma was used, while in the highest range, any staining with the antibody was considered positive. Ramondetta et al[37] also demonstrated expression of Abl and platelet-derived growth factor receptor β (PDGFR-β) in some MMMTs, providing another possible avenue of therapy with tyrosine kinase inhibitors such as imatinib (Gleevec/Glivec). In the same study, nearly 25% of MMMTs expressed estrogen and progesterone receptors, suggesting that at least some tumors may respond favorably to hormonal manipulation.[37]

Pathology at the MD Anderson Cancer Center

For completion, as well as to address the multitude of potential prognostic indicators, in pathology reports from our institution we include the composition of the tumor, including the histologic subtype of the carcinoma and sarcoma, along with the approximate percentage of each component. The depth of myometrial invasion, the presence or absence of vascular involvement, and the presence or absence of cervical involvement are also included. Although it is accepted that heterologous elements do not adversely affect prognosis and the question of carcinoma subtype influencing prognosis is yet to be fully proven, these features are reported in order that possible recurrences can be more easily recognized as related to the MMMT.

USE OF PROGNOSTIC PREDICTIVE FACTORS IN THE MANAGEMENT OF MMMT

Role of radiotherapy

Regardless of the presence or absence of the above-mentioned prognostic factors, the role of radiotherapy in the treatment of MMMT is controversial. Postoperative pelvic irradiation appears to have little impact on overall survival.[26] There are multiple single-institution studies showing that pelvic radiotherapy improves local control. The European Organization for Research and Treatment of Cancer (EORTC) Trial 55874 is an important randomized trial directly addressing the benefit of adjuvant pelvic irradiation. In this study, patients with early-stage uterine sarcoma were randomized to receive either surgery alone or surgery followed by adjuvant irradiation. This study included all types of uterine sarcomas, not just MMMT. The results of this study are still pending. Another study that may help address the question of the importance of radiotherapy is GOG 150, which is a phase III randomized study of whole-abdominal radiotherapy (WAI) versus combination chemotherapy with cisplatin–ifosfamide and mesna (CIM) in optimally debulked stage I, II, III, or IV uterine MMMT. The abstract reports that compared to WAI, adjuvant CIM reduces the recurrence rate and significantly prolongs overall survival in optimally debulked MMMT patients.[39] The final report is pending.

In a retrospective study performed at the MD Anderson Cancer Center, patients treated with pelvic radiotherapy had a lower rate of pelvic recurrence than patients treated with surgery alone (28% vs 48%; $p = 0.0002$), but the overall 5-year survival rates (36% vs 27%; $p = 0.10$) and distant metastasis rates (57% vs 54%; $p = 0.96$) were not significantly different.[40] However, patients treated with pelvic radiotherapy had a longer mean time to any distant relapse (17.3 vs 7.0 months; $p = 0.001$) than patients treated with surgery alone. Only one study has suggested that therapeutic advantage may be gained from postoperative pelvic irradiation in the treatment of surgical stage I or II uterine MMMT.[41]

The GOG has evaluated its experience with pelvic radiotherapy for all uterine sarcomas, including MMMT, endometrial stromal sarcomas, and leiomyosarcomas.[42] In this study, patients with stage I or II uterine disease were randomly assigned to receive doxorubicin or no chemotherapy after surgery. The use of adjuvant pelvic radiotherapy was not mandated, but was left to the discretion of the individual investigator, and the study was not stratified on the basis of use of radiotherapy. In a subset analysis, the authors demonstrated a reduction in pelvic recurrences in patients who received pelvic radiotherapy compared with those who did not; however, irradiated patients had a higher rate of distant metastasis, and there was no significant difference between the two groups in the 2-year survival rate.[42] At the MD Anderson Cancer Center, patients with stage I or II uterine MMMT are offered pelvic radiotherapy to improve local control, but are clearly told that it may not improve survival. The pelvis is treated adjuvantly with a four-field technique to a total dose of 45–50 Gy. Presently, we are conducting a phase II trial evaluating adjuvant pelvic radiotherapy concurrent with weekly cisplatin, followed by four courses of carboplatin and paclitaxel in patients with stage I, II, or IIIA uterine MMMT. In patients with extensive pelvic disease who are poor candidates for surgery, palliative radiotherapy followed by chemotherapy off protocol is also considered.

Role of adjuvant chemotherapy

Over the past two decades, standard adjuvant treatment of uterine MMMT at the MD Anderson Cancer Center has shifted from primarily locoregional radiotherapy to chemotherapy. Unfortunately, chemotherapy has shown only minimal evidence of improved survival. Hannigan et al[43] showed no difference in 5-year survival between patients treated with adjuvant vincristine, dactinomycin (actinomycin D), and cyclophosphamide (VAC) and those who did not receive adjuvant chemotherapy. The aforementioned GOG trial did not show any survival benefit from chemotherapy when patients with stage I or II disease were randomized to adjuvant doxorubicin or no further treatment after hysterectomy.[42] More recently, the GOG has investigated adjuvant ifosfamide and cisplatin in patients with completely resected stage I or II disease. The impact of the treatment on survival

was indeterminate.[44] There is no definitive proof for any survival benefit of adjuvant chemotherapy in uterine sarcomas. However, better agents and molecular targeting may improve outcomes in the future.

TREATMENT SUMMARY

Ultimately, the ideal treatment for uterine MMMT may be combined radiotherapy and chemotherapy after optimal surgical debulking. However, the best treatment for uterine MMMT has yet to be determined. Because current therapies are associated with poor response rates and high recurrence rates, molecular evaluation of these tumors should continue through research endeavors, in order to continue to learn about options for further therapies. Because of the rarity of uterine MMMT, we believe that patients with these tumors should be referred to major cancer treatment centers, where larger and more informative trials can be conducted to help answer these questions more efficiently and effectively.

REFERENCES

1. George E, Lillemoe TJ, Twiggs LB, Perrone T. Malignant mixed mullerian tumor versus high grade endometrial carcinoma and aggressive variants of endometrial carcinoma: a comparative analysis of survival. Int J Gynecol Pathol 1995;14:39–44.

2. Inthasorn P, Beale P, Dalrymple C, Carter J. Malignant mixed mullerian tumour of the ovary: prognostic factor and response of adjuvant platinum-based chemotherapy. Aust NZ J Obstet Gynaecol 2003;43:61–4.

3. Sreenan JJ, Hart WR. Carcinosarcomas of the female genital tract: a pathologic study of 29 metastatic tumors: further evidence for the dominant role of the epithelial component

and the conversion theory of histogenesis. Am J Surg Pathol 1995;19:666–74.

4. Nielsen S, Podratz K, Scheithauer B, O'Brien P. Clinicopathologic analysis of uterine malignant mixed mullerian tumors. Gynecol Oncol 1989;34:372–8.

5. Bitterman P, Chun B, Kurman RJ. The significance of epithelial differentiation in mixed mesodermal tumors of the uterus: a clinicopathologic and immunohistochemical study. Am J Surg Pathol 1990;14:317–28.

6. Silverberg S, Major FJ, Blessing JA, Fetter B, et al. Carcinosarcoma (malignant mixed mesodermal tumors) of the uterus. A Gynecologic

Oncology Group pathologic study of 203 cases. Int J Gynecol Pathol 1990;9:1–19.

7. Tavassoli FA, Devilee P. World Health Organization: Pathology and Genetics of Tumours of the Breast and Female Genital Organs (WHO/IARC Classification of Tumours). Lyon: IARC Press, 2003.

8. Norris HJ, Roth E, Taylor HB. Mesenchymal tumors of the uterus: II. A clinical and pathologic study of 31 mixed mesodermal tumors. Obstet Gynecol 1966;28:57–63.

9. Barwick KW, LiVolsi VA. Malignant mixed mullerian tumors of the uterus: a clinicopathologic assessment of 34 cases. Am J Surg Pathol 1979;3:125–35.

10. Macasaet MA, Waxman M, Fruchter RG, Boyce J, et al. Prognostic factors in malignant mesodermal (müllerian) mixed tumors of the uterus. Gynecol Oncol 1985;20:32–42.

11. Dinh TV, Slavin RE, Bhagavan BS, Hannigan EV, et al. Mixed müllerian tumor of the uterus: a clinicopathologic study. Obstet Gynecol 1989;74:388–92.

12. Ho SP, Ho TH. Malignant mixed müllerian tumours of the uterus – a ten year experience. Singapore Med J 2002;43:452–6.

13. Nordal RR, Thoresen SO. Uterine sarcomas in Norway 1956–1992: incidence, survival and mortality. Eur J Cancer 1997;33:907–11.

14. George E, Manivel JC, Dehner LP, Wick MR. Malignant mixed mullerian tumors: an immunohistochemical study of 47 cases, with histogenetic considerations and clinical correlation. Hum Pathol 1991;22:215–23.

15. DiSaia PJ, Castro JR, Rutledge FN. Mixed mesodermal sarcoma of the uterus. AJR Am J Roetgenol 1973;117:632–6.

16. DiSaia PJ, Creasman WT. Clinical Gynecologic Oncology, 6th edn. St Louis, MO: Mosby, 2002.

17. Chuang JT, Van Velden JJ, Graham JB. Carcinosarcoma and mixed mesodermal tumor of the uterine corpus: review of 49 cases. Obstet Gynecol 1970;35:769–80.

18. Sartori E, Bazzurini L, Gadducci A, et al. Carcinosarcoma of the uterus: a clinicopathological multicenter CTF study. Gynecol Oncol 1997;67:70–5.

19. Iwasa Y, Haga H, Konishi I, et al. Prognostic factors in uterine carcinosarcoma: a clinicopathologic study of 25 patients. Cancer 1998;82:512–19.

20. Wolfson A, Wolfson DJ, Sittler SY, et al. A multivariate analysis of clinicopathologic factors for predicting outcome in uterine sarcomas. Gynecol Oncol 1994;52:56–62.

21. Bodner-Adler B, Bodner K, Obdrmair A, et al. Prognostic parameters in carcinosarcomas of the uterus: a clinico-pathologic study. Anticancer Res 2001;21:3069–84.

22. Schweizer W, Demopoulos R, Beller U, Dubin N. Prognostic factors for malignant mixed mullerian tumors of the uterus. Int J Gynecol Pathol 1990;9:129–36.

23. Pautier P, Genestie C, Rey A, et al. Analysis of clinicopathologic prognostic factors for 157 uterine sarcomas and evaluation of grading score validated for soft tissue sarcoma. Cancer 2000;88:1425–31.

24. Marth C, Windbichler G, Petru E, et al. Parity as an independent prognostic factor in malignant mixed mesodermal tumors of the endometrium. Gynecol Oncol 1997;64:121–5.

25. Peters WA, Kumar NB, Flemin WP, Morley G. Prognostic features of sarcomas and mixed tumors of the endometrium. Obstet Gynecol 1984;63:550–6.

26. Yamada SD, Burger RA, Brewster WR, et al. Pathologic variables and adjuvant therapy as predictors of recurrence and survival for patients with surgically evaluated carcinosarcoma of the uterus. Cancer 2000;88:2782–6.

27. Major FJ, Blessing JA, Silverberg SG, et al. Prognostic factors in early-stage uterine sarcoma. A Gynecologic Oncology Group study. Cancer 1993;71:1702–9.

28. Kanbour AI, Buchsbaum HJ, Hall A. Peritoneal cytology in malignant mixed mullerian tumors of the corpus uteri. Gynecol Oncol 1989;33:91–5.

29. Muntz HG, Jones MA, Goff BA, et al. Malignant mixed mullerian tumors of the ovary: experience with surgical cytoreduction and combination chemotherapy. Cancer 1995;76:1209–13.

30. Barakat RR, Rubin SC, Wong G, et al. Mixed mesodermal tumor of the ovary: analysis of prognostic factors in 31 cases. Obstet Gynecol 1992;80:660–4.

31. Kohorn EI, Schwartz PE, Chambers JT, et al. Adjuvant therapy in mixed mullerian tumors of the uterus. Gynecol Oncol 1986;23:212–21.

32. Costa MJ, Khan R, Judd R. Carcinosarcoma (malignant mixed mullerian [mesodermal] tumor) of the uterus and ovary: correlation of clinical, pathologic, and immunohistochemical features in 29 cases. Arch Pathol Lab Med 1991;115:583–90.

33. DeBrito PA, Silverberg SG, Orenstein JM. Carcinosarcoma (malignant mixed mullerian [mesodermal] tumor) of the female genital tract: immunohistochemical and ultrastructural analysis of 28 cases. Hum Pathol 1993;24:132–42.

34. Kahanpaa KV, Wahlstrom T, Grohn P, et al. Sarcomas of the uterus: a clinicopathologic study of 119 patients. Obstet Gynecol 1986;67:417–24.

35. Larson B, Silfversard C, Nilsson B, Pettersson F. Mixed mullerian tumours of the uterus – prognostic factors: a clinical and histopathologic study of 147 cases. Radiother Oncol 1990;17:123–32.

36. Reid-Nicholson M, Iyengar P, Hummer AJ, et al. Immunophenotypic diversity of endometrial adenocarcinomas: implications for differential diagnosis. Mod Pathol 2006;9: 1091–100.

37. Ramondetta LM, Burke TW, Jhingran A, et al. A phase II trial of cisplatin, ifosfamide, and mesna in patients with advanced or recurrent uterine malignant mixed mullerian tumors with evaluation of potential molecular markers. Gynecol Oncol 2003;90:529–36.

38. Nasu K, Kawano Y, Hirota Y, et al. Immunohistochemical study of c-erb B-2 expression in malignant mixed mullerian tumors of the female genital tract. J Obstet Gynaecol Res 1996;22:347–51.

39. Wolfson AH, Brady MF, Rocereto TF, et al. A Gynecologic Oncology Group randomized trial of whole abdominal irradiation (WAI) vs. cisplatin–ifosfamide + mesna (CIM) in optimally debulked stage I–IV carcinosarcoma (CS) of the uterus. ASC. Annual Meeting Abstracts. J Clin Oncol 2006;24(Suppl):5001.

40. Callister M, Ramondetta LM, Jhingran A, et al. Malignant mixed mullerian tumors of the uterus: analysis of patterns of failure, prognostic factors, and treatment outcome. Int J Radiat Oncol Biol Phys 2004;58:786–96.

41. Molpus KL, Redlin-Frazier S, Reed G, et al. Postoperative pelvic irradiation in early stage uterine mixed mullerian tumors. Eur J Gynaecol Oncol 1998;19:541–6.

42. Omura GA, Blessing JA, Major F, et al. A randomized clinical trial of adjuvant Adriamycin in uterine sarcoma: a Gynecologic Oncology Group study. J Clin Oncol 1985;3: 1240–5.

43. Hannigan EV, Freedman RS, Rutledge FN. Adjuvant chemotherapy in early uterine sarcomas. Gynecol Oncol 1983;15:56–64.

44. Sutton G, Kauderer J, Carson LF, et al. Adjuvant ifosfamide and cisplatin in patients with completely resected stage I or II carcinosarcomas (mixed mesodermal tumors) of the uterus: a Gynecologic Oncology Group study. Gynecol Oncol 2005;96:630–4.

Section III
Cervical

Section Editor: Robert L Coleman

Clinical–pathologic predictors in patients with cervical cancer

16

Devansu Tewari and Bradley J Monk

INTRODUCTION

Progress made in the understanding and treatment of cervical cancer has made the dream of eradicating this disease a potential reality. Advances in research have led to the development of effective screening programs, treatment options, and a vaccine that may eliminate the suffering and death due to this cancer for future generations. The USA has seen mortality rates decline nearly 80% in just the last 50 years, with an estimated 11 150 new cases of invasive cervical cancer and 3670 cancer-related deaths expected in 2007.[1] These numbers reflect the 4% annual reduction in the overall death rate as the majority of cases continue to be diagnosed in the early stages of disease.[2]

The global perspective of cervical cancer, however, is much different. Cervical cancer is a worldwide pandemic, with nearly 500 000 new cases annually, and half of these women are expected to die.[3] It is second overall only to breast cancer as the major cause of cancer death, while being the leading cause of cancer mortality in developing countries where effective screening programs have not been implemented. As a result, a majority of cases diagnosed are locally advanced and not amenable to current surgical and radiotherapy protocols.[4] Despite the many successes in the battle against this cancer, there is still much to learn if more women are to be cured of this disease. A better understanding of the clinical–pathologic factors associated with prognosis is imperative if individually tailored effective treatment strategies are to be implemented.

FIGO STAGING AND TREATMENT

Prognostic predictors for cervical cancer are strongly predicated on the stage of the disease, which is based upon clinical assessment and follows the guidelines outlined by the International Federation of Gynecology and Obstetrics (FIGO) (Table 16.1).[5] Although early-stage cancers are associated with high cure rates, prognosis declines significantly when more advanced lesions are encountered. General guidelines for treatment vary, depending upon the clinical stage, and are outlined in Table 16.2.[6] For microscopic stage IA1 lesions, either an extrafascial hysterectomy may be performed or close observation may be maintained in a woman desiring fertility, so long as negative margins are identified on a cervical conization specimen.[7] In this group, overall survival rates of 95–98% have been reported.[8] The treatment options for stages IA2, IB1, and IIA (<4 cm) tumors include a radical hysterectomy and pelvic lymphadenectomy, which is associated with an 80–90% survival rate and can be similarly achieved with primary radiotherapy.[9] The standard of care for bulky stage IB2 (≥4 cm) to IVA cancers is concurrent use of radio- and chemotherapy.

Table 16.1 FIGO staging nomenclature for cervical carcinoma[5,9]

Stage	Description
0	Carcinoma in situ
IA1	Invasive cancer identified only microscopically, measured stromal invansion is ≤3 mm in depth and ≤7 mm in horizontal spread
IA2	Invasive cancer identified only microscopically, measured stromal invasion is >3 mm but <5 mm in depth and ≤7 mm in horizontal spread
IB1	Clinically visible lesions confined to the cervix ≤4 cm
IB2	Clinically visible lesions confined to the cervix >4 cm
IIA	Cancer involves the vagina, excluding the lower third of the vagina, with no parametrial invasion
IIB	Cancer involves the vagina, excluding the lower third of the vagina, with parametrial invasion
IIIA	Cancer involves the lower third of the vagina
IIIB	Cancer extends to the pelvic wall and/or causes hydronephrosis or nonfunctioning kidney
IVA	Cancer involves the mucosa of the bladder or rectum
IVB	Distant metastasis

It is for these larger and more advanced lesions, particularly stages IIB–IVA, where survival rates decline, with reported ranges of 20–70%, as a result of local or in-field treatment failure.[4]

LIMITATIONS OF CLINICAL STAGING

The problem with the current FIGO staging system for cervical cancer is that it is not an accurate reflection of the spread and extent of disease. It does not incorporate many of the clinical–pathologic parameters that affect prognosis and are associated with an increased risk of recurrence. For example, disease metastatic to the pelvic and para-aortic lymph nodes negatively

Table 16.2 Primary treatment for early-stage cervical cancer[6,9]

Clinical stage	Primary treatment
IA1	Extrafascial hysterectomy OR Observation if cone biospy has negative margins and patient desires future fertility
IA2	Radical hysterectomy, pelvic lymph node dissection ± para-aortic lymph node sampling OR Brachytherapy and RT (point A dose: 75–80 Gy)
IB1 and IIA (≤4 cm)	Radical hysterectomy, pelvic lymph node dissection + para-aortic lymph node sampling + tailored postoperative adjuvant therapy OR Concurrent cisplatin-based CT[a] + RT + brachytherapy (point A dose: 80–85 Gy)
IB2 and IIA (>4 cm), and IIB–IVA	Concurrent cisplatin-based CT[a] + RT + brachytherapy (point A dose: ≥85 Gy)

CT, chemotherapy; RT, pelvic radiotherapy.
[a]40 mg/m^2 intravenously (maximum dose 70 mg) weekly × 6.

impacts survival and increases with each stage of disease (Table 16.3).[8,10] Higher rates of metastasis also correlate with the volume of the primary tumor, independently of clinical stage.[8,11] But current FIGO standards do not reflect these issues. This has contributed to the debate that the surgical evaluation of the pelvic and para-aortic lymph nodes should be included in the staging of cervical cancer, as their removal may have both diagnostic and therapeutic value.

Table 16.3 Influence of FIGO stage on prevalence of para-aortic metastases in cervical carcinoma. Reproduced from Berman et al. Gynecol Oncol 1984;19:8–16[10] with permission from Elsevier.

Stage	Percentage
I–II	12.3
III–IV	24.4

SURGICALLY MANAGED PATIENTS

Surgical staging of cervical cancer

The Gynecologic Oncology Group (GOG) experience with surgical staging in 436 patients with stage IIB–IVA disease noted that the rate of para-aortic metastasis was 20% and increased with each stage of disease: 5% of stage IB; 16% of stage II; and 25% of stage III.[8,10] A survival probability of 25% at 3 years was seen in patients with para-aortic metastases, with a median survival of 15.2 months in this group, while the median duration of survival upon recurrence was only 5 months.[10] Five-year survival rates of 20–50% have been reported elsewhere.[12,13] Surgical evaluation of the lymph nodes can be performed with minimal morbidity through a retroperitoneal approach without entry into the peritoneum to determine the need for extended-field radiation to the para-aortic region. This technique reduces the toxicity of radiotherapy on the small bowel and has identified more extensive disease in nearly 34% of patients than that suspected from their FIGO stage alone.[11,12]

The ability to remove diseased lymph nodes prior to the start of radiotherapy has also been reported to confer a survival advantage.[14] In one review, 266 patients surgically staged prior to radiotherapy were categorized into four groups based upon the status of the lymph nodes: negative nodes; microscopic disease; macroscopic disease; and unresectable macroscopic lymph nodes. Both the 5- and 10-year disease-free survival rates were similar between the microscopically and macroscopically resected lymph node groups (43% and 35% vs 50% and 46%, respectively). At 3 years, all patients with unresectable lymph nodes had recurred, with 0% survival. Although the role of surgical staging is still controversial, it is clear that the identification of para-aortic involvement with cervical cancer with the purpose of administering extended-field radiation can lead to increased survival in some patients.

Pathologic risk factors for lymph node metastasis

The GOG sought to investigate the independent risk factors associated with nodal metastasis in surgically managed patients with stage I disease. GOG 49 was a large prospective surgical–pathologic study of 1125 patients with squamous cell carcinoma of the cervix who underwent radical hysterectomy and pelvic and para-aortic lymphadenectomy.[15,16] Five major risk factors were identified that were statistically significant for pelvic nodal metastasis: depth of invasion ($p = 0.0001$); parametrial involvement ($p = 0.0001$); lymphovascular space invasion (LVSI) ($p = 0.0001$); tumor grade ($p = 0.01$); and gross versus occult primary tumor ($p = 0.009$). The multivariate analysis identified LVSI ($p < 0.0001$), depth of invasion ($p < 0.0001$), parametrial involvement ($p = 0.0005$), and age ($p = 0.02$) as independent risk factors.[15] Differences in disease-free interval did not identify age as a significant risk factor in follow-up data from GOG 49.[15,16] Although tumor grade was independently related to nodal metastasis and disease-free survival, it was not found to be effective in predicting nodal spread or progression-free survival when submitted slides were evaluated by independent review in GOG 49.[8,15,17] However, depth of invasion and LVSI were still important predictors of behavior.[17]

Parametrial invasion in the absence or presence of diseased lymph nodes is a poor prognostic factor.[18] GOG 49 confirmed the importance of this in nodal metastasis and showed a statistically significant decrease in disease-free interval when it was identified in the surgical specimen.[15,16] In one study, a decline in 5-year survival rate from 86% to 62% was seen in 270 surgically managed patients in whom parametrial invasion was identified.[19] The status of tumor margins in surgical specimens is an important finding. In one study of 23 cases of close (≤0.5 cm) or positive margins, the 5-year survival rate was 28.6%.[20] Although GOG 49 did not find an association between surgical margin status and either nodal metastasis or disease-free interval, many still regard this

as an issue of concern and would consider adjuvant therapy.[15,16,21]

Tumor volume, lymphovascular space, depth of invasion

A subset analysis of stage IB lesions from GOG 49 identified clinical tumor size, LVSI, and depth of tumor invasion as independent prognostic factors for nodal spread and disease-free intervals (Figure 16.1).[16] The disease-free interval at 3 years was 85.6% for patients with negative

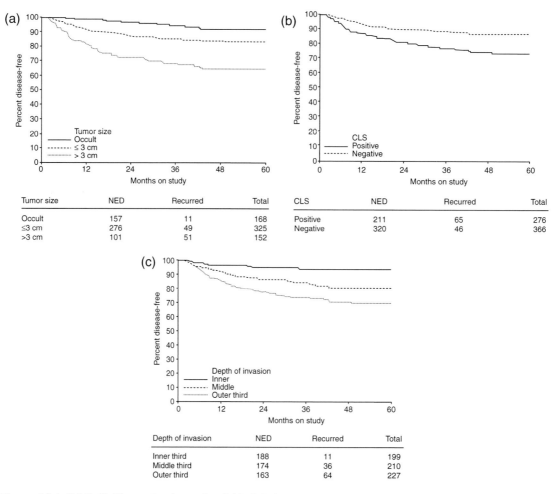

Tumor size	NED	Recurred	Total
Occult	157	11	168
≤3 cm	276	49	325
>3 cm	101	51	152

CLS	NED	Recurred	Total
Positive	211	65	276
Negative	320	46	366

Depth of invasion	NED	Recurred	Total
Inner third	188	11	199
Middle third	174	36	210
Outer third	163	64	227

Figure 16.1 GOG 49. Disease-free interval and: (a) clinical tumor size; (b) lymphovascular space invasion; (c) depth of invasion. NED, no evidence of disease; CLS, capillary/lymphatic space. Reproduced from Delgado et al. Gynecol Oncol 1990;38:352–7[16] with permission from Elsevier.

nodes, compared with 74.4% for those with lymph node metastasis. This correlated with depth of tumor invasion in fractional thirds (p <0.0001), clinical tumor size (p <0.0001), and LVSI (p = 0.0001). For occult tumors ≤3 cm in size, the interval was 85.5%, compared with 68.4% for lesions >3 cm. Based upon these results, GOG 49 was able to construct a model of the risk of recurrence. The relative risk of

each of these three variables was used to construct disease-free survival curves to classify patients into low-, intermediate-, or high-risk categories (Table 16.4). Based upon these survival curves, cases can be plotted to determine the category of individual risk (Figure 16.2).

The main difficulty in the surgical management of cervical cancer is deciding when to recommend adjuvant radiotherapy in patients

Table 16.4 GOG 49: proportional hazards modeling of disease-free interval. Reproduced from Delgado et al. Gynecol Oncol 1990;38:352–7[16] with permission from Elsevier.

Variable	Regression coefficient	Relative risk	Significance test[a]
Depth of tumor penetration			
Superficial			
mm	1.86	–	11.3 (p = 0.0008)
mm^2	−0.110	–	10.9 (p = 0.001)
3[b]	0.000	1.0	
4	1.09	3.0	
5	1.97	7.2	
6	2.62	14.0	
7	3.06	21.0	
8	3.27	26.0	
10	3.04	21.0	
Middle			
mm	0.0781	–	1.71 (p = 0.19)
mm^2	−0.000841	–	0.773 (p = 0.38)
5	3.02	20.0	
6	3.09	22.0	
7	3.16	23.0	
8	3.22	25.0	
10	3.35	28.0	
12	3.47	32.0	
14	3.58	36.0	
Deep			
mm	0.071	–	4.74 (p = 0.03)
mm^2	−0.000818	–	3.19 (p = 0.07)
7	3.35	28.0	
8	3.40	30.0	
10	3.52	34.0	
12	3.62	37.0	
14	3.72	41.0	
16	3.81	45.0	
18	3.90	49.0	
20	3.98	54.0	

Continued

Table 16.4 (*cont*) GOG 49: proportional hazards modeling of disease-free interval. Reproduced from Delgado et al. Gynecol Oncol 1990;38:352–7[16] with permission from Elsevier.

Variable	Regression coefficient	Relative risk	Significance test[a]
Clinical tumor size			
Occult tumor	0.000	1.0	
Size (cm)	0.204	–	8.95 (*p* = 0.003)
1 cm	0.456	1.6	
2 cm	0.659	1.9	
3 cm	0.863	2.4	
4 cm	1.07	2.9	
6 cm	1.47	4.4	
8 cm	1.88	6.6	
Capillary/lymphatic space involvement	0.554	1.7	7.47 (*p* = 0.006)

[a]Likelihood ratio test.

[b]Arbitary reference for depth of invasion.

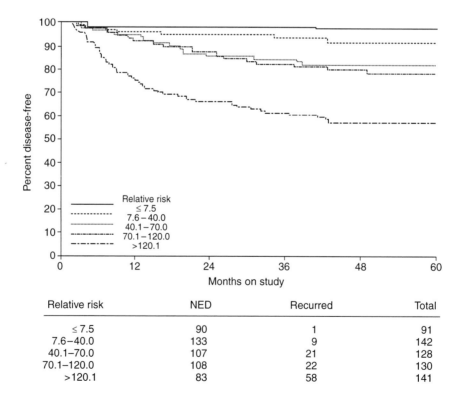

Relative risk	NED	Recurred	Total
≤ 7.5	90	1	91
7.6–40.0	133	9	142
40.1–70.0	107	21	128
70.1–120.0	108	22	130
>120.1	83	58	141

Figure 16.2 GOG 49: disease-free survival curves. NED, no evidence of disease. Reproduced from Delgado et al. Gynecol Oncol 1990;38:352–7[16] with permission from Elsevier.

Table 16.5 GOG 92: eligibility criteria. Reproduced from Sedlis et al. Gynecol Oncol 1999;73:177–83[22] with permission from Elsevier.

CLSI[a]	Stromal invasion	Tumor size (cm)
Positive	Deep third	Any
Positive	Middle third	≥2
Positive	Superficial third	≥5
Negative	Deep or middle third	≥4

[a]Capillary lymphatic space tumor involvement.

with node-negative disease. GOG 92 was a prospective randomized study designed to address the potential benefits and risks of adjuvant radiotherapy for stage IB cervical cancer patients surgically treated with the variables of risk identified in GOG 49.[22] The rationale was to determine which patients with node-negative disease should be treated with adjuvant radiation, as 50% of cervical cancer recurrences are in patients with negative lymph nodes after radical surgery.[23] Eligibility included patients with squamous, adenocarcinoma, or adenosquamous lesions who had undergone a radical hysterectomy and pelvic lymphadenectomy with pathologic findings consistent with two of the

three risk factors of large tumor diameter, LVSI, and depth of invasion (Table 16.5). Patients were randomized to receive external-beam irradiation without brachytherapy or no adjuvant therapy. This study was designed to determine the rate of recurrence and decrease in mortality for stage IB patients, as GOG 49 had reported that a 31% risk of recurrence was seen in patients with any of the poor-prognostic risk factors.[16] Results from GOG 92 showed a statistically significant 47% reduction in risk of recurrence in the patients who received radiotherapy (relative risk 0.53) with recurrence-free rates of 88% for this group at 3 years, compared with 79% for the observation group (Figure 16.3). At the time of this report, the survival analysis had not matured. Follow-up data have since shown, however, that progression-free survival is still significantly increased with radiation but that the increase in overall survival (hazard ratio 0.70; $p = 0.074$) did not reach statistical significance (Figure 16.4).[24] This is surprising, as advantages in progression-free survival usually parallel overall survival in cervix cancer. One explanation for this is that the sample size may have been too low and the 80% power did not

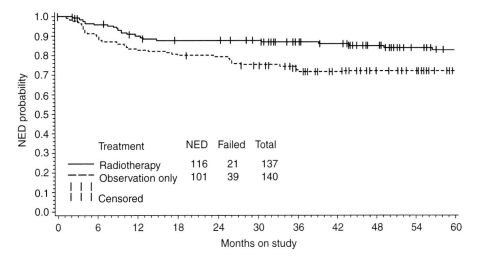

Figure 16.3 GOG 92: recurrence-free intervals. NED, no evidence of disease. Reproduced from Sedlis et al. Gynecol Oncol 1999;73:177–83[22] with permission from Elsevier.

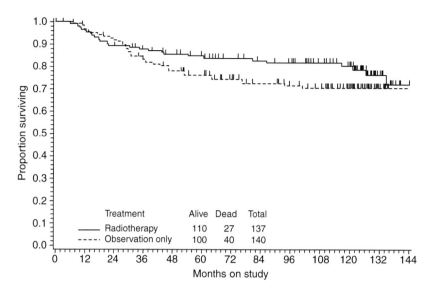

Figure 16.4 GOG 92: survival curves. Reproduced from Rotman et al. Int J Radiat Oncol Biol Phys 2006;65:169–176[24] with permission from Elsevier.

find significance in the 26–30% hazard reductions that were reported.[24] The importance of this has to be balanced by the understanding that although GOG 92 seemed to define standards in which adjuvant therapy might be implemented, it was conducted in a period in which the impact of chemotherapy had not been accounted for.

CHEMORADIOTHERAPY

The era of platinum-based therapy

The era of chemoradiotherapy for cervical cancer began in April 1999, when the results of three randomized phase III trials were published in the *New England Journal of Medicine*. These three trials and the publication of two additional phase III studies within a year prompted the US National Cancer Institute (NCI) to issue a national clinical alert that combination chemotherapy with radiation should be the treatment for cervical cancer when radiotherapy is the preferred option.[8,25–29]

The data from these five prospective randomized phase III trials demonstrated a decrease in the risk of death from cervical cancer by 30–50%.

GOG 120 randomized 526 women with stage IIB–IVA squamous cell carcinoma, adenocarcinoma and adenosquamous carcinoma of the cervix undergoing radiotherapy to three treatment arms for six cycles: weekly cisplatin $(40 \, mg/m^2)$; cisplatin $(50 \, mg/m^2,$ days 1 and 29) followed by 5-fluorouracil (5-FU, $4 \, g/m^2$ 96-hour infusion, days 1 and 29) and oral hydroxyurea $(2 \, g/m^2,$ weekly); and oral hydroxyurea $(2 \, g/m^2,$ twice weekly).[25] In each of the cisplatin-based regimens a statistically significant improvement in progression-free survival $(p <0.001)$ as well as overall survival $(p = 0.004$ and $0.002)$ was demonstrated compared with single-agent oral hydroxyurea, with less local and distant recurrence (Figure 16.5). However, the three-drug regimen was much more toxic than single-agent cisplatin, leading the authors to recommend weekly cisplatin in conjunction with radiotherapy as the standard

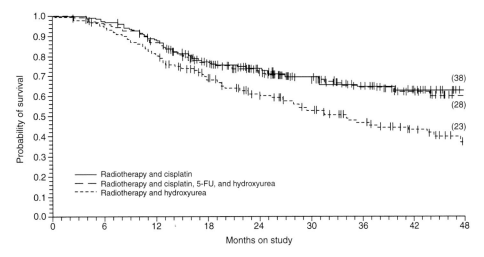

Figure 16.5 GOG 120: survival curves. Reproduced from Rose et al. N Engl J Med 1999;340:1144–53[25] with permission from Massachusetts Medical Society. © 1999. All rights reserved.

drug for locally advanced cervical cancers. But the impact was not limited to advanced cancers alone.

GOG 123 was a phase III study that randomized stage IB cervical cancers (≥4 cm) to treatment with pelvic radiation with or without weekly cisplatin (40 mg/m^2) for 6 cycles followed by an extrafascial hysterectomy.[26] Progression-free and overall survival (p <0.001

and p <0.008, respectively) were statistically significant, favoring the chemoradiotherapy group at 4 years (Figure 16.6). There was no added value in performing an extrafascial hysterectomy, and the authors concluded that the exclusion of this procedure would not affect the survival advantage seen with cisplatin.

Radiation Therapy Oncology Group (RTOG) Protocol 9001 studied 403 patients

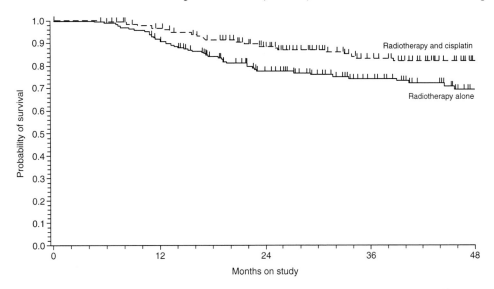

Figure 16.6 GOG 123: survival curves. Reproduced from Keys et al. N Engl J Med 1999;340:1154–61[26] with permission from Massachusetts Medical Society. © 1999. All rights reserved.

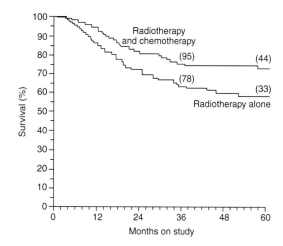

Figure 16.7 RTOG 9001: survival curves (numbers in parentheses are the numbers of patients alive and included in a follow-up assessment at 3 and 5 years.) Reproduced from Morris et al. N Engl J Med 1999; 340:1137–43[27] with permission from Massachusetts Medical Society. © 1999. All rights reserved.

between 1990 and 1997 with stage IIB–IVA disease or stage IB or IIA lesions >5 cm or with involvement of the pelvic lymph nodes.[27] Patients were randomized to 45 Gy irradiation to the pelvic and para-aortic nodes or to 45 Gy to the pelvis alone plus two 5-day cycles of cisplatin (75 mg/m^2, day 1) and 5-FU

(4000 mg/m^2, days 2–5) during radiotherapy. The 5-year cumulative rates of survival were 73% in the chemotherapy arm, compared with 58% in the radiation-alone group ($p = 0.004$) (Figure 16.7). Disease-free survival at 5 years was 67% versus 40% favoring the chemotherapy arm ($p < 0.001$), while rates of distant metastasis ($p < 0.001$) and locoregional recurrence ($p < 0.001$) were higher in the group not receiving chemotherapy. Moreover, an update of RTOG 9001 confirms the trend in favor of the chemotherapy group, with overall survival rates of 67% versus 41% at 8 years ($p < 0.0001$) and no increase in the rate of late treatment-related side-effects.[30]

GOG 85 randomized 388 patients between 1986 and 1990 with stage IIB–IVA squamous cell carcinoma, adenocarcinoma, or adenosquamous cancer of the cervix to either treatment with standard whole-pelvic radiation with concurrent 5-FU infusion and cisplatin (50 mg/m^2 intravenously) or radiation with oral hydroxyurea.[28] The differences in progression-free survival ($p = 0.033$) and overall survival were statistically significant ($p = 0.018$), favoring the cisplatin-based treatment arm (Figure 16.8).

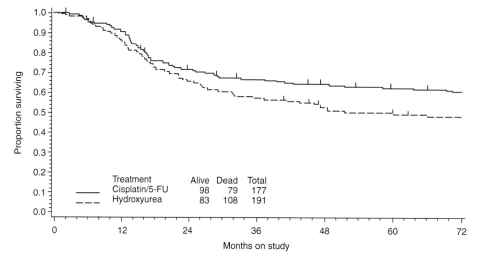

Figure 16.8 GOG 85: survival curves. Reproduced from Whitney et al. J Clin Oncol 1999;17:1334–5[28] with permission from the American Society of Clinical Oncology.

GOG 109 was the defining chemoradiotherapy for surgically managed patients. It randomized stage IA2–IIA cervical cancer patients initially treated with radical hysterectomy and pelvic lymphadenectomy who had positive pelvic lymph nodes and/or positive margins and/or parametrial invasion. The two arms of the study were radiation versus radiation and cisplatin (70 mg/m², q3wks) and a 96-hour infusion of 5-FU (1 g/m²/day q3wks) for four cycles.[29] Again, the chemotherapy arm demonstrated a statistically significant ($p = 0.003$) advantage in progression-free survival at 4 years of 80% versus 63% for radiation alone. In addition, the projected overall survival at 4 years was 71% versus 81%, favoring the chemoradiotherapy arm ($p = 0.007$) (Figure 16.9).

The results from these five randomized phase III trials all support the concomitant use of chemotherapy with radiation in the treatment of locally advanced cervical cancer. Although 5-FU infusion was a significant part of the chemotherapy arms in several of the studies, it has not been shown to have an advantage over single-agent cisplatin. GOG 165 randomized patients with stage IIB, IIIB, and IVA cervical cancers who were receiving radiotherapy to either weekly cisplatin (40 mg/m²) or

a protracted infusion of 5-FU (225 mg/m²/day ×5 days) for six cycles.[31] The study was closed prematurely when a 35% higher treatment failure rate was seen in the 5-FU arm.

Neoadjuvant chemotherapy

The positive impact of chemotherapy in the treatment of cervical cancer has led many to consider its use in the neoadjuvant setting. The rationale of this approach is that it might be able to diminish the size of a large primary lesion to a level at which it can be resected. Unfortunately, the results of neoadjuvant chemotherapy have not been impressive. No randomized clinical trials incorporating the results of GOG 92 and GOG 109 have supported this treatment approach. A meta-analysis of 21 randomized trials investigating neoadjuvant chemotherapy in cervical cancer did not show any improvement in survival or increased operability and did not decrease the need for postoperative therapy.[32] GOG 141 was a neoadjuvant chemotherapy trial with vincristine and cisplatin with bulky stage IB lesions in which patients undergoing radical hysterectomy and pelvic lymphadenectomy were randomized to either neoadjuvant chemotherapy or nothing. The study was terminated after an interim analysis showed no increased feasibility of performing surgery and no improvement in survival when compared with GOG 92 or GOG 109. In addition, there was no reduction in need for postoperative therapy, and greater toxicity was encountered in the chemotherapy arm.

Clinical–pathologic issues in the chemoradiotherapy era

The era of chemoradiotherapy may potentially change the importance of certain clinical and pathologic factors established during the period

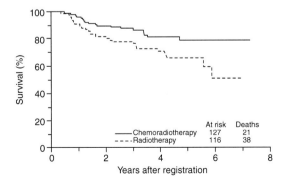

Figure 16.9 GOG 109: survival curves. Reproduced from Peters et al. J Clin Oncol 2000;18:1606–13[29] with permission from the American Society of Clinical Oncology.

when radiotherapy was administered alone. For example, studies such as GOG 92 were designed to answer questions regarding the role of adjuvant radiotherapy. But, with the importance of chemotherapy in current treatment protocols, it is unclear whether these previous standards are applicable in this new era.

This is exemplified in stage IB2 lesions, where controversy continues on the issue of the role of primary surgery followed by tailored postoperative radiotherapy based upon surgical risk factors versus that of primary chemoradiotherapy.[33] The importance of this debate is that these tumors have higher local failure and survival when compared with smaller lesions. In a retrospective review of 600 radical hysterectomies primarily performed prior to the 1999 clinical alert, criteria from GOG 92 and GOG 109 were applied and compared with the outcomes of 58 stage IB2 lesions identified within this group. If criteria from GOG 92 and GOG 109 were used, 30 (52%) should have received adjuvant radiotherapy and 21 (36%) chemoradiotherapy (Table 16.6). In the study set, 35 (60%) received adjuvant radiotherapy and 1 patient was given chemoradiotherapy. The estimated 5-year survival rate was 62.1%, as 21 (38%) women recurred. This tailored

approach to postoperative therapy resulted in survival rates in this high-risk group comparable to those with primary chemoradiotherapy.

The GOG has conducted exploratory analyses of several of their chemoradiotherapy studies. A review of the data from GOG 109 was performed to assess the benefits from chemoradiotherapy in certain subgroups of patients and to identify common histopathologic and clinical factors that might predict recurrence.[34] Although this was a retrospective analysis of a previously prospective randomized trial, several interesting results were identified. There appeared to be a smaller absolute benefit in 5-year survival with chemoradiotherapy compared with adjuvant radiotherapy alone in patients with a single positive node (83% vs 79%) compared with findings of at least two positive nodes (75% vs 55%) (Figures 16.10 and 16.11). In addition, in tumors ≤2 cm in size, the benefit in 5-year survival rate was less pronounced (82% vs 77%) when compared with lesions >2 cm (77% vs 58%) (Figure 16.12). Retrospective analyses of GOG 120 and GOG 165 have also been completed.[35] The findings from these reports have shown that FIGO stage and tumor grade were predictive of prognosis in patients with locally advanced cervical cancer treated with cisplatin and radiation. Ethnicity and age were also identified as having significant roles, with non-Caucasian/non-African-American patients between the ages of 51 and 60 years having better outcomes than their older/younger Caucasian/African-American counterparts. In addition, a poorer prognosis was associated with clinical versus surgical staging.

These findings are a reminder that previously established clinical–pathologic factors that have influenced practice management may not have the same impact with the addition of chemotherapy to radiation protocols. Many of the studies that were the foundation for determining the clinical and pathologic predictors of response

Table 16.6 Nodal status and likelihood of receiving postsurgical adjuvant therapy based on GOG 92 and 109/SWOG 8797 protocol criteria in the study population. Reproduced from Monk et al. Gynecol Oncol 2007;105:427–33[35] with permission from Elsevier.

	No. of patients	
Treatment	Negative pelvic nodes	Positive pelvic nodes
GOG 92-like (adjuvant radiotherapy)	30	0
GOG 109-like (adjuvant chemoradiotherapy)	5	16
None	7	0

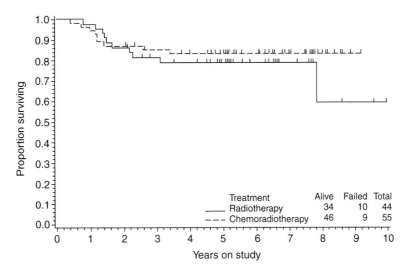

Figure 16.10 Clinicopathologic analysis of GOG 109: survival curves for single nodal metastasis. Reproduced from Monk et al. Gynecol Oncol 2005;96:721–8[34] with permission from Elsevier.

and prognosis were based upon studies that did not incorporate chemoradiotherapy into their protocols. As a result, these factors may not apply in the new era of chemoradiotherapy. The future development of prospective trials involving chemoradiotherapy in cervical cancer will need to address these issues.

RECURRENT CERVICAL CANCER

The unfortunate truth about cervical cancer is that it can be prevented but is not because of a lack of commitment to women's health in many parts of the world. As a result, the disease is too often found in the advanced stages. The consequence

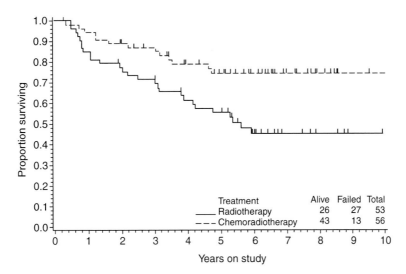

Figure 16.11 Clinicopathologic analysis of GOG 109: survival curves for ≥2 nodal metastasis. Reproduced from Monk et al. Gynecol Oncol 2005;96:721–8[34] with permission from Elsevier.

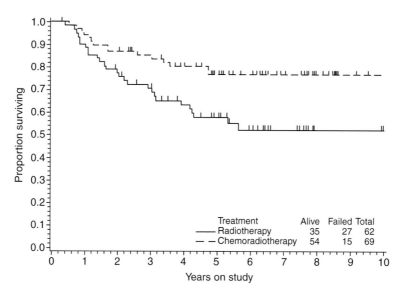

Figure 16.12 Clinicopathologic analysis of GOG 109: survival curves for tumor size >2 cm. Reproduced from Monk et al. Gynecol Oncol 2005;96:721–8[34] with permission from Elsevier.

is that cure rates are lower and patients with either recurrent or persistent disease can expect a fatal outcome with few clinically meaningful responses ever attained. Unless disease is limited to a central recurrence and a patient is a candidate for pelvic exenteration, few treatment options exist. The GOG experience with cervical cancer has been quite successful in frontline therapy, but has yielded only minimal responses in the recurrent setting. There is an incredible toll on the quality of life in this setting, which makes this group a key focus of study. It is for this reason that the NCI identifies patients in this setting as ideal candidates for clinical trials, as few active treatment options exist.

Systemic chemotherapy

Treatment of recurrent or persistent cervical cancer is a systemic problem and therefore has to be drug-based, as few situations exist in which radiation can play a salvage role. Multiple phase II studies have determined that cisplatin is

the single most active agent in the treatment of recurrent cervical cancer. Since a response rate of 44% with cisplatin was originally reported by the GOG, this agent has been the foundation against which to compare new drugs and combination therapy.[36] GOG 43 was a randomized study that set as the standard the treatment dose of 50 mg/m². Although a dose of 100 mg/m² was associated with a greater response rate, no differences in complete remission rate, progression-free survival, or overall survival were seen.[37]

Phase III trials

GOG 110 was a major phase III chemotherapy trial in patients with advanced, recurrent, or persistent squamous cell carcinoma of the cervix.[38] This study randomized patients to three different treatment arms every 3 weeks for six cycles: cisplatin (50 mg/m²); cisplatin (50 mg/m², day 1) and mitolactol (180 mg/m², days 2–6); and cisplatin (50 mg/m², day 1) plus ifosfamide

(5 g/m², 24-hour infusion) with mesna. Although the combination of cisplatin and ifosfamide when compared with single-agent cisplatin demonstrated a statistically significant higher response rate (31.1% vs 17.8%; $p = 0.004$) and progression-free survival (4.6 months vs 3.2 months; $p = 0.003$), more toxicity was seen, with no significant difference in overall survival (Figure 16.13). Moreover, the combination of cisplatin and mitolactol had no advantage over single-agent cisplatin.

GOG 149 was a randomized phase III trial that sought to compare the combination of cisplatin and ifosfamide studied in GOG 110 with combination bleomycin (30 units over 24 hours, day 1) followed by cisplatin (50 mg/m²) and ifosfamide (5 g/m², 24-hour infusion) with mesna in patients with advanced, recurrent, and persistent disease.[39] The data showed no differences in response rate (32% vs 31.2%), progression-free survival rate, or overall survival rate with the addition of bleomycin (Figure 16.14).

As the search continued for combination therapies that could result in clinically meaningful responses better than with single-agent cisplatin, the GOG conducted another phase III trial, GOG 169.

GOG 169 compared single-agent cisplatin (50 mg/m², day 1) with the combination of paclitaxel (135 mg/m², 24-hour infusion) followed by cisplatin (50 mg/m²) every 3 weeks for six cycles.[40] The data obtained demonstrated that the combination therapy was associated with a greater objective response rate (36% vs 19%; $p = 0.002$) (Table 16.7) and longer progression-free survival (4.8 months vs 2.8 months; $p < 0.001$). However, no statistically significant differences in overall survival (9.7 months vs 8.8 months) were seen (Figure 16.15). This study was also important in that it was the first phase III trial by the GOG in which quality-of-life (QOL) data were obtained, and the QOL was sustained in the combination-treatment arm.

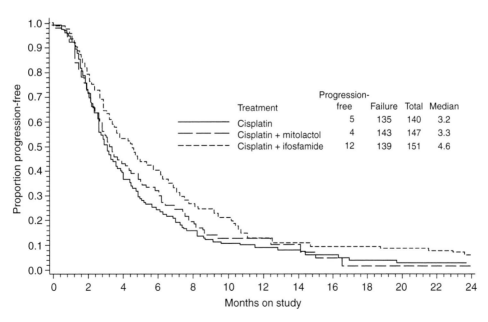

Figure 16.13 GOG 110: survival curves. Reproduced from Omura et al. J Clin Oncol 1997;15:165–71[38] with permission from the American Society of Clinical Oncology.

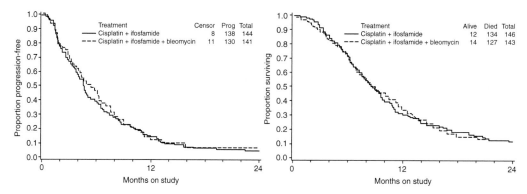

Figure 16.14 GOG 149: survival curves. Reproduced from Bloss et al. J Clin Oncol 2002;20:1832–7[39] with permission from the American Society of Clinical Oncology.

The most successful outcome to date with chemotherapy in the recurrent setting was established in GOG 179.[41,42] This trial was initially developed with three treatment arms in patients with stage IVB, recurrent, or persistent cervical cancer: cisplatin (50 mg/m²); cisplatin (50 mg/m², day 1) plus topotecan (0.75 mg/m², days 1–3); and MVAC (methotrexate, vinblastine, doxorubicin, and cisplatin). The MVAC treatment arm was discontinued after an interim analysis revealed significant toxicity with four treatment-related deaths and the study analysis continued with the two arms for six cycles. Outcome data showed that cisplatin in combination with topotecan resulted in a statistically

superior outcome over single-agent cisplatin in terms of median survival (9.4 months vs 6.5 months; $p = 0.017$), progression-free survival (4.6 months vs 2.9 months; $p = 0.014$), and overall response rate (27% vs 13%; $p = 0.004$) (Figure 16.16). This was the first randomized phase III trial to demonstrate a survival advantage with combination chemotherapy over single-agent cisplatin in patients with recurrent disease. Equally important was that the QOL assessment up to 9 months showed there was no significant reduction on the combination arm despite increased hematologic toxicity. The baseline scores of the QOL assessments the FACT-Cx (Functional Assessment of Cancer

Table 16.7 GOG 169: objective response by treatment group. Reproduced from Moore et al. J Clin Oncol 2004; 22:3113-19[40] with permission from the American Society of Clinical Oncology.

	C (n – 134)		C+P (n – 130)		
	No. of patients	%	No. of patients	%	Total
Responders	26	19	47	36	73
Complete	8	6	20	15	28
Partial	18	13	27	21	45
Nonresponders	108	81	83	64	91

C, cisplatin; C+P, cisplatin plus paclitaxel.

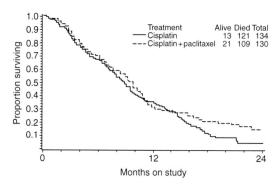

Figure 16.15 GOG 169: survival curves. Reproduced from Moore et al. J Clin Oncol 2004;22:3113–19[40] with permission from the American Society of Clinical Oncology.

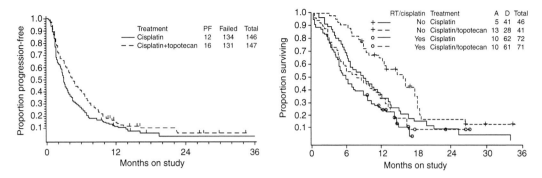

Figure 16.16 GOG 179: progression-free (PF) and overall survival curves. RT, radiotherapy; A, alive; D, dead. Reproduced from Long et al. J Clin Oncol 2005;23:4626–33[41] with permission from the American Society of Clinical Oncology.

Therapy–General + Cervix subscale were associated with survival and may serve as an important prognostic tool in future trials.[42]

The results of GOG 169 and GOG 179 are interesting to look at from the perspective of the era in which they were designed. GOG 169 had a higher response rate with combination cisplatin and paclitaxel (37%) than the cisplatin-plus-topotecan arm of GOG 179 (27%). But no survival advantage was demonstrated despite the higher response rate. What makes this perplexing is that GOG 169 was conducted before the new era of chemoradiotherapy had been firmly established. As a result, nearly 27% of patients in GOG 169 had received chemoradiotherapy, compared with 57% in GOG 179, when the role of chemotherapy in cervical cancer was more widely accepted. This might explain the reason why cisplatin plus topotecan resulted in similar response rates (39%) in patients not previously treated with platinum-based therapy, and might be representative of greater activity from topotecan.

The results of these four randomized phase III trials in recurrent metastatic cervical cancer are summarized in Table 16.8.[43] Based upon the inconclusive data with minimal improvements in clinical outcomes in these studies, the GOG is currently conducting an additional phase III randomized clinical trial. GOG 204 was developed to determine the optimal combination therapy in patients with stage IVB, recurrent, or persistent disease: paclitaxel and cisplatin from GOG 169; cisplatin plus topotecan from GOG 179; combination vinorelbine (30 mg/m^2, days 1 and 8) and cisplatin (50 mg/m^2, day 1); and gemcitabine (1000 mg/m^2, days 1 and 8) plus cisplatin (50 mg/m^2, day 1). The winning arm from this study will serve as the standard treatment in cervical cancer against which future therapies will need to be compared.

FUTURE DIRECTIONS AND CONTROVERSIES

The story of cervical cancer continues to evolve. Despite the many successes achieved in the fight against this cancer, its future management will need to focus on the unanswered issues that still need to be addressed. These issues will shape the manner in which this disease is prevented, primarily treated, and managed in the recurrent setting in order to maximize the quality of life for women worldwide.

Table 16.8 Phase III GOG trials in metastatic cervical cancer

GOG protocol	Ref	Year	Arms	n	Response rate (%) PR	CR	Overall	Median PFS (months)	Median survival (months)
110	38	1997	Cisplatin 50 mg/m² IV q21d	140	11.4	6.4	17.8	3.2	8.0
			Cisplatin 50 mg/m² IV + mitolactol 180 mg/m² PO days 2, 6 q21d	147	11.6	9.5	21.1	3.3	7.3
			Cisplatin 50 mg/m² IV + ifosfamide 5 g/m² 24-h infusion plus mesna 6 g/m² q21d	151	18.5	12.6	31.1 ($p = 0.004$)	4.6 ($p = 0.003$)	8.3
149	39	2002	Cisplatin 50 mg/m² IV + ifosfamide 5 g/m² 24-h infusion plus mesna 6 g/m² q21d	146	NS	NS	32.2	4.6	8.5
			Bleomycin 30 units 24-h infusion, followed by cisplatin 50 mg/m² IV + ifosfamide 5 g/m² 24-h infusion plus mesna 6 g/m² q21d	141	NS	NS	32.1	5.1	8.4
169	40	2004	Cisplatin 50 mg/m² IV q21d	134	13	6	19	2.8	8.8
			Paclitaxel 135 mg/m² 24-h infusion + cisplatin 50 mg/m² IV q21d	130	21	15	36 ($p = 0.002$)	4.8 ($p < 0.001$)	9.7
179	41	2005	Cisplatin 50 mg/m² IV q21d	145	10	13	13	2.9	6.5
			Topotecan 0.75 mg/m² IV days 1–3 + cisplatin 50 mg/m² IV q21d	148	16	10	26 ($p = 0.004$)	4.6 ($p = 0.00048$)	9.4 ($p = 0.015$)
			MVAC q4wk (analysis forthcoming)	63	9	13	22	4.4	9.4

PR, partial response; CR, complete response; PFS, progression-free survival; IV, intravenously; PO, orally; MVAC, methotrexate, vinblastine, doxorubicin, and cisplatin; NS, not significant. Reproduced from Tewari and Monk, Curr Oncol Rep 2005;7:419–34[43] with permission from Current Medicine Group, LLC.

Positron emission tomography

Positron emission tomography (PET) is one of the most important new imaging techniques that are taking on added importance in cervical cancer. The increased role of PET in the clinical evaluation of cervical cancer centers on the importance of identifying nodal metastasis. Prospective reports on the use of PET in the evaluation of para-aortic metastasis show that it has a sensitivity of 75%, a specificity of 92%, a positive predictive value of 75% and a negative predictive value of 92%.[43] A retrospective comparison of PET and computed tomography (CT) in cervical cancer reported a greater detection of lymph node metastasis and prediction of survival with PET.[44] A review of the literature for the Centers for Medicare and

Medicaid Services investigating the diagnostic accuracy of PET compared with conventional imaging techniques has been published.[45] The pooled sensitivity and specificity of PET for the pretreatment staging of retroperitoneal lymph nodes in cervical cancer was higher than that of magnetic resonance imaging (MRI) or CT.[45] With increasing evidence supporting the use of PET in cervical cancer, the Centers for Medicare and Medicaid Services agreed in April 2005, to implement the coverage of PET in newly diagnosed cervical cancer in which a clinical suspicion of nodal metastasis existed but MRI and CT findings were negative. The contribution of this technology to the accurate assessment of disease in cervical cancer has the ability to further direct appropriate treatment fields to areas in which disease might otherwise reside unnoticed.

Human papillomavirus types

The issue of human papillomavirus (HPV) type as a clinical risk factor remains debatable. HPV is associated with >99% of all cervical cancers and is the etiologic factor for this disease.[46] There is no greater association between a malignancy and a virus than that seen with HPV. Although >100 genotypes of HPV have been identified, a select few, including HPV-16, -18, -31, and -45, are considered high-risk and most frequently associated with cervical cancer. There has been debate centering on the role that these individual viruses play in the aggressiveness of this disease. In particular, the controversy surrounds the virulency of HPV-16 and HPV-18.

It has been suggested that HPV-18-related cervical cancers are more aggressive than HPV-16 tumors and are associated with a poorer prognosis. In a study of 247 HPV-related cervical tumors of all stages, HPV-18 DNA was identified as an independent negative prognostic factor in patients treated with radical hysterectomy and

pelvic lymphadenectomy.[47] In addition, a study of stage IB cervical cancers containing HPV-18 treated with radical hysterectomy and pelvic lymphadenectomy showed that HPV-18 was associated with deeper cervical stromal invasion and more nodal metastases, suggesting that these HPV-related tumors are more aggressive.[48]

Histology

The clinical issue with regard to histologic risk factors for cervical cancer is also controversial. Neuroendocrine small cell carcinomas of the cervix are rare, and it is generally accepted these tumors have an extremely poor prognosis. (see Chapter 21).[8,49] But the data are less clear with regard to the prognosis of squamous and nonsquamous (adenocarcinoma and adenosquamous) cell carcinomas.[21] Both adenocarcinoma and adenosquamous lesions have been reported to be independent prognostic factors for reduced recurrence-free survival when all other confounding variables are controlled for.[50] It is suggested by some that these nonsquamous lesions are more often associated with HPV-18, and this may therefore account for the presumed aggressiveness of these histologies. There are, however, conflicting reports on the overall prognosis of these lesions. The suggestion that adenocarcinomas are more aggressive and radioresistant than their squamous cell counterparts may reflect the bulky nature of these tumors and their occupation of the endocervical canal.[8] However, as already mentioned, recent follow-up data from GOG 92 have shown a statistically significant reduction in recurrence rate with adjuvant radiation versus no treatment of stage IB node-negative adenocarcinomas and adenosquamous cancers of the cervix when compared with squamous lesions.[24] Nonsquamous lesions had higher recurrence rates in the observation group (44.0%) than in the radiotherapy arm (8.8%), with a statistically significant ($p = 0.019$) decrease in risk of recurrence. This report suggests an added benefit with adjuvant radiotherapy in these histologies because of the higher risk of recurrence.

Radiation resistance

The majority of deaths in cervical cancer are in the advanced stages of disease, when the use of high-dose radiotherapy and radiosensitizing chemotherapy is the primary treatment option. Inability to control the primary tumor deposit in the radiation field is a result of the intrinsic ability of the cancer to develop radiation resistance.[4] In many ways, understanding the factors that lead to such resistance may be the critical step in ensuring cure in all women with this disease.

The added benefit from chemotherapy with standard radiation protocols is purported to be due to the radiosensitizing property of cisplatin. As a result, the search continues for additional radiosensitizers that may be added to standard chemoradiation protocols. One of these agents is tirapazamine, which is cytotoxic to hypoxic cells while sparing oxygenated cells and has been shown to synergistically interact to potentiate the effects of cisplatin. The presence of hypoxic cells within solid tumors such as cervical cancer have been known to contribute to radiation resistance through a multitude of molecular pathways.[51] Similarly, anemia contributes to tumor hypoxia. The GOG has reported that hemoglobin levels are independent predictors of treatment outcome in patients with advanced cervical cancer treated with primary chemoradiotherapy.[52] It is for these reasons that GOG 219, a randomized phase III trial, was developed to study the addition of tirapazamine during concurrent chemoradiotherapy for stage IB2–IV cervical cancer. This study is intended to determine if the addition of agents targeting

hypoxia to platinum-based therapy targeting hypoxia can even better sensitize these cancers to radiation. This approach to enhancing therapy will be a key focus of study in the future.

Biologic therapy

The failure of current treatment strategies to result in clinically meaningful responses in patients with recurrent and advanced disease will naturally lead to the search for more effective agents. Identifying these agents is critical to the overall strategy against cervical cancer, and will likely come about from a better understanding of the biologic pathways involved with the disease. One of the key processes being recognized in the growth and spread of solid tumors such as cervical cancer is tumor angiogenesis. Targeting of this pathway is one of great interest in oncology, with the success of bevacizumab, a monoclonal antibody that targets the proangiogenic protein vascular endothelial growth factor (VEGF) and has had promising results in the inhibition of tumor growth in a multitude of cancers. GOG 227-C is currently studying bevacizumab in the phase II setting in the treatment of persistent or recurrent squamous cell carcinoma of the cervix. In addition, another biologic agent that targets the epidermal growth factor receptor (EGFR), OSI-774, is also being investigated in the same setting in GOG 227-D. This drug targets the tyrosine kinase pathway that promotes cell growth and is highly expressed in cervical cancer. Both of these studies illustrate the new approaches to biologic therapy toward which future investigations are being directed in the treatment of this disease.

CONCLUSIONS

The advances made in the understanding of cervical cancer have been sufficiently significant that eradication of this disease is now considered possible. Public health screening programs have proven successful when implemented, and high cure rates are seen in the early stages of disease. In addition, early vaccination trials are proving promising. But, despite these successes, many issues remain unresolved and the standard of care continues to evolve. Clinical prognostic factors previously established may not necessarily apply in the new era of chemoradiotherapy. And the lack of effective treatment options in the recurrent setting and the inability to prevent radiation resistance in frontline therapy are reminders that there is still much research to be done. Cervical cancer is a preventable disease. However, if it is not treated properly when it develops, the outcome is fatal. It is clear that the progress made has been exceptional. But, with a little more, cervical cancer will be cancer therapy's poster of success.

REFERENCES

1. Jemal A, Siegel R, Ward E, et al. Cancer Statistics 2007. CA Cancer J Clin 2007;57: 43–66.

2. Kosary CL. FIGO stage, histology, histologic grade, age and race as prognostic factors in determining survival for cancers of the female gynecological system: an analysis of 1973–87 SEER cases of cancers of the endometrium, cervix, ovary, vulva, and vagina. Semin Surg Oncol 1994;10:31–46.

3. World Health Organization. Cervical Cancer Screening in Developing Countries. Report of a WHO Consultation. Geneva: WHO, 2002.

4. Lanciano RM, Won M, Coia LR, Hanks GE. Pretreatment and treatment factors associated with improved outcome in squamous cell carcinoma of the uterine cervix: a final report of the 1973 and 1978 patterns of care studies. Int J Radiat Oncol Biol Phys 1991;20: 667–76.

5. Pecorelli S, Benedet JL, Creasman WT, Shepherd JH. FIGO staging of gynecologic cancer. 1994–1997 FIGO Committee on Gynecologic Oncology. International Federation of Gynecology and Obstetrics. Int J Gynaecol Obstet 1999;64:5–10.

6. National Comprehensive Cancer Network. NCCN Practice Guidelines in Oncology: Cervical Cancer, Version 1.2004. Jenkintown, PA: NCCN.

7. Stehman FB, Rose PG, Greer BE, et al. Innovations in the treatment of invasive cervical cancer. Cancer 2003;98(9 Suppl):2052–63.

8. DiSaia PJ, Creasman WT. Clinical Gynecological Oncology, 6th edn. St Louis, MO: Mosby, 2002.

9. duPont NC, Monk BJ. Chemotherapy and chemoradiotherapy in the current management of cervical carcinoma. Oncology Special Edition 2005;8:1–7.

10. Berman ML, Keys H, Creasman W, et al. Survival and patterns of recurrence in cervical cancer metastatic to periaortic lymph nodes (a Gynecologic Oncology Group study). Gynecol Oncol 1984;19:8–16.

11. Ballon SC, Berman ML, Lagasse LD, Petrilli ES, Castaldo TW. Survival after extraperitoneal pelvic and paraaortic lymphadenectomy and radiation therapy in cervical carcinoma. Obstet Gynecol 1981;57:90–5.

12. Berman ML, Lagasse LD, Watring WG, et al. The operative evaluation of patients with cervical carcinoma by an extraperitoneal approach. Obstet Gynecol 1977;50:658–64.

13. Rubin SC, Brookland R, Mikuta JJ, et al. Para-aortic nodal metastases in early cervical carcinoma: long-term survival following extended-field radiotherapy. Gynecol Oncol 1984;18:213–17.

14. Cosin JA, Fowler JM, Chen MD, et al. Pretreatment surgical staging of patients with cervical carcinoma: the case for lymph node debulking. Cancer 1998;82:2241–8.

15. Delgado G, Bundy BN, Fowler WC Jr, et al. A prospective surgical pathological study of stage I squamous carcinoma of the cervix: a Gynecologic Oncology Group study. Gynecol Oncol 1989;35:314–20.

16. Delgado G, Bundy B, Zaino R, et al. Prospective surgical–pathological study of disease-free interval in patients with stage IB squamous cell carcinoma of the cervix: a Gynecologic Oncology Group study. Gynecol Oncol 1990;38:352–7.

17. Zaino RJ, Ward S, Delgado G, et al. Histopathologic predictors of the behavior of surgically treated stage IB squamous cell carcinoma of the cervix. A Gynecologic Oncology Group study. Cancer 1992;69:1750–8.

18. Zreik TG, Chambers JT, Chambers SK. Parametrial involvement, regardless of nodal status: a poor prognostic factor for cervical cancer. Obstet Gynecol 1996;87:741–6.

19. Burghardt E, Baltzer J, Tulusan AH, Haas J. Results of surgical treatment of 1028 cervical cancers studied with volumetry. Cancer 1992;70:648–55.

20. Averette HE, Nguyen HN, Donato DM, et al. Radical hysterectomy for invasive cervical cancer. A 25-year prospective experience with the Miami technique. Cancer 1993; 71(4 Suppl):1422–37.

21. Singh N, Arif S. Histopathologic parameters of prognosis in cervical cancer – a review. Int J Gynecol Cancer 2004;14:741–50.

22. Sedlis A, Bundy BN, Rotman MZ, et al. A randomized trial of pelvic radiation therapy versus no further therapy in selected patients with stage IB carcinoma of the cervix after radical hysterectomy and pelvic lymphadenectomy: a Gynecologic Oncology Group study. Gynecol Oncol 1999;73:177–83.

23. Smiley LM, Burke TW, Silva EG, et al. Prognostic factors in stage IB squamous cervical cancer patients with low risk for recurrence. Obstet Gynecol 1991;77:271–5.

24. Rotman M, Sedlis A, Piedmonte MR, et al. A phase III randomized trial of postoperative pelvic irradiation in stage IB cervical carcinoma with poor prognostic features: follow-up of a Gynecologic Oncology Group study. Int J Radiat Oncol Biol Phys 2006;65: 169–76.

25. Rose PG, Bundy BN, Watkins EB, et al. Concurrent cisplatin-based radiotherapy and chemotherapy for locally advanced cervical cancer. N Engl J Med 1999;340:1144–53 [Erratum 1999;341:708].

26. Keys HM, Bundy BN, Stehman FB, et al. Cisplatin, radiation, and adjuvant hysterectomy compared with radiation and adjuvant hysterectomy for bulky stage IB cervical carcinoma. N Engl J Med 1999;340:1154–61 [Erratum 1999;341:708].

27. Morris M, Eifel PJ, Lu J, et al. Pelvic radiation with concurrent chemotherapy compared with pelvic and para-aortic radiation for high-risk cervical cancer. N Engl J Med 1999;340:1137–43.

28. Whitney CW, Sause W, Bundy BN, et al. Randomized comparison of fluorouracil plus cisplatin versus hydroxyurea as an adjunct to radiation therapy in stage IIB–IVA carcinoma of the cervix with negative para-aortic lymph nodes: a Gynecologic Oncology Group and Southwest Oncology Group study. J Clin Oncol 1999;17:1334–5.

29. Peters WA 3rd, Liu PY, Barrett RJ 2nd, et al. Concurrent chemotherapy and pelvic radiation therapy compared with pelvic radiation therapy alone as adjuvant therapy after radical surgery in high-risk early-stage cancer of the cervix. J Clin Oncol 2000;18:1606–13.

30. Eifel PJ, Winter K, Morris M, et al. Pelvic irradiation with concurrent chemotherapy versus pelvic and para-aortic irradiation for high-risk cervical cancer: an update of Radiation Therapy Oncology Group trial (RTOG) 90-01. J Clin Oncol 2004;22:872–80.

31. Lanciano R, Calkins A, Bundy BN, et al. Randomized comparison of weekly cisplatin or protracted venous infusion of fluorouracil in combination with pelvic radiation in advanced cervix cancer: a Gynecologic Oncology Group study. J Clin Oncol 2005;23:8289–95.

32. Neoadjuvant Chemotherapy for Locally Advanced Cervical Cancer Meta-analysis Collaboration. Neoadjuvant chemotherapy for locally advanced cervical cancer: a systematic review and meta-analysis of individual patient data from 21 randomised trials. Eur J Cancer 2003;39:2470–86.

33. Yessaian A, Magistris A, Burger RA, Monk BJ. Radical hysterectomy followed by tailored postoperative therapy in the treatment of stage IB2 cervical cancer: feasibility and indications for adjuvant therapy. Gynecol Oncol 2004;94:61–6.

34. Monk BJ, Wang J, Im S, et al. Rethinking the use of radiation and chemotherapy after radical hysterectomy: a clinical–pathologic analysis of a Gynecologic Oncology Group/Southwest Oncology Group/Radiation Therapy Oncology Group trial. Gynecol Oncol 2005;96:721–8.

35. Monk BJ, Tian C, Rose PG, Lanciano R. Which clinical/pathologic factors matter in the era of chemoradiation as treatment for locally advanced cervical carcinoma? Analysis of two Gynecologic Oncology Group (GOG) trials. Gynecol Oncol 2007;105:427–33.

36. Thigpen T, Shingleton H, Homesley H, LaGasse L, Blessing J. cis-Dichlorodiammine-platinum(II) in the treatment of gynecologic malignancies: phase II trials by the Gynecologic Oncology Group. Cancer Treat Rep 1979; 63:1549–55.

37. Bonomi P, Blessing JA, Stehman FB, et al. Randomized trial of three cisplatin dose schedules in squamous-cell carcinoma of the cervix: a Gynecologic Oncology Group study. J Clin Oncol 1985;3:1079–85.

38. Omura GA, Blessing JA, Vaccarello L, et al. Randomized trial of cisplatin versus cisplatin plus mitolactol versus cisplatin plus ifosfamide in advanced squamous carcinoma of the cervix: a Gynecologic Oncology Group study. J Clin Oncol 1997;15:165–71.

39. Bloss JD, Blessing JA, Behrens BC, et al. Randomized trial of cisplatin and ifosfamide with or without bleomycin in squamous carcinoma of the cervix: a Gynecologic Oncology Group study. J Clin Oncol 2002;20:1832–7.

40. Moore DH, Blessing JA, McQuellon RP, et al. Phase III study of cisplatin with or without paclitaxel in stage IVB, recurrent, or persistent squamous cell carcinoma of the cervix: a Gynecologic Oncology Group study. J Clin Oncol 2004;22:3113–19.

41. Long HJ 3rd, Bundy BN, Grendys EC Jr, et al. Randomized phase III trial of cisplatin with or without topotecan in carcinoma of the uterine cervix: a Gynecologic Oncology Group Study. J Clin Oncol 2005;23:4626–33.

42. Monk BJ, Huang HQ, Cella D, Long HJ 3rd. Quality of life outcomes from a randomized phase III trial of cisplatin with or without topotecan in advanced carcinoma of the cervix: a Gynecologic Oncology Group Study. J Clin Oncol 2005;23:4617–25 [Erratum:8549].

43. Tewari KS, Monk BJ. Gynecologic oncology group trials of chemotherapy for metastatic and recurrent cervical cancer. Curr Oncol Rep 2005;7:419–34.

44. Rose PG, Adler LP, Rodriguez M, et al. Positron emission tomography for evaluating para-aortic nodal metastasis in locally advanced cervical cancer before surgical staging: a surgicopathologic study. J Clin Oncol 1999; 17:41–5.

45. Grigsby PW, Siegel BA, Dehdashti F. Lymph node staging by positron emission tomography in patients with carcinoma of the cervix. J Clin Oncol 2001;19:3745–9.

46. Havrilesky LJ, Kulasingam SL, Matchar DB, Myers ER. FDG–PET for management of cervical and ovarian cancer. Gynecol Oncol 2005;97:183–91.

47. Walboomers JM, Jacobs MV, Manos MM, et al. Human papillomavirus is a necessary

cause of invasive cervical cancer worldwide. J Pathol 1999;189:12–19.

48. Burger RA, Monk BJ, Kurosaki T, et al. Human papillomavirus type 18: association with poor prognosis in early stage cervical cancer. J Natl Cancer Inst 1996;88:1361–8.

49. Im SS, Wilczynski SP, Burger RA, Monk BJ. Early stage cervical cancers containing human papillomavirus type 18 DNA have more nodal metastasis and deeper stromal invasion. Clin Cancer Res 2003;9:4145–50.

50. Chan JK, Loizzi V, Burger RA, Rutgers J, Monk BJ. Prognostic factors in neuroendocrine small cell cervical carcinoma: a multivariate analysis. Cancer 2003;97:568–74.

51. Lai CH, Hsuch S, Hong JH, et al. Are adenocarcinomas and adenosquamous carcinomas different from squamous carcinomas in stage IB and II cervical cancer patients undergoing primary radical surgery? Int J Gynecol Cancer 1999;9:28–36.

52. Hockel M, Vaupel P. Tumor hypoxia: definitions and current clinical, biologic, and molecular aspects. J Natl Cancer Inst 2001; 93:266–76.

53. Winter WE 3rd, Maxwell GL, Tian C, et al. Association of hemoglobin level with survival in cervical carcinoma patients treated with concurrent cisplatin and radiotherapy: a Gynecologic Oncology Group study. Gynecol Oncol 2004;94:495–501.

Predictors of radiation sensitivity and resistance

17

Anuja Jhingran

INTRODUCTION

Local control of tumor is a very important predictor of outcome in all cancer patients, including quality of life and survival. Local tumor failure is the cause of 40–60% of cancer deaths, and may occur in 60–80% of cancer patients at the time of death. Any process that enhances tumor cell kill for a given radiation dose (sensitization) is important, and investigators have focused on three tumor parameters that are likely to influence local tumor control after radiotherapy: intrinsic radiosensitivity, the degree of tumor hypoxia, and the rate of repopulation of tumor cells. In this chapter, we will discuss these three parameters as well as modifiers of radiation effects. Any factor that decreases the relative amount of normal tissue injury is also important and can affect the therapeutic benefit of treatment. We will discuss these factors as well (Figure 17.1).

Intrinsic radiosensitivity

Cells in tissue culture exhibit a wide variation in radiosensitivity despite being irradiated under standard conditions, suggesting the presence of inherent factors influencing the radiation response of mammalian cells. This was clearly demonstrated by the discovery that both lymphocytes and fibroblasts from patients with the genetic disorder ataxiatelangiectasia (AT)

were a factor of 2–3 times more radiosensitive than their normal counterparts.[1] This suggests, that under standard conditions, tumors comprising cells that are found to be inherently resistant to radiation will be more difficult to cure with radiotherapy than those comprising radiosensitive cells and also that tumors comprising radiosensitive cells may be overtreated with conventional doses of radiation. Therefore, it would be reasonable to try to predict for inherent radiosensitivity in tumors so that one can tailor the treatment for better cure rates and lower toxicity.

Several methods for measuring radiosensitivity for predictive purposes have been tested in human tumors; however, the most reliable and relevant measure is based on the fraction of cell surviving a particular radiation dose. This is done using a clonogenic assay. Two aspects of the initial region of the cell survival curves seem to correlate best with clinical radiosensitivity: SF_2, the fraction of cells surviving 2 Gy, and the $\alpha{:}\beta$, the initial slope. The most convincing study to date is that of West et al[2] on cervical carcinomas treated by radiotherapy alone. In vitro tumor SF_2 values from fresh biopsy material using colony formation in agar were found to correlate highly with outcome. Patients with tumors exhibiting SF_2 values higher than the median value had significantly worse local control and significantly worse survival rates than did those with tumors with SF_2

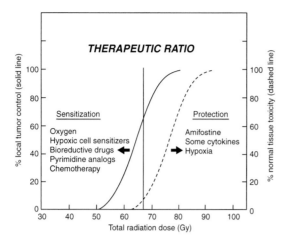

Figure 17.1 Schematic diagram showing tumor response (solid line) and normal tissue toxicity (dashed line) as a function of total radiation dose. Sensitization is produced by chemicals that shift the tumor response curve selectively to the left, and protection results from chemicals that can shift the toxicity curve selectively to the right. Reproduced from Wasserman TH, Chapman JD. Radiation response modulation. In: Perez AC et al, eds. Principles and Practice of Radiation Oncology. Philadelphia: Lippincott Williams and Wilkins, 2004:664 with permission.

values below the median. This trend was the same for all tumor stages (I–III). In 88 patients, the absolute differences in local control and survival rates between the high- and low-radiosensitivity groups were around 30% at 2 years. However, no matter how promising these results are, colony assays are highly unlikely to be used routinely for clinical application, since they need 3–4 weeks to complete and are not simple to perform, requiring a highly skilled laboratory team with extensive experience.

Other methods are being evaluated that are quicker, including assays based on cell growth rather than clonogenicity, in which cells are cultured in microplates and exposed to radiation, after which their viability is assessed by staining for ability to reduce compounds or by estimating total DNA or RNA content.

These endpoints are surrogates for reproductive integrity. These assays are rapid, easy, and amenable to automation; they are suitable for screening drugs for their cytotoxic activity, but are not suitable for predicting radiosensitivity. Another type of nonclonogic assay assesses the ability of tumor cells to adhere and grow on a specially prepared matrix; the ability of this assay to predict tumor cell radiosensitivity also has yet to be proven.

Rate of tumor repopulation

Radiation is usually given in a series of fractions. These are usually separated by 1 day but can be separated by up to 3 days (weekends), giving time for cells to repopulate. This is good if normal cells are repopulating and repairing, but bad if tumor cells are growing, since more cells will need to be killed with the subsequent radiation fraction, leading to a higher chance of recurrence. The rate of tumor repopulation can be expressed in terms of its T_{pot}, which takes into account cell cycle time and growth fraction but not cell loss. T_{pot} is commonly measured by labeling tumor biopsy specimens with bromodeoxyuridine (BrdU) and then using flow cytometry to estimate the doubling time. In a phase III trial by the European Organization for Research and Treatment of Cancer (EORTC) in head and neck cancer,[3] T_{pot} was measured prior to the start of treatment. In this trial, local control of fast-growing tumors (T_{pot} <4 days) was better after accelerated fractionation than after conventional therapy, but no difference was found in local control of slow-growing tumors from either type of therapy. Two other studies have also shown that T_{pot} is a significant predictor of outcome for radiotherapy schedules longer than 6 weeks;[4,5] however, another large multicenter trial found no correlation between T_{pot} and outcome after radiotherapy.[6] In short, predictive assays show promise: although none of the markers explored so far has proven reliable for predicting the response of a tumor to radiotherapy, some may show promise for identifying groups of patients who may benefit from altered treatment protocols such as accelerated treatment, hyperfractionation, bioreductive drugs, or neutron therapy.

Tumor hypoxia

The importance of hypoxia in human tumors has been suggested by several findings, including the existence of tumor necrosis, known to be often associated with hypoxia,[7] by direct measurement of hypoxia in human tumors using several techniques, by the clinically observed correlation between anemia and outcome,[8,9] and by the limited success of trials combining hyperbaric oxygen or hypoxic cell radiosensitizers with radiotherapy. Significant advances in reliable methods for measuring the oxygenation status of individual human tumors have been made. One of the quickest and easiest ways is the use of the Eppendorf probe. This is a computer-driven microelectrode device that obtains direct readings of tissue partial oxygen pressure (pO_2) along a track in the tumor. Significant correlations between low oxygen levels and radiotherapy failures in cervical cancer, head and neck carcinoma, prostate carcinoma, and sarcomas have been reported. Specifically in cervical cancer, a clinical trial in Germany of patients with advanced carcinoma of the cervix treated with radiotherapy has shown lower overall and recurrence-free survival in patients whose tumors exhibited median pO_2 values ≤ 10 mmHg as measured with the Eppendorf probe.[10] This study suggested that hypoxia leads to radioresistance; later studies indicate that hypoxia may also lead to more aggressive and malignant tumors.[11]

Other methods for measuring hypoxia in tumor cells include deposition of labeled nitroimidazoles in the tumor or with polarographic oxygen probes. Compounds labeled with the short-lived γ-emitting isotope 123I can also be used in regions of low oxygen tension. The presence of hypoxia can be visualized by single photon emission computed tomography (SPECT), but recently investigators have been looking at magnetic resonance imaging (MRI), magnetic resonance spectroscopy (MRS), and electron paramagnetic resonance (EPR) to yield more information on the status of tumor oxygenation. More exciting is the development of histopathologic assays of tumor hypoxia using antibody staining of molecular factors that are thought to be directly or indirectly proportional to hypoxic microenvironments within tumors. These molecular expressions include vascular endothelial growth factor (VEGF), hypoxia-inducing factor 1α (HIF-1α), CD31, Ki-67, carbonic anhydrase IX, and several others. These histopathologic assays of tumor hypoxia and associated molecular factors have been useful for establishing important correlations between tumor vasculature and a hypoxic microenvironment.

MODIFIERS OF RADIATION EFFECTS

Oxygen

Hyperbaric oxygen

As discussed above, the sensitivity of biologic material to sparsely ionizing radiation is critically dependent on the presence or absence of molecular oxygen. For oxygen to act as a sensitizer, it must be present during the radiation exposure – or at least during the lifetime of the free radicals that are involved in the indirect action of radiation. Oxygen was the first radiation sensitizer to be clinically tested. Clinical trials using hyperbaric oxygen were performed; however, the results are difficult to interpret given the small numbers of subjects and the use of unconventional fractionation schemes involving a few large fractions being given over short periods. The largest multicenter trials of hyperbaric oxygen, performed by the UK Medical Research Council (MRC), showed significant benefits in local control and survival for patients with carcinoma of the cervix or advanced head and neck cancer, but not for those with bladder cancer. Another overview of these trials revealed a 6.6% improvement in local control and perhaps an increase in late normal-tissue damage.[12,13] However, hyperbaric oxygen treatment is very cumbersome, and therefore fell into disuse when it was felt that drugs could achieve the same results more easily.

Chemical radiosensitizers

Where as the hyperbaric oxygen approach was to 'force' oxygen into tissue, the aim of chemical radiosensitization is to focus on the use of oxygen substitutes that will diffuse into poorly vascularized areas of tumors and hopefully penetrate further than oxygen, reaching all of the hypoxic cells in the tumor by chemical means. Three nitroimidazole-type radiosensitizers have been tested in clinical trials. The first to be used in clinical trials was misonidazole. Not one of the 20 or more randomized prospective controlled clinical trials performed in the USA by the Radiation Therapy Oncology Group (RTOG), including a trial in cervical cancer, showed a statistically significant advantage for misonidazole, although several suggested a slight benefit. The Danish Head and Neck Cancer Study (DAHANCA) performed the largest single randomized trial,[14] using misonidazole in

626 patients with advanced head and neck cancers. They found no significant advantage when all patients were analyzed as a group; however, in a subgroup analysis, male patients with high hemoglobin levels and cancer of the pharynx derived the most benefit from the addition of misonidazole. The dose-limiting toxicity of misonidazole was peripheral neuropathy, which progressed to central nervous system toxicity if use of the drug continued. Due to this toxicity, evaluation of etanidazole was undertaken. Etanidazole showed equivalent sensitization but much less toxicity than misonidazole; however, all clinical studies again showed no benefit of adding this drug to radiotherapy. Another compound, nimorazole, which is much less toxic than the other two drugs and therefore can be given with each treatment, is being used in Denmark. The DAHANCA conducted a phase III trial in head and neck cancers using nimorazole and found a statistically significant improvement in locoregional tumor control but not in overall survival,[15] and nimorazole has become the standard of care in Denmark.

A number of groups in Europe are evaluating the used of nicotinamide (a vitamin B_3 analogue) and carbogen in the clinic, with either conventional or accelerated radiotherapy. This is referred to as ARCON therapy and has been applied to the treatment of nonsmall cell lung cancers (NSCLC) and of head and neck cancers, and trials are presently underway.

Hypoxia cytotoxic agents

A different approach from designing drugs that preferentially radiosensitize hypoxic cells is to develop drugs that selectively kill such cells. There are three classes of these agents: quinine antibiotics, nitroaromatic compounds and benzotriazine di-N-oxides. The nitroaromatic class has included dual-function agents, but thus far toxicity to normal tissues has precluded clinical trials of these compounds. Mitomycin-C is the most common compound from the quinine antibiotic class, and has been used for many years. Weissberg et al[16] reported on a randomized clinical trial of mitomycin-C with radiotherapy in patients with head and neck cancers compared with standard radiotherapy alone, and found an increase in disease-free survival rate at 5 years from 49% to 75% with mitomycin-C, as well as an improvement in local control (49% vs 75%). A phase III randomized study of radiotherapy alone or radiotherapy plus mitomycin-C was performed in 160 patients with locally advanced cervical cancer,[17] and an interim analysis showed a significant difference in favor of the patients receiving mitomycin-C in terms of disease-free survival but not overall survival or local control. The study is still ongoing. The largest trial looking at mitomycin-C in cervical cancer comes from Thailand.[18] In a phase III randomized trial, 926 patients were randomized to four arms: arm 1, conventional radiation; arm 2, conventional radiation and adjuvant chemotherapy; arm 3, conventional radiation plus concurrent chemotherapy; arm 4, conventional radiation plus concurrent chemotherapy and adjuvant chemotherapy. The concurrent chemotherapy consisted of mitomycin-C and oral 5-fluorouracil (5-FU) and the adjuvant chemotherapy was oral 5-FU. The results of this study showed that patients who received concurrent mitomycin-C and 5-FU with radiotherapy had better 5-year disease-free survival compared with patients receiving radiotherapy alone (48.2% vs 64.5%). Mitomycin-C has been used in other tumors as well with radiotherapy and seems to be promising, and future studies are presently underway in multiple sites, especially the head and neck.

The lead compound in the third class of drugs is tirapazamine, which shows highly selective toxicity towards hypoxic cells both in vitro and in vivo. Several phase I and II trials of single and multiple doses of tirapazamine have been performed in multiple sites, including head and neck and cervical cancer. A phase II study showed that it was feasible to give cisplatin and tirapazamine together in patients with advanced or recurrent cervical cancer.[19] In a phase III trial comparing cisplatin or cisplatin combined with tirapazamine for advanced (stage IIIB and IV) NSCLC,[20] patients given the combination had twice the response rate and significantly longer survival than patients given cisplatin alone (Figure 17.2). Several phase III trials are looking at combination of chemotherapy and tirapazamine with radiotherapy particularly, in cervical cancer and head and neck cancer. The Gynecologic Oncology Group (GOG) has a phase III trial currently accruing patients that randomizes patients with locally advanced cervical cancer to two arms consisting of concurrent cisplatin and radiation versus concurrent cisplatin plus tirapazamine and radiation.

Summary

Of the numerous clinical trials that have been performed in attempts to overcome the perceived problem of hypoxic cells in tumors, most have shown inconclusive or borderline results. In 1996, Overgaard and Horsman[21] published the results of a meta-analysis of 10602 patients treated in 82 randomized clinical trials involving hyperbaric oxygen, chemical sensitizers, carbogen breathing, or blood transfusions; the tumor sites studied included bladder, uterine cervix, central nervous system, head and neck, and lung. Overall, anti-hypoxic cell treatments were found to improve local tumor control by

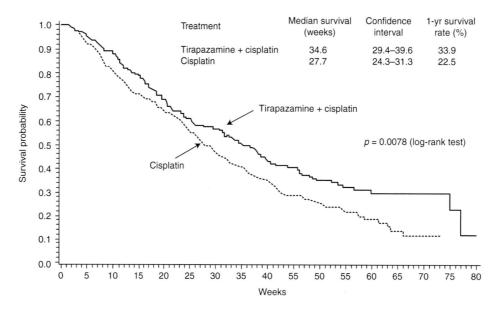

Figure 17.2 Overall survival (in weeks) of nonsmall cell lung cancer patients treated with cisplatin alone (*n* = 219) versus cisplatin plus tirapazamine (*n* = 219). Reproduced from von Pawel et al. Clin Oncol 2000;18:1351–9[20] with permission from the American Society of Clinical Oncology.

4.6% and survival rate by 2.8%. The largest number of trials involved head and neck tumors, which also showed the greatest benefit. Overgaard and Horsman[21] concluded from the meta-analysis that the problem of hypoxia may be marginal in most adenocarcinomas and most important in squamous cell carcinomas.

RADIOPROTECTORS

The rationale behind the use of radioprotectors in clinical trials is the need for improvement in local control with reduction of normal tissue complications. One class of compounds, the thiophosphates, have shown differential protection of normal tissue compared with tumor tissue. After extensive animal testing, one of these compounds, amifostine (WR-2721) came into clinical use. Amifostine is a prodrug; the presence of a terminal phosphorothioic acid group makes it relatively unreactive, and it does not readily permeate cell membranes. Dephosphorylation by

alkaline phosphatase, which is present in high concentrations in normal tissues and capillaries, converts amifostine to its active form, WR-1065. This metabolite readily enters normal cells by facilitated diffusion, where it scavenges free radicals generated by ionizing radiation or by some alkylating chemotherapeutic agents. Whatever the underlying mechanism, the compound quickly floods normal tissues but penetrates tumors more slowly. The extent to which amifostine protects normal tissues from radiation effect varies considerably among tissue types (Table 17.1). The hematopoietic system, the gut lining, and the salivary glands are generally well protected; however, the drug does not cross the blood–brain barrier and therefore it provides no protection to the brain, nor does if provide much provide protection to the lung.

Amifostine has been used for nearly a quarter of a century. Initial phase I toxicity trials conducted in the USA have shown that the dose-limiting toxicity is hypotension; this and other

Table 17.1 Summary of normal tissue responsiveness to protection by amifostine (WR-2721)

Protected tissues[a]	Unprotected tissues
Bone marrow (2.4–3.0)	Brain
Immune system (1.8–3.4)	Spinal cord
Skin (2.0–2.4)	
Small intestine (1.8–2.0)	
Colon (1.8)	
Lung (1.2–1.8)	
Esophagus (1.4)	
Kidney (1.5)	
Liver (2.7)	
Salivary gland (2.0)	
Oral mucoas (>1)	
Testis (2.1)	

[a]Numbers in parentheses are the dose-reduction factors or factor in resistance associated with amifostine injection.

Reprinted from Yuhus JM, Spellman JM, Culo F. The role of WR-2721 in radiotherapy and/or chemotherapy. In: Brady L, ed. Radiation Sensitizers. New York: Masson, 1980.

adverse effects such as sneezing and somnolence have tended to limit the amount of drug given to less than the dose needed to achieve maximum protection according to animal experiments. However, over the two decades of its use, several phase II and III trials in multiple sites have found some advantage in the use of amifostine. In a phase III randomized trial in 315 patients with local advanced head and neck tumors,[22] patients who received amifostine had a significantly reduced incidence of acute grade 2 xerostomia than patients who did not receive amifostine (76% vs 54%, $p = 0.004$), and more importantly a significantly higher dose of radiation could be administered as a median dose yielding xerostomia. This effect on xerostomia from amifostine also translated into a better quality of life for the patients.

Phase III studies in lung cancer have shown that amifostine combined with chemotherapy and radiation reduces the incidence of esophagitis and pneumonitis compared with patients who did not receive amifostine.[23,24] Data from a New York Gynecology Oncology Group study of patients with cervical cancer[25] who received amifostine before cisplatin and whole-pelvic radiation suggest that, relative to historic controls, patients treated with amifostine had less radiation toxicity to the pelvic mucosa, in particular late toxicities such as rectovaginal fistula and proctitis. Recently, with the development of the subcutaneous form of amifostine, there has been even more interest in its use. The RTOG presently has a phase II trial accruing patients with locally advanced cervical cancer and positive para-aortic nodes. Patients in the initial phase were treated with weekly cisplatin and extended-field radiotherapy and in the second phase are being treated with subcutaneous amifostine, weekly cisplatin, and extended-field radiotherapy. The trial is still accruing patients.

In a review by the American Society of Clinical Oncology of clinical practice guidelines for the use of chemotherapy and radiotherapy protectants,[26] it was concluded that there was no evidence that the use of amifostine protected tumors and that it did protect from acute and late xerostomia in patients receiving fractionated radiotherapy for head and neck cancers. The data for protection against mucositis was marginal but insufficient to recommend amifostine at this time, and further trials are needed to achieve a more definitive conclusion regarding protection from radiation-induced mucositis in the head and neck, thorax, and pelvic areas. As new radiotherapy delivery techniques, such as three dimensional conformal radiotherapy and intensity-modulated radiotherapy (IMRT), lead to higher doses of radiation, protection of normal tissues will become more important, and it is anticipated that additional clinical studies will identify new indications for amifostine and other radioprotectors.

REFERENCES

1. Taylor AMR, Harnden DG, Arlett CF, et al. Ataxia–telangiectasia: a human mutation with abnormal radiation sensitivity. Nature 1975; 528:427.

2. West CM, Davidson SE, Roberts SA, Hunter RD. Intrinsic radiosensitivity and prediction of patient response to radiotherapy for carcinoma of the cervix. Br J Cancer 1993;68:819.

3. Begg AC, Hofland I, Moonen I, et al. The predictive value of cell kinetic measurements in a European trial of accelerated fractionation in head and neck tumors: an interm report. Int J Radiat Oncol Biol Phys 1990;19:1449–53.

4. Corvo R, Giaretti W, Sanguineti G, et al. Potential doubling time in head and neck tumors treated by primary radiotherapy: preliminary evidence for a prognostic significance in local control. Int J Radiat Oncol Biol Phys 1993;27:1165.

5. Bourhis J, Wilson G, Wibault P, et al. In vivo measurement of potiential doubling time by flow cytometry in oropharyngeal cancer treated by conventional radiotherapy. Int J Radiat Oncol Biol Phys 1993;27:1165.

6. Begg AC, Haustermans K, Hart AAM, et al. The value of pretreatment cell kinetic parameters as predictors for radiotherapy outcome in head and neck cancer: a multicenter analysis. Radiother Oncol 1999;50:13–23.

7. Thomlinson, RH, Gray LH. The histological structure of some human lung cancers and the possible implication for radiotherapy. Br J Cancer 1955;9:539.

8. Disch S. Radiotherapy and anaemia: the clinical experience. Radiother Oncol 1991; 20(Suppl):35.

9. Bush RS: The significance of anemia in clinical radiation therapy. Int J Radiat Oncol Biol Phys 1986:12:2047.

10. Hockel M, Knoop C, Schlenger K, et al. Intramural pO$_2$ predicts survival in advanced cancer of the uterine cervix. Radiother Oncol 1993;26:45–50.

11. Hockel M, Schelenger K, Aral B, et al. Association between tumor hypoxia and malignant progression in advanced cancer of the uterine cervix. Cancer Res 1996;56:4509–15.

12. Henk JM, Smith CW. Radiotherapy and hyperbaric oxygen in head and neck cancer. Lancet 1997;ii:104.

13. Watson ER, Halnan KE, Dische S, et al. Hyperbaric oxygen and radiotherapy: a Medical Research Council trial in carcinoma of the cervix. Br J Radiol 1978;51:879.

14. Overgaard J, Hansen HS, Anderson AP. Misonidazole combined with split course radiotherapy in the treatment of invasive carcinoma of the larynx and pharynx. Int J Radiat Oncol Biol Phys 1989;16:1065–8.

15. Overgaard J, Hansen HS, Overgaard M, et al. A randomized double-blind phase III study of minorazole as a hypoxic radiosensitizer of primary radiotherapy in supraglottic larynx and pharynx carcinoma. Results of the Danish Head and Neck Cancer Study (DAHANCA) Protocol 5–85. Radiother Oncol 1998;46:135–46.

16. Weissberg JB, Son YH, Papac RJ, et al. Randomized clinical trial of mitomycin C as an adjunct to radiotherapy in head and neck cancer. Int J Radiat Oncol Biol Phys 1989;17:3–9.

17. Roberts KB, Urdaneta N, Vera R, et al. Interim results of a randomized trial of mitomycin C as an adjunct to radical radiotherapy in the treatment of locally advanced squamous-cell carcinoma of the cervix. Int J Cancer 2000;90:206–23.

18. Lorvidhaya V, Chitapanarux I, Sangruchi S, et al. Concurrent mitomycin C, 5-fluorouracil and radiotherapy in the treatment of locally advanced carcinoma of the cervix: a randomized trial. Int J Radiat Oncol Biol Phys 2003; 55:1226–32.

19. Maluf FC, Leiser AL, Aghajanian C, et al. Phase II study of tirapazamine plus cisplatin in patients with advanced or recurrent cervical cancer. Int J Gynecol Cancer 2006;16:1165–71.

20. von Pawel J, von Roemeling R, Gatzemeier U, et al. Tirapazimine plus cisplatin in advanced non-small cell lung cancer: a report of the international CATAPULT I Study Group. Cisplatin And Tirapazamine in subjects with Advanced Previously Untreated non-small-cell Lung Tumors. J Clin Oncol 2000;18:1351–9.

21. Overgaard J, Horsman MR. Modification of hypoxia-induced radioresistance in tumours by the use of oxygen and sensitizers. Semin Radiat Oncol 1996;6:10–21.

22. Brizel DM, Wasserman TH, Henke M, et al. Phase III randomized trial of amifostine as a radioprotector in head and neck cancer. J Clin Oncol 2000;18:3339–45.

23. Antonadou D, Coliarakis N, Synodinou M, et al. Randomized phase III trial of radiation ± amifostine in patients with advanced stage lung cancer. Int J Radiat Oncol Biol Phys 1999;45:113.

24. Komaki R, Lee JS, Kaplan B, et al. Randomized phase III study of chemoradiation with or without amifostine for patients with favorable performance status inoperable stage II–III non-small cell lung cancer: preliminary results. Semin Radiat Oncol 2002;12:46–9.

25. Wadler S, Goldberg G, Fields A, et al. The potential role of amifostine in conjunction with cisplatin in the treatment of locally advanced carcinoma of the cervix. Semin Oncol 1996;23:64–8.

26. Hensley ML, Schuchter LM, Lindley C, et al, for the American College of Clinical Oncology. American Society of Clinical Oncology Clinical Practice Guidelines for the Use of Chemotherapy and Radiotherapy Protectants. J Clin Oncol 1999;17:3333–55.

Molecular prognostic and predictive factors in cervical cancer

18

Jayanthi S Lea and Carolyn Y Muller

INTRODUCTION

The molecular alterations involved in cervical carcinogenesis are complex and not fully understood. The human papillomavirus (HPV) is universally accepted as the causative agent of nearly all cervical cancers worldwide and serves as the prototype molecular marker for clinical diagnostic utility.[1] However, uncovering additional common molecular events has been difficult, with studies demonstrating vast heterogeneity, likely a result of interactive effects between environmental insults, host immunity, and somatic cell genomic variations (Figure 18.1). Advances in molecular biologic techniques in concert with technology have generated a plethora of studies geared at understanding altered pathways in cervical cancer progression, and subsequent identification of clinically useful biomarkers for diagnostic, prognostic, and therapeutic endpoints. This chapter will review the current progress in biomarker development for both preinvasive and invasive cervical cancer.

BIOMARKERS OF CERVICAL DYSPLASIA AND CANCER: TRANSLATIONAL APPLICATIONS

Biomarker studies in preinvasive cervical disease and transition to invasive cancer are geared to understanding the biologic consequence of HPV infection in relation to clinically relevant cervical disease. There are two critical endpoints on the spectrum of cervical dysplasia. (Figure 18.2). The initial point (A) represents the cell at risk due to active HPV infection, whereas the second point (B) represents the clinically relevant preinvasive lesion, cervical intraepithelial neoplasia (CIN) 3 or carcinoma in situ (CIS). The latter lesion is the immediate precursor to invasive cervical cancer (C), and is the target for molecular diagnostic strategies, chemoprevention targeted at reversing aberrant molecular pathways in the preinvasive cells and vaccine strategies aimed at preventing the initiation step. The following sections will highlight some of the progress made in this translational science.

HUMAN PAPILLOMAVIRUS – THE PROTOTYPE MOLECULAR MARKER

As molecular techniques have developed, it is clear that nearly all invasive cervical cancers and relevant preinvasive disease are associated with one or more oncogenic HPV types.[1,2] HPV appears to play a major role in the development of cervical cancers, and increasing evidence

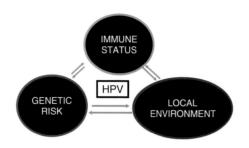

Figure 18.1 Schematic demonstration of the interplay between gene, environment, and host factors to modulate human papillomavirus infection and pathologic expression.

suggests that the presence of HPV oncoproteins may also be a critical component of continued cancer cell proliferation (Table 18.1).[3,4] Oncogenic HPV early replication proteins E1 and E2 enable the virus to replicate within the cervical cell and are expressed in high levels early in an HPV infection, which can lead to cytologic changes detected as a 'low-grade' or an LSIL (low-grade squamous intraepithelial lesion) Pap diagnosis. Unlike the low-risk subtypes, oncogenic HPV can integrate into the human genome, ramping up viral replication

and subsequent transformation of normal cells into tumor cells.[3] The ability of the *E7* gene product to hyperphosphorylate the retinoblastoma protein (pRb), resulting in simultaneous activation of the E2F transcription factor and the effect of E6 on p53 degradation is well studied and implicated in the proliferation and immortalization of cervical cells.[3–5] It is understandable that E6 and E7 remain viral-specific diagnostic and therapeutic targets for CIN3, CIS, and invasive cancer.

HPV detection via CLIA (Clinical Laboratory Improvement Amendments)-approved molecular assays such as hybrid capture is the prototype of a successful molecular marker and is now used widely in clinical practice. Identification of oncogenic HPV in association with other clinical endpoints triages the risk of clinically relevant cervical disease. For example, results from the ASCUS–LSIL Triage Study (ALTS) and other clinical trials have established the utility of reflex HPV testing to determine the risk of prevalent high-grade dysplasia in women who have an ASCUS

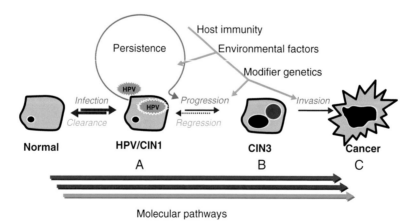

Figure 18.2 The stepwise progression from a normal phenotype to cancer involves the collaboration of several factors. For most early infections, viral clearance returns the cell to its normal constitution. With persistent infection, there must be a series of molecular alterations to achieve a malignant phenotype; this process may be influenced by a myriad of factors and cofactors (see text). The end-product, not uncommonly following several years, is an invasive process – cancer – if regression and/or clearance is not realized.

Table 18.1 Genetic alterations in cervical cancer

Genetic alterations	Mechanism	Function
Overexpression of HPV E6 and E7 oncoproteins	Integration into host genome	Cell cycle deregulation; inhibition of apoptosis
Chromosomal aberrations	Regional gains and, losses and global aneuploidy	Loss or gain of gene function
Epigenetic modification	Aberrant methylation	Loss of gene function

(atypical squamous cells of undetermined significance) Pap smear.[6–9] HPV testing in combination with cytology in women over age 30 carries a high negative predictive value and is an approved strategy for cervical cancer screening in this population.[10] Correlations with disease prevalence and HPV viral load have not been reproducible.[11–14] Recent studies have targeted the development of type-specific HPV identification, particularly HPV-16 and -18, as additional means of triaging the risk of high-grade cervical neoplasia.[15–18] The established expertise in these clinical trial designs to evaluate the molecular marker HPV alone and in combination with cervical cytology sets the groundwork for the validation of other putative biomarkers. The following sections of this chapter will address some of the other non-HPV prognostic and predictive biomarker developments.

Despite a great depth of knowledge regarding the life cycle of the common oncogenic HPV viruses and their effect on normal cellular machinery, targeted HPV therapeutic interventions aimed at eradicating active infection or preinvasive disease have been disappointing. There has been recent optimism, however, with regard to vaccines targeting E6/E7 due to preliminary phase II trials of three different E6/E7 vaccine approaches to the treatment of CIN2/3.[19] Based on the design and inherent baseline regression rate of these lesions, large phase III randomized trials will be needed to confirm the efficacy of such approaches. The greatest advance to date has been the success of the preventive vaccine, which utilizes a viral-like capsid composed of the HPV L1 viral protein as an inducer of high levels of neutralizing antibodies that have nearly 100% prevention of type-specific HPV infection.[20] Successful clinical trials have supported the recent recommendation by its US Food and Drug Administration (FDA) for vaccine use in women 9–26 years of age.[21–23]

Oncogenic HPV E6 and/or E7 have evolved as the key molecular targets for treatment of invasive cervical cancer. Strategies to inhibit E6/E7 such as antisense, ribozymes, and RNA interference can significantly decrease established cervical cancer growth both in vitro and in vivo, suggesting an effective method of disease control.[24,25] Inhibition of HPV E6 and E7 augments cisplatin activity in cervical cancer cells, probably secondary to the increase in p53 levels leading to increased apoptosis when radiotherapy was combined with *TP53* gene transfection.[26] The oncoproteins E6 and E7 continue to be expressed during later stages of disease, and are the primary targets of therapeutic vaccines designed to treat invasive cervical cancer. The goal of such therapeutic HPV vaccines is to prompt cell-mediated immunity, since antibodies cannot reach and eliminate the virus once it has been incorporated into host cells. Clinical trials are in early phase I and II development.[27] The Gynecologic Oncology Group (GOG) trial using antigen-presenting cell (APC) pulsed vaccination with synthetic E6 and E7 peptides with granulocyte–macrophage colony-stimulating factor (GM-CSF) stimulation is not yet mature, but will report on specific immunologic endpoints.

CHROMOSOMAL ABERRATIONS

Chromosomal instability is a hallmark of carcinogenesis, leading to regional gains and losses and to global aneuploidy. Although the actual mechanisms responsible for these DNA replication or migration errors are not well understood, the physical identification of common disrupted regions can be applied to diagnosis and prognosis in cervical preinvasive disease. Comparative genomic hybridization (CGH) has identified regional loss of 2q, 3p, 11q, 13q, 6q, and 4p, and gains of 3q, 5q, 15q, and 5p.[28–30] Gain of 3q is reported to be a switchpoint for CIS progression to invasive cancer.[31] In situ hybridization techniques can be performed on liquid-based cytology, which can survey both HPV activity and targeted chromosomal aberrations, which would have the greatest clinical application.[32] One such study shows that DNA ploidy analysis has comparative sensitivity, specificity, and positive and negative predictive value to cervical cytology and HPV by the Hybrid Capture 2 (HC2) test.[33] A large effort is underway to develop and validate assays that successfully define panels of lost or duplicated chromosomal regions that diagnose high-grade lesions and predict which lesions have the greatest risk for rapid progression to invasive cancer.

The frequency and average number of genetic alterations corresponded directly to the extent to which the cervical carcinoma had progressed. The most frequent heterogeneous aberrations reported are loss of 4p14–q25, and gain of 2p22, 11qcen–q13, and 8q, suggesting that these events are integral to the progression of cervical cancer at a later stage correlating with poorer prognosis. Many of the heterogeneous regions contain genes that have been correlated with the prognosis of cervical cancer, such as 7p (*EGFR*), 8q (*MYC*), 11qcen–q13 (*CCND1*), and 17q (*ERBB2*).[34] The emergence of these chromosomal aberrations may give rise to treatment-resistant subpopulations responsible for the poor prognosis of certain cervical cancers. In addition, identifying the target genes within the regions of gain and loss will direct targeted therapeutics in treating primary or recurrent disease.

CELL CYCLE CONTROL AND APOPTOSIS

Abrogation of the homeostatic balance between cell senescence, mitosis, and programmed cell death (apoptosis) results in heightened cell turnover and accumulation of additional genetic changes leading to invasive cancer (Table 18.2). The major checkpoint regulator, pRb, is inactivated early by oncogenic HPV E7, and therefore fails as a good biomarker of progression. Other immediate cell cycle-regulating proteins such as cyclin D1 and p16[INK4A] have better predictive utility. Decreased or lost protein expression of cyclin D1 is seen in most CINs. In contrast, immunohistochemical analyses reveal that a significant proportion of invasive cancers of the cervix overexpress cyclin D1 and may be associated with the downstream effect of the HPV oncoproteins E6 and E7.[35,36] Accordingly, overexpression of cyclin D1 in cervical cancers has been shown to confer poorer disease-free and overall survival, indicating that anti-cyclin D1 therapy may be highly specific in the treatment

Table 18.2 Molecular predictors in cervical cancer

Molecular predictors	Function	Expression and impact on prognosis
Cyclin D1 (*CCND1*)	Cell cycle regulation	Decreased expression in CIN. Increased expression in cancers
p16[INK4A](*CDKN2A*)	Cell cycle regulation	Overexpressed in dysplasias and cervical cancers
PTEN	Candidate tumor suppressor gene	Epigenetic changes and loss of gene expression in cervical cancers
		Gene mutations indicative of advanced-stage disease
cIAP1 (*BIRC2*)	Suppression of apoptosis	Overexpression in cancer cells is an independent predictor of disease-free survival
COX-2	Induces cyclooxygenase activity	Overexpressed in CIN3
		Overexpression in cancers is associated with decreased overall survival
EGFR	Tyrosine kinase receptor	Overexpression is associated with lower disease-free survival when associated with overexpression with COX-2
HLA	HLA*A201, -B7 and -DQB1*0302	Altered host immune response

of all human cancers expressing high-risk HPV subtypes.[36] The p16[INK4A] cyclin-dependent kinase inhibitor (encoded by the *CDKN2A* gene) is the most advanced non-HPV molecular biomarker for the detection of clinically relevant dysplasia. Overexpression of p16[INK4A] results as a compensatory response to persistent increasing HPV E7 expression. Diffuse immunohistochemical staining for p16[INK4A] in paraffin-embedded cervical tissues selected from the Guanacaste Project demonstrated a sensitivity and specificity of 100% and 95%, respectively, for detection of CIN3.[37] Subsequent studies have successfully applied this immunohistochemical technique to liquid-based cytology.[38,39] Interestingly, other molecular markers can mimic the same patterns of overexpression of p16[INK4A], such as the heat-shock proteins HSP40 and HSP70.[40] Larger well-controlled studies are needed to validate this and other potential markers as predictors of CIN3, either alone or in a triage strategy with cytology and/or HPV.

PTEN (*MMAC/TEP*), a candidate tumor suppressor gene located at chromosome 10q23.3, is found to be abnormally expressed in cervical cancer. *PTEN* has important roles in controlling cell growth, inducing cell cycle arrest, promoting apoptosis, and downregulating adhesion and cell migration. Epigenetic changes, including promoter methylation of *PTEN*, has corresponded to loss of gene expression in cervical cancer. Losses of *PTEN* expression are early events in cervical cancer development, and have also been correlated with poor disease-free and overall survival in patients with cervical cancer.[41,42] In addition, *PTEN* gene mutation rate also increases with tumor progression. Mutations within the *PTEN* gene, detected by polymerase chain reaction (PCR)-based assay, single-strand conformation polymorphism (SSCP), and direct sequencing are significantly increased in patients with advanced-stage disease compared with early-stage.[42] Targeting *PTEN* in advanced disease may have a positive impact on treatment outcome.

Overexpression of the *BIRC2* gene (encoding cIAP1) has been implicated in the prognosis of cervical squamous cell carcinomas.[43] Among several molecules implicated in the deregulation of apoptosis in cancer cells, cIAP1 is thought to be one of the more important contributors to carcinogenesis. Suppression of apoptosis is believed to contribute to tumorigenesis by abnormally prolonging cellular lifespan, enhancing growth factor-dependent cell survival, developing resistance to immunobased cytotoxicity, and allowing cells to miss cell cycle checkpoints that would normally induce apoptosis.[44] cIAP1 has been shown to be overexpressed in cervical cancer cell lines, and cell lines overexpressing cIAP1 are resistant to radiation-induced cell death.[43] Immunohistochemical analysis of primary squamous carcinomas of the cervix from patients treated only with radiotherapy has demonstrated that both overall and local recurrence-free survival were significantly poorer among patients with tumors showing high levels of nuclear cIAP1 staining than among patients whose tumors revealed little or no nuclear cIAP1. Multivariate analysis showed nuclear cIAP1 staining to be an independent predictive factor for local recurrence-free survival after radiotherapy among patients with cervical squamous carcinoma.

SIGNAL TRANSDUCTION PATHWAYS

Genes involved in several complex signal transduction pathways are of great clinical interest, as there are several drug targets to interfere with receptor-based signaling. For example, overexpression of epidermal growth factor receptor (EGFR), a tyrosine kinase receptor, has frequently been observed in cervical cancers and correlates with poor prognosis. Multivariate analyses have revealed that overexpression of EGFR as measured by enzyme-linked immunosorbent assay (ELISA) provides prognostic information with respect to disease-free and overall survival.[45] Knowledge of these prognostic factors leads to specific drug targets with growth factor inhibitors such as cetuximab, bevacizumab, and lapatinib. Patients with positive immunoreactivity for both EGFR and cyclooxygenase-2 (COX-2) and advanced-stage cervical cancer also have a higher likelihood of locoregional recurrence than those with either EGFR or COX-2 overexpression alone.[45] Preliminary data suggest that elevated COX-2 expression is mediated by an activated EGFR, which causes downstream signaling to induce COX-2 promoter activation.[46] Overexpression of COX-2 alone as determined by immunohistochemical analysis has also been associated in more adenocarcinomas than in squamous carcinomas, with decreased overall survival.[47] In addition, COX-2 staining intensity correlates positively with tumor size. COX-2 overexpression has been found in CIN3 lesions, thus making it an attractive target for chemoprevention trials with COX-2 inhibitors.[48,49] Such a phase II trial is ongoing within the Gynecologic Oncology Group.

Angiogenic markers have recently become popular targets in the context of various solid tumors. In support of this concept, a large number of in vitro and in vivo studies have demonstrated aberrant expression of microvessel density (MVD) and vascular endothelial growth factor (VEGF) in preinvasive and invasive cervical cancer. Clinically, increased MVD is seen in colposcopic progression from punctation to mosaic patterns in progressive dysplastic lesions. MVD is significantly increased in intratumoral cervix and peritumoral cervix in comparison with benign cervix.[50] A mono-clonal anti-CD34 antibody with reactivity for tumor-associated microvessels is associated with poorer prognosis.[51] Both lymphatic invasion and peritumoral neoangiogenesis have been correlated with high expression of the vascular endothelial growth factor (VEGF) C isoform. VEGF-A splicing variants were increased in malignant compared with normal cervical samples, but were not associated with the invasive activity of the cells. Although over-expression of VEGF isoforms alone does not correlate with cervical cancer prognosis, their contribution to the malignant and invasive process of cervical cancer make them attractive molecular targets.[52]

EPIGENETIC MODIFICATIONS

Epigenetic modifications are common in cervical cancer and are means of deregulating genes and pathways in cervical carcinogenesis. Aberrant methylation is one of the most actively studied for clinical utility. Although cervical cancer undergoes global hypomethylation, key gene promoter regions undergo hypermethylation, thus resulting in predominantly tumor suppressor gene silencing. The mechanism of promoter methylation is not well understood; however, some genes seem to be targets of certain carcinogens – such as with methylation of CDKN2A and tobacco exposure.[53] Methylation of some genes may be associated with HPV infection early in the process and therefore not predictive of any relevant disease.[54] Wide variations in targeted genes exist; therefore, panels of predictive genes are under active investigation. Several promising panels have been described using as few as 3 genes to ≥11 genes as the predictive panel.[40,53–55] One study has reported high specificity and sensitivity.[55] Large validation

trials will be necessary to validate the assays for clinical utility.

MODIFIER GENETICS AND ENVIRONMENT

The interaction with the underlying somatic cell (cervical cell) genetics and its local environment, compounded by host immunity, all interact to modify disease risk. No single gene overexpression or loss or abrogated pathway will definitely correlate with invasive cancer. However, gene–environment interactions still play an important role in the progression of cancer and can serve as additional predictive markers. Perhaps the most debated in the literature is the role of the TP53 codon 72 polymorphism as a biomarker of cancer risk as first described by Storey et al,[56] which demonstrated associated functional gene consequence. Although this is still controversial and subject to study design flaws, a meta-analysis found no correlation in cervical dysplasia and a possible weak association in specific invasive cancers.[57] Host response to the initiating HPV infection and prediction of persistent infection is associated with host human leukocyte antigen (HLA) type; therefore, studies have assessed HLA typing as a biomarker for HPV persistence leading to CIN3. In one study, the HLA*A201 allele was predictive of CIN2/3 regression in non-HPV-16 infections.[58] Alternatively, in a nested case–control study using the well-characterized Portland Kaiser Permanente cohort, HLA-B7 and -DQB1*0302 alleles were confirmed to be associated with cervical neoplasia.[59]

SUMMARY

The molecular events that occur within a normal cervical cell concerning HPV infection with subsequent development of cervical dysplasia are confounded by heterogeneity driven by the field carcinogenesis theory. Subpopulations bearing an increasing number of aberrations successively emerge, leading to increasing genetic heterogeneity within the tissue. This heterogeneity is a major challenge in using molecular markers as predictors and prognosticators of disease. Markers in study samples may not represent all tumors present. Markers used as treatment guides may not predict treatment success, since different subpopulations may have different capacities for growth, differentiation, and metastasis, as well as sensitivity to radiation and chemotherapeutic agents. Evolution of technology and better tumor sampling will provide increasingly useful biomarker information for translational application.

REFERENCES

1. Bosch FX, de Sanjose S. Chapter 1: Human papillomavirus and cervical cancer – burden and assessment of causality. J Natl Cancer Inst Monogr 2003:3–13.

2. Schiffman MH, Castle P. Epidemiologic studies of a necessary causal risk factor: human papillomavirus infection and cervical neoplasia. J Natl Cancer Inst 2003;95:2.

3. Mantovani F, Banks L. The human papillomavirus E6 protein and its contribution to malignant progression. Oncogene 2001;20: 7874–87.

4. Munger K, Basile JR, Duensing S, et al. Biological activities and molecular targets of the human papillomavirus E7 oncoprotein. Oncogene 2001;20:7888–98.

5. Jones DL, Thompson DA, Munger K. Destabilization of the RB tumor suppressor protein and stabilization of p53 contribute to HPV type 16 E7-induced apoptosis. Virology 1997;239:97–107.

6. The Atypical Squamous Cells of Undetermined Significance/Low-Grade Squamous Intraepithelial Lesions Triage Study (ALTS) Group. Human papillomavirus testing for triage of women with cytologic evidence of low-grade squamous intraepithelial lesions: baseline data from a randomized trial. J Natl Cancer Inst 2000; 92:397–402.

7. Kiatpongsan S, Niruthisard S, Mutirangura A, et al. Role of human papillomavirus DNA testing in management of women with atypical squamous cells of undetermined significance. Int J Gynecol Cancer 2006; 16:262–5.

8. Kulasingam SL, Kim JJ, Lawrence WF, et al. Cost-effectiveness analysis based on the Atypical Squamous Cells of Undetermined Significance/Low-Grade Squamous Intraepithelial Lesion Triage Study (ALTS). J Natl Cancer Inst 2006;98:92–100.

9. Schiffman M, Castle PE. When to test women for human papillomavirus. BMJ 2006;332:61–2.

10. Sherman ME, Lorincz AT, Scott DR, et al. Baseline cytology, human papillomavirus testing, and risk for cervical neoplasia: a 10-year cohort analysis. J Natl Cancer Inst 2003; 95:46–52.

11. Castle PE, Schiffman M, Scott DR, et al. Semiquantitative human papillomavirus type 16 viral load and the prospective risk of cervical precancer and cancer. Cancer Epidemiol Biomarkers Prev 2005;14:1311–14.

12. Kovacic MB, Castle PE, Herrero R, et al. Relationships of human papillomavirus type, qualitative viral load, and age with cytologic abnormality. Cancer Res 2006;66: 10112–19.

13. Lorincz AT, Castle PE, Sherman ME, et al. Viral load of human papillomavirus and risk of CIN3 or cervical cancer. Lancet 2002; 360:228–9.

14. Sherman ME, Schiffman M, Cox JT. Effects of age and human papilloma viral load on colposcopy triage: data from the randomized Atypical Squamous Cells of Undetermined Significance/Low-Grade Squamous Intraepithelial Lesion Triage Study (ALTS). J Natl Cancer Inst 2002;94:102–17.

15. Castle PE, Sadorra M, Garcia F, et al. Pilot study of a commercialized human papillomavirus (HPV) genotyping assay: comparison of HPV risk group to cytology and histology. J Clin Microbiol 2006;44:3915–17.

16. Castle PE, Solomon D, Schiffman M, et al. Human papillomavirus type 16 infections and 2-year absolute risk of cervical precancer in women with equivocal or mild cytologic abnormalities. J Natl Cancer Inst 2005;97: 1066–71.

17. Khan MJ, Castle PE, Lorincz AT, et al. The elevated 10-year risk of cervical precancer and cancer in women with human papillomavirus (HPV) type 16 or 18 and the possible utility of type-specific HPV testing in clinical practice. J Natl Cancer Inst 2005;97:1072–9.

18. Wheeler CM, Hunt WC, Schiffman M, et al. Human papillomavirus genotypes and the cumulative 2-year risk of cervical precancer. J Infect Dis 2000;194:1291–9.

19. McNeil C. Search for HPV treatment vaccine heats up, researchers optimistic. J Natl Cancer Inst 2006;98:954–5.

20. Lowy DR, Schiller JT. Prophylactic human papillomavirus vaccines. J Clin Invest 2006; 116:1167–73.

21. Koutsky LA, Ault KA, Wheeler CM, et al. A controlled trial of a human papillomavirus type 16 vaccine. N Engl J Med 2002;347: 1645–51.

22. Mao C, Koutsky LA, Ault KA, et al. Efficacy of human papillomavirus-16 vaccine to prevent cervical intraepithelial neoplasia: a randomized controlled trial. Obstet Gynecol 2006;107:18–27.

23. Villa LL, Costa RL, Petta CA, et al. Prophylactic quadrivalent human papillomavirus (types 6, 11, 16, and 18) L1 virus-like particle vaccine in young women: a randomised double-blind placebo-controlled multicentre phase II efficacy trial. Lancet Oncol 2005;6:271–8.

24. Butz K, Ristriani T, Hengstermann A, et al. siRNA targeting of the viral E6 oncogene efficiently kills human papillomavirus-positive cancer cells. Oncogene 2003;22:5938–45.

25. Jiang M, Milner J. Selective silencing of viral gene expression in HPV-positive human cervical carcinoma cells treated with siRNA, a primer of RNA interference. Oncogene 2002; 21:6041–8.

26. Putral LN, Bywater MJ, Gu W, et al. RNA interference against human papillomavirus oncogenes in cervical cancer cells results in increased sensitivity to cisplatin. Mol Pharmacol 2005;68:1311–19.

27. Mahdavi A, Monk BJ. Vaccines against human papillomavirus and cervical cancer: promises and challenges. Oncologist 2005;10:528–38.

28. Kirchhoff M, Rose H, Petersen BL, et al. Comparative genomic hybridization reveals a recurrent pattern of chromosomal aberrations in severe dysplasia/carcinoma in situ of the cervix and in advanced-stage cervical carcinoma. Genes Chromosomes Cancer 1999;24: 144–50.

29. Rao PH, Arias-Pulido H, Lu XY, et al. Chromosomal amplifications, 3q gain and deletions of 2q33–q37 are the frequent genetic changes in cervical carcinoma. BMC Cancer 2004;4:5.

30. Allen DG, White DJ, Hutchins AM, et al. Progressive genetic aberrations detected by comparative genomic hybridization in squamous cell cervical cancer. Br J Cancer 2000; 83:1659–63.

31. Heselmeyer K, Schrock E, du Manoir S, et al. Gain of chromosome 3q defines the transition from severe dysplasia to invasive carcinoma of the uterine cervix. Proc Natl Acad Sci USA 1996;93:479–84.

32. Cheung AN, Chiu PM, Tsun KL, et al. Chromosome in situ hybridisation, Ki-67, and telomerase immunocytochemistry in liquid based cervical cytology. J Clin Pathol 2004; 57:721–7.

33. Guillaud M, Benedet JL, Cantor SB, et al. DNA ploidy compared with human papilloma virus testing (Hybrid Capture II) and conventional cervical cytology as a primary screening test for cervical high-grade lesions and cancer in 1555 patients with biopsy confirmation. Cancer 2006;107:309–18.

34. Lyng H, Beigi M, Svendsrud DH, et al. Intratumor chromosomal heterogeneity in advanced carcinomas of the uterine cervix. Int J Cancer 2004;111:358–66.

35. Al Moustafa AE, Foulkes WD, Wong A, et al. Cyclin D1 is essential for neoplastic transformation induced by both E6/E7 and E6/E7/ErbB-2 cooperation in normal cells. Oncogene 2004;23:5252–6.

36. Wisman GB, Knol AJ, Helder MN, et al. Telomerase in relation to clinicopathologic prognostic factors and survival in cervical cancer. Int J Cancer 2001;91:658–64.

37. Wang SS, Trunk M, Schiffman M, et al. Validation of p16INK4a as a marker of oncogenic human papillomavirus infection in cervical biopsies from a population-based cohort in Costa Rica. Cancer Epidemiol Biomarkers Prev 2004;13:1355–60.

38. Bose S, Evans H, Lantzy L, et al. p16INK4A is a surrogate biomarker for a subset of human papilloma virus-associated dysplasias of the uterine cervix as determined on the Pap smear. Diagn Cytopathol 2005;32:21–4.

39. Nieh S, Chen SF, Chu TY, et al. Is p16INK4A expression more useful than human papillomavirus test to determine the outcome of atypical squamous cells of undetermined significance-categorized Pap smear? A comparative analysis using abnormal cervical smears with follow-up biopsies. Gynecol Oncol 2005; 97:35–40.

40. Castle PE, Ashfaq R, Ansari F, et al. Immunohistochemical evaluation of heat shock proteins in normal and preinvasive lesions of the cervix. Cancer Lett 2005;229:245–52.

41. Cheung TH, Lo KW, Yim SF, et al. Epigenetic and genetic alternation of PTEN in cervical neoplasm. Gynecol Oncol 2004;93:621–7.

42. Lee JS, Choi YD, Lee JH, et al. Expression of PTEN in the progression of cervical neoplasia and its relation to tumor behavior and angiogenesis in invasive squamous cell carcinoma. J Surg Oncol 2006;93:233–40.

43. Imoto I, Tsuda H, Hirasawa A, et al. Expression of cIAP1, a target for 11q22 amplification, correlates with resistance of cervical cancers to radiotherapy. Cancer Res 2002;62:4860–6.

44. LaCasse EC, Baird S, Korneluk RG, et al. The inhibitors of apoptosis (IAPs) and their emerging role in cancer. Oncogene 1998;17: 3247–59.

45. Kim GE, Kim YB, Cho NH, et al. Synchronous coexpression of epidermal growth factor receptor and cyclooxygenase-2 in carcinomas of the uterine cervix: a potential predictor of poor survival. Clin Cancer Res 2004;10:1366–74.

46. Kim MH, Seo SS, Song YS, et al. Expression of cyclooxygenase-1 and -2 associated with expression of VEGF in primary cervical cancer and at metastatic lymph nodes. Gynecol Oncol 2003;90:83–90.

47. Kim YB, Kim GE, Pyo HR, et al. Differential cyclooxygenase-2 expression in squamous cell carcinoma and adenocarcinoma of the uterine cervix. Int J Radiat Oncol Biol Phys 2004; 60:822–9.

48. Gaffney DK, Haslam D, Tsodikov A, et al. Epidermal growth factor receptor (EGFR) and vascular endothelial growth factor (VEGF) negatively affect overall survival in carcinoma

of the cervix treated with radiotherapy. Int J Radiat Oncol Biol Phys 2003;56:922–8.

49. Gaffney DK, Holden J, Davis M, et al. Elevated cyclooxygenase-2 expression correlates with diminished survival in carcinoma of the cervix treated with radiotherapy. Int J Radiat Oncol Biol Phys 2001;49:1213–17.

50. Gombos Z, Xu X, Chu CS, et al. Peritumoral lymphatic vessel density and vascular endothelial growth factor C expression in early-stage squamous cell carcinoma of the uterine cervix. Clin Cancer Res 2005;11:8364–71.

51. Vieira SC, Silva BB, Pinto GA, et al. CD34 as a marker for evaluating angiogenesis in cervical cancer. Pathol Res Pract 2005;201: 313–18.

52. Bachtiary B, Selzer E, Knocke TH, et al. Serum VEGF levels in patients undergoing primary radiotherapy for cervical cancer: impact on progression-free survival. Cancer Lett 2002; 179:197–203.

53. Lea JS, Coleman R, Kurien A, et al. Aberrant p16 methylation is a biomarker for tobacco exposure in cervical squamous cell carcinogenesis. Am J Obstet Gynecol 2004;190: 674–9.

54. Virmani AK, Muller C, Rathi A, et al. Aberrant methylation during cervical carcinogenesis. Clin Cancer Res 2001;7:584–9.

55. Feng Q, Balasubramanian A, Hawes SE, et al. Detection of hypermethylated genes in women with and without cervical neoplasia. J Natl Cancer Inst 2005;97:273–82.

56. Storey A, Thomas M, Kalita A, et al. Role of a p53 polymorphism in the development of human papillomavirus-associated cancer. Nature 1998;393:229–34.

57. Koushik A, Platt RW, Franco EL. p53 codon 72 polymorphism and cervical neoplasia: a meta-analysis review. Cancer Epidemiol Biomarkers Prev 2004;13:11–22.

58. Trimble CL, Piantadosi S, Gravitt P, et al. Spontaneous regression of highgrade cervical dysplasia: effects of human papillomavirus type and HLA phenotype. Clin Cancer Res 2005; 11:4717–23.

59. Hildesheim A, Schiffman M, Scott DR, et al. Human leukocyte antigen class I/II alleles and development of human papillomavirus-related cervical neoplasia: results from a case–control study conducted in the United States. Cancer Epidemiol Biomarkers Prev 1998;7:1035–41.

Virology in the prevention and management of cervical cancer

19

Jason D Wright

INTRODUCTION

Since the introduction of cervical cancer screening with the Pap smear, the incidence of cervical cancer has decreased dramatically. Despite these advances, cervical cancer remains an important cause of morbidity and mortality in women. In 2005, it was estimated that over 490 000 new cases of cervical cancer would be diagnosed worldwide.[1] The importance of human papillomavirus (HPV) in the pathogenesis of cervical cancer is now well recognized.[2] The necessity for HPV in the development of cervical cancer provides an optimal target for diagnostic testing as well as an important target for vaccines and other interventions aimed at reducing the burden of cervical cancer in women.

VIROLOGY OF HUMAN PAPILLOMAVIRUS

HPVs are small, nonenveloped double-stranded DNA tumor viruses. The viruses were first demonstrated in condyloma accuminata, while later experiments elucidated the association between HPV and cervical cancer.[3,4] To date, more than 200 HPV types been characterized and described.[5] The papillomaviruses are classified based upon the DNA sequence homology and their biologic properties. New HPV types must have a gene sequence that differs by at least 10% from other known types.[5] Based upon their disease association, the genital tract HPVs have been categorized into low-risk and high-risk groups (Table 19.1). The low-risk viruses are the causative agents of condyloma accuminata. The prototypic low-risk viruses are HPV-6 and HPV-11. In contrast, the high-risk viruses cause cervical dysplasia and cervical cancer. High-risk viral types include HPV-16, -18, -31, -33, -35, -39, -45, -51, -52, -56, -58, -59, -68, -73, and -82.[6] Among the high-risk viruses documented in squamous intraepithelial lesions (SIL) and cervical cancer, HPV-16 and HPV-18 are the most frequently isolated. In a pooled analysis of 1918 women with squamous cell carcinomas, the overall prevalence of HPV-16 was 59%, while HPV-18 was detected in 15% of the tumors. The odds ratio for cervical cancer based on the presence of HPV DNA is 158.[6] While HPV-16 appears to be the most common viral type in most countries, worldwide distribution studies have suggested that non-European populations have a higher relative infection rate with HPV types other than HPV-16.[7]

Table 19.1 Human papillomavirus (HPV) classification

Classification	Viral types
Low-risk	6, 11, 40, 42, 43, 44, 54, 61, 70, 72, 81, CP6108
High-risk	16[a], 18[a], 31[a], 33[a], 35[a], 39[a], 45[a], 51[a], 52[a], 56[a], 58[a], 59[a], 68[a], 73, 82

[a]Included in Hybrid Capture 2 (HC 2) high-risk probe cocktail.

The HPV genome consists of a circular DNA molecule of approximately 8000 bp. The genome is divided functionally into two open reading frames (ORFs): an early (E) and a late (L) region (Figure 19.1). The early region encodes the nonstructural protein responsible for viral replication and transformation, while the late region encodes the two major viral capsid proteins, L1 and L2. In addition, the HPV genome contains a noncoding region referred to as the long control region (LCR) that contains elements that regulate viral replication. The E1 and E2 proteins both function in viral replication. E2 functions as a transcription factor and has the ability to both activate and repress gene expression.[3,8] An important function of intact E2 is transcriptional repression of the E6 and E7 oncoproteins. As described below, viral integration often results in disruption of E2 and consequent increased transcriptional activity of E6 and E7.[9] E4 produces intermediate filaments that localize with cytokeratin. E4 may play a role in disruption of the normal cellular matrix. E5 appears to play a minor role in viral transformation. The E5 protein associates with the cell membrane and enhances growth factor-mediated signal transduction from epidermal growth factor (EGF) and platelet-derived growth factor (PDGF) receptors.[10] The major transforming properties of HPV are attributed to the E6 and E7 proteins. E7 is a 100-amino-acid protein that interacts with and inactivates the retinoblastoma tumor suppressor protein (pRb). A conserved region within the C-terminus of E7 is responsible for interaction with pRb. Variations in this region of E7 are in part responsible for differences in the oncogenic potential of various HPV types. E7 from high-risk HPV types interacts with pRb with more affinity than E7 proteins encoded by the low-risk viruses.[11] In addition to pRb, E7 targets the related cellular tumor suppressors p107 and p130. E6 is a 150-amino-acid protein. It complexes with the cellular protein E6-activating protein (E6-AP). The E6/E6-AP complex then targets p53 for ubiquitination and ultimately proteosomal degradation. In addition to inactivation of p53, E6 induces transcription of the catalytic subunit of telomerase, hTERT. Activation of hTERT prevents telomere shortening and contributes to cellular immortalization.[12] Finally, emerging evidence suggests that E6 and E7

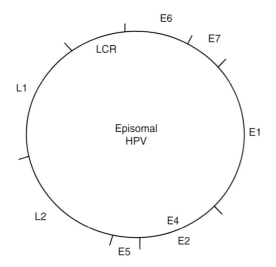

Figure 19.1 HPV viral genome. The early (E) genes encode proteins for viral replication while the late (L) genes encode the viral capsid proteins. The long control region (LCR) is a segment of regulatory DNA.

contribute to genomic instability. In conjunction, the oncoproteins induce centrosomal abnormalities that lead to mitotic defects and chromosomal abnormalities.[3]

Despite the transforming capabilities of HPV, the normal viral life cycle is tightly regulated. HPV is highly epitheliotrophic and only infects epithelial cells of the skin, oral and genital tracts, and anus. HPV infects the basal keratinocytes of the squamous epithelium. The basal keratinocytes represent the only replicating cell population within normal squamous epithelium. The viral DNA is initially maintained in episomal form within the nucleus at a relatively low copy number. As the squamous cells undergo terminal differentiation and traverse toward the cell surface, the latent virus begins to increase its copy number and expression of the L1 and L2 capsid proteins begins. The viral particles are then packaged into mature virions and shed as the epithelial cells desquamate.[13] A sentinel event in viral transformation is the integration of the viral genome into the host cell's chromosomal complement (Figure 19.2). Integration of the HPV genome can occur anywhere in the cellular genome. While there do not appear to be any hotspots for integration, HPV does preferentially integrate into fragile sites – genomic regions that are prone to chromosomal breaks that facilitate the insertion of DNA.[9] A comprehensive review of genomic integration sites

was unable to demonstrate a role for insertional mutagenesis (disruption of cellular genes) in the pathogenesis of HPV infection.[9] Viral insertion usually results in disruption of the E2 ORF, which allows increased expression of E6 and E7. While E6 and E7 immortalize infected cells, the oncoproteins alone are not tumorigenic. Additional genetic events such as *RAS* expression are required for malignant progression.[14]

Cervical carcinogenic progression is dependent on the presence and persistence of HPV. The incidence of HPV positivity increases with progressive dysplasia. The transition to invasive cervical cancer is a gradual process that takes years from the time of initial HPV infection. Careful analysis has revealed that >99% of invasive cervical tumors are positive for HPV.[2] Progression from dysplasia to cancer is facilitated by other environmental and molecular cofactors (Figure 19.3). Dysplastic lesions in which the HPV genome has integrated into the host chromosome appear to be a critical factor for the development of high-grade dysplasia.[15] The long preinvasive phase of cervical dysplasia provides an ideal opportunity for cancer screening and intervention prior to the development of cervical cancer. The near-universal association between cervical cancer and HPV provides an ideal target for molecular diagnostic testing to aid in prognostication and treatment planning.

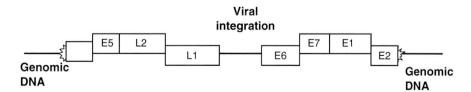

Figure 19.2 Integration of HPV in to the host cellular DNA. The upper panel depicts HPV in episomal form while the lower displays the integrated viral genome.

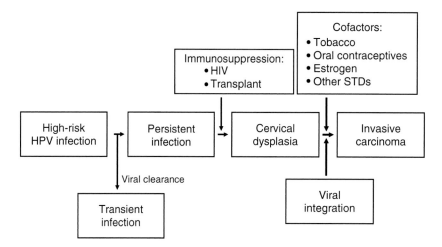

Figure 19.3 Model of multistage cervical carcinogenesis.

VIRAL FACTORS IN THE MANAGEMENT OF CERVICAL DYSPLASIA

Qualitative HPV testing

Methods for HPV detection

A number of methodologies have been evaluated for the detection and quantitation of HPV. Given that serologic tests are unreliable and HPV culture is technically challenging, currently available assays for HPV rely upon direct detection of the HPV genome. The two most commonly utilized modalities are Hybrid Capture 2 (HC 2; Digene Diagnostics, Gaithersburg, MD) and the polymerase chain reaction (PCR).

HC 2 is a commercially available assay that relies on the detection of HPV DNA-RNA hybrids. It was originally approved by the US Food and Drug Administration (FDA) in 1999. HC 2 requires collection of a sample of cervical cells. The cells are then lysed in solution and the HPV DNA is denatured. The DNA is then mixed with an RNA probe cocktail.

The high-risk probe cocktail detects HPV -16, -18, -31, -33, -35, -39, -45, -51, -52, -56, -58, -59, and -68 while the low-risk probe cocktail detects HPV, -6, -11, -42, -43, and -44. There is currently little clinical utility for the low-risk probe set. After the RNA probe cocktail has been added, HPV DNA–RNA hybrids form. These hybrids are then immobilized by antibodies bound to the microplate wells. Anti-hybrid antibodies conjugated with alkaline phosphatase are then added. Finally, the well is washed with substrate that produces a chemoluminescent reaction that can be detected. The reaction intensity is measured in relative light units (RLU) and is semiquantitative. The currently recommended threshold for a positive test is 1.0 RLU, which corresponds to approximately 1 pg of viral DNA.[16,17] HPV typing cannot be performed with HC 2.

While not currently in commercial use, PCR-based assays are the most sensitive modality for the detection of HPV. PCR can detect as few as 10 copies of the HPV genome.[16] A sample of cervical cells is collected and heated to allow DNA strand separation.

Oligonucleotide primers that hybridize to complementary DNA strands are then added. A thermostabile DNA polymerase is added, and allows replication of the DNA segments defined by the primers. The sequence is repeated for several cycles to allow exponential expansion of the original DNA. The PCR products are then analyzed by gel electrophoresis or enzyme-linked immunosorbent assay (ELISA). DNA sequencing or type-specific hybridization may be performed to elucidate the specific HPV type.[18] The most commonly utilized PCR primers target the highly conserved *L1* region of the viral genome. The PGMY09/11 primers amplify an approximately 450 bp region. These primers contain a pool of nucleotides that recognize a number of HPV types.[19] The GP5+/6+ primer amplifies a 150 bp region, and has been utilized in a number of epidemiologic studies.[20]

Primary screening

Over the past decade, HPV testing has been evaluated in several settings, including primary screening for cervical dysplasia and cancer, the triage of abnormal cervical cytology, and post-procedure follow-up after treatment for cervical dysplasia.

The goal of primary screening is to detect cervical cancer and its precursor lesions in asymptomatic women. Strategies that rely on HPV testing as a screening modality are particularly appealing in developing countries, where high-quality cytology laboratories are rare and where the cost of the evaluation and follow-up of cervical cytologic screening is prohibitive.[21] A number of studies have been performed that have compared HPV testing with traditional cervical cytology as a screening test. These studies have been performed in a number of different populations in both developed and

developing countries.[22–24] Compared with cytology, HPV testing has a higher sensitivity but a lower specificity. In a review of 13 published studies on the use of HPV testing as primary screening, the sensitivity of HPV testing was 27% higher than that of cytology, while its specificity was 8% lower than that of cytology.[22] The average sensitivity for HPV testing was 85% compared with 60% for cytology, while the mean specificity was 84% for HPV testing, versus 95% for cytology.[22] In addition to a high sensitivity, HPV testing is consistently associated with a high negative predictive value.[22]

Despite the encouraging performance of HPV testing as a primary screening tool, implementation of this strategy would result in the referral of a large number of women with no underlying cervical abnormalities. To overcome this limitation, programs that focus on women at higher risk have been examined. Transient HPV infections are common in young women. These infections are typically short-lived and often associated with no or only mild cytologic changes.[25] The rate of HPV positivity consistently declines with age. In one study, the prevalence of HPV was 36% in women under the age of 25, compared with 3% in women older than 45.[26] A positive HPV test in women over the age of 30 is more likely to be associated with underlying pathology than a similar test in younger women. Current HPV screening strategies in the US focus on implementing HPV testing in women over the age of 30.[27,28] In the meta-analysis described above, the sensitivity of HPV testing improved to 89% and the specificity to 90% when the analysis was limited to women over age 30.[22]

Currently available consensus guidelines for HPV testing are displayed in Table 19.2. It is recommended that if HPV testing is utilized for primary screening, it should be combined with cytology.[27–29] Women with negative

Table 19.2 Screening guidelines incorporating HPV testing

Organization	Guideline
American Cancer Society (ACS)	Reasonable to consider cytology in combination with HPV testing in women aged 30 and over. The frequency of combined screening should not be more than every 3 years
American College of Obstetricians and Gynecologists (ACOG)	Combined screening with cytology and HPV testing in women aged 30 years and older. Any women who receives negative test results on both should not be rescreened more frequently than every 3 years

cytology and a negative HPV test are at extremely low risk for high-grade cervical disease and should not be rescreened for 3 years.[27,28,30] In a cohort of >20 000 HPV- and cytology-negative subjects, the incidence of cervical intraepithelial neoplasia (CIN) 3 or cancer was < 0.5% over a 45-month follow-up period.[31] Among women who are HPV-positive with negative cytology, the incidence of underlying high-grade disease is low; however, these patients are at increased risk for the development of cervical dysplasia.[32] Approximately 15% of these women will develop a cytologic abnormality within 5 years.[32] Based upon the reliability of HPV testing, alternative, sequential testing approaches have been proposed.[23] In this schema, HPV testing alone would serve as primary screening, and those women with a positive HPV test would be further evaluated with cytology.[23,33]

Evaluation of cytologic abnormalities

HPV testing is highly predictive for the detection of high-grade cervical lesions and has now been incorporated into management schemas for the evaluation of cytologic abnormalities. HPV DNA testing is currently the preferred management strategy for women with a cytologic diagnosis of atypical squamous cells of undetermined significance (ASCUS).[34–37]

The ASCUS–LSIL Triage Study (ALTS) compared three management strategies for women with ASCUS and low-grade squamous intraepithelial lesions (LSIL): repeat cytology, HPV testing with HC 2, and immediate colposcopy.[34,38] For the management of ASCUS, HPV testing had a sensitivity of 96% and required colposcopy for a positive test in 56% of women. Cytology had a sensitivity of 85% when women with a repeat sample of ASCUS or greater were referred for colposcopic examination. This strategy required referral of 59% of subjects for colposcopy.[34] In a meta-analysis of 15 studies comparing HPV testing and cytology for the management of ASCUS, the performance of HPV testing was superior to that of repeat cytology. The sensitivity and specificity of HC 2 for the detection of CIN2 or greater were 95% and 67%, respectively. In contrast, repeat cytology with referral to colposcopy for any repeat sample that revealed ASCUS or greater had a sensitivity of 82% and specificity of 58% for the detection of CIN2 or greater.[35] While HPV DNA testing has a high sensitivity for the detection of high-grade cervical disease, it should be noted that only 15–25% of HPV-positive women with ASCUS who undergo colposcopy will have underlying CIN2 or worse.[16,34] Based upon these findings, reflex HPV testing is currently the recommended strategy for the evaluation of ASCUS cytology.[29]

Despite the utility of HPV DNA testing for the management of ASCUS, such a strategy has not found utility for the management of LSIL. In the National Cancer Institute (NCI)-sponsored LSIL arm of the ALTS trial, 83% of women with a cytologic diagnosis of LSIL were HPV-positive. The high incidence of HPV in this cohort limits the utility and cost–effectiveness of HPV testing.[38] The current recommendation for the management of women with LSIL is immediate colposcopy.[29]

Post-cervical-excision surveillance

HPV testing has been proposed as a post-treatment management strategy for women who undergo cervical excision or ablation for cervical dysplasia.[16,39,40] Up to 50% of women will develop persistent or recurrent dysplasia, and treated women remain at elevated risk for the development of invasive cervical cancer.[41] Women who test positive for HPV after treatment would be expected to be at higher risk for persistent or recurrent dysplasia, while the risk of persistent disease should be negligible in those who test negative. In a meta-analysis of 11 studies that included 900 women, post-treatment HPV testing appeared to be useful. Among women in whom treatment was considered successful, the post-treatment HPV test was negative in 84% and positive in 16%. In contrast, among the treatment failures, the post-procedure HPV test was negative in only 17% and positive in 83%. The sensitivity of HPV testing varied in the studies reviewed. Four studies reported a sensitivity of 100%, while two studies reported sensitivities of 47–67%. Specificity ranged from 44% to 95%.[39] Clearly, further study is required, but post-treatment HPV positivity may be predictive of women at high risk for treatment failure and subsequent recurrent/persistent dysplasia.

Quantitative HPV testing

It is recognized that viral persistence is a requisite for the development and progression of cervical neoplasia.[42] Given the importance of viral persistence, identifying women with a high HPV viral burden may allow for the identification of a subset of patients at high risk for the development of high-grade cervical dysplasia. Several studies have evaluated the influence of HPV viral load on the progression of cervical neoplasia, with conflicting results.[43-45] In one of the largest studies, investigators performed a nested case–control study of 478 women with carcinoma in situ (CIS) and 608 controls. Quantitative real-time PCR was performed on nearly 4000 previously collected cytologic samples. The median HPV-16 viral load was significantly higher at all time points in the CIS cases. For women with a high viral load the probability of developing CIS was 23%, compared with 7% in women with a low viral load.[44] Other investigators have not confirmed the utility of HPV viral load assessment. In an evaluation of the ALTS data, HPV viral load varied greatly among cases of CIN3. Viral load appeared to correlate with the extent of surrounding dysplasia (CIN1), then with the number of HPV types and the number of ASCUS and LSIL cells present in the sample. These findings were based upon semiquantitative data provided by HC 2.[43] Currently, quantitative HPV viral load testing is not routinely employed in clinical practice. While theoretically appealing, technical issues will require standardization prior to widespread implementation.

HPV typing

Interest has emerged in further quantitating the risk of high-grade cervical disease based upon the specific viral type present. HC 2, which remains the standard diagnostic test in clinical practice, merely distinguishes whether one of 13 high-risk viral types is present. Certain viral types such as HPV-16 and HPV-18 are associated with a higher risk of carcinogenic progression.[6] This concept was demonstrated in a report describing 20 810 women in whom HPV testing with HC 2 was performed as a screening test. Women who tested positive with HC 2 underwent specific testing for HPV-16 and HPV-18. After 10 years of follow-up, the rate of CIN3 or greater was 17% in the HPV-16 positive group, 14% in the HPV-18-positive, group, only 3% in the HC 2-positive/HPV-16- and HPV-18-negative group, and 0.8% in the HC 2-negative group. Based on these findings, it would appear that women with HPV-16 or -18 are at a much higher risk for ultimately developing CIN3 or cancer.[46] A similar experimental design was performed on women with ASCUS and LSIL cytology. For subjects with ASCUS, who were HPV-16-positive, the 2-year risk of CIN3 or greater was 33%, compared with 8% for ASCUS with other HPV types. For women with LSIL with HPV-16, the 2-year CIN3-positivity risk was 39%, compared with 10% for subjects with other HPV types.[47] While these findings require validation, the results suggest that future HPV screening and triage strategies may focus on the detection of those women at highest risk (HPV-16- or HPV-18-positive).

VIRAL FACTORS IN THE MANAGEMENT OF INVASIVE CERVICAL CANCER

HPV typing

HPV is now accepted as the major etiologic agent of cervical cancer. The majority of invasive cervical tumors harbor HPV DNA.[2] Several investigations have indicated that HPV genotype influences tumor progression and outcome. A number of studies have now documented that HPV-18 is associated with particularly aggressive cervical carcinomas.[48-50] Early reports were unable to demonstrate a survival difference for women with HPV-18-containing neoplasms.[51,52] These early reports often included small sample sizes and failed to account for other known prognostic factors. More recent data have consistently shown that HPV-18 has an important impact on outcome. HPV-18 is associated with tumors in younger women and is more commonly associated with adenocarcinomas.[48,50,53,54] It has been associated with other pathologic risk factors, including lymph node metastasis and deep stromal invasion.[50] Most importantly, the presence of HPV-18 increases the risk of disease recurrence and is associated with decreased overall and cervical cancer-specific survival.[48-50,53,54] In a large population-based study, the hazard ratio for death from cervical cancer in women with HPV-18-containing tumors was 2.5.[49] The effect of HPV-18 on survival appears to be strongest for women with early-stage disease.[48-50] In one report, HPV-45, an HPV type closely related phylogenetically to HPV-18, conveyed the same impact on survival as HPV-18.[48] While not currently a part of standard clinical care, HPV typing may have a role in women with newly diagnosed cervical cancer, particularly those with early-stage disease. Knowledge of the underlying HPV genotype provides important prognostic information, and may aid in the selection of women at high risk for recurrence who could be offered adjuvant therapy.

HPV and other cofactors

Despite the prevalence of HPV in most populations, only a small fraction of women who harbor the virus develop clinically significant cervical disease. In addition to HPV, a number of environmental, genetic, and molecular cofactors have been implicated in cervical carcinogenesis. In addition to enhancing carcinogenesis, a number of these factors play an important role in prognosis, particularly when examined in the context of underlying HPV infection.

A well-known environmental cofactor for the development of cervical cancer is tobacco smoking.[55] Smoking is associated with decreased survival for women with early- as well as advanced-stage disease.[48] The adverse effects of smoking appear to be compounded in the presence of HPV-18. Compared with nonsmokers with HPV-18, current smokers who harbored HPV-18 had a hazard ratio of 4.1 for death from cervical cancer.[48]

A number of genetic and molecular risk factors have also been shown to function in conjunction with HPV as prognostic factors for the development of cervical cancer. While controversial, several authors have demonstrated that polymorphisms in codon 72 of the *TP53* gene appear to influence the development of cervical cancer. Single-nucleotide polymorphisms at this codon are believed to determine the efficiency by which E6 interacts with and degrades the *TP53* gene product, p53. Codon 72 polymorphisms are more frequent among women with invasive carcinomas than in those with dysplasia or normal cervical cytology.[56] These findings appear to be population-specific and have not been confirmed in several studies.[57] A second molecular marker that has received attention is p16^{INK4A}. This is a regulatory protein that influences cell cycle progression and is upregulated in response to pRb inactivation. Studies have suggested that it is useful in predicting preinvasive lesions and cytologic samples that are likely to progress.[58] In an analysis evaluating p16^{INK4A} levels in normal cervical epithelium, dysplastic epithelium, and invasive cancer, the levels of p16^{INK4A} were higher in the malignant samples. Likewise, women with biopsy that stained strongly for p16^{INK4A} had a shorter time to progression to CIN3/cancer than women with low-level p16^{INK4A} expression (64 months vs 122 months).[58] A variety of other molecular markers are under investigation, and will likely serve as important prognostic markers in the future.

REFERENCES

1. Parkin DM, Bray F, Ferlay J, Pisani P. Global cancer statistics, 2002. CA Cancer J Clin 2005;55:74–108.

2. Walboomers JM, Jacobs MV, Manos MM, et al. Human papillomavirus is a necessary cause of invasive cervical cancer worldwide. J Pathol 1999;189:12–19.

3. Munger K, Baldwin A, Edwards KM, et al. Mechanisms of human papillomavirus-induced oncogenesis. J Virol 2004;78:11451–60.

4. Durst M, Gissmann L, Ikenberg H, zur Hausen H. A papillomavirus DNA from a cervical carcinoma and its prevalence in cancer biopsy samples from different geographic regions. Proc Natl Acad Sci USA 1983; 80:3812–15.

5. Bernard HU. The clinical importance of the nomenclature, evolution and taxonomy of human papillomaviruses. J Clin Virol 2005; 32(Suppl 1):S1–6.

6. Munoz N, Bosch FX, de Sanjose S, et al. Epidemiologic classification of human papillomavirus types associated with cervical cancer. N Engl J Med 2003;348:518–27.

7. Clifford GM, Gallus S, Herrero R, et al. Worldwide distribution of human papillomavirus types in cytologically normal women in the International Agency for Research on Cancer HPV prevalence surveys: a pooled analysis. Lancet 2005;366:991–8.

8. Demeret C, Desaintes C, Yaniv M, Thierry F. Different mechanisms contribute to the E2-mediated transcriptional repression of human papillomavirus type 18 viral oncogenes. J Virol 1997;71:9343–9.

9. Wentzensen N, Vinokurova S, von Knebel Doeberitz M. Systematic review of genomic integration sites of human papillomavirus genomes in epithelial dysplasia and invasive cancer of the female lower genital tract. Cancer Res 2004;64:3878–84.

10. Leechanachai P, Banks L, Moreau F, Matlashewski G. The *E5* gene from human papillomavirus type 16 is an oncogene which enhances growth factor-mediated signal transduction to the nucleus. Oncogene 1992;7:19–25.

11. Munger K, Basile JR, Duensing S, et al. Biological activities and molecular targets of the human papillomavirus E7 oncoprotein. Oncogene 2001;20:7888–98.

12. Klingelhutz AJ, Foster SA, McDougall JK. Telomerase activation by the *E6* gene product of human papillomavirus type 16. Nature 1996;380:79–82.

13. Stubenrauch F, Laimins LA. Human papillomavirus life cycle: active and latent phases. Semin Cancer Biol 1999;9:379–86.

14. Durst M, Gallahan D, Jay G, Rhim JS. Glucocorticoid-enhanced neoplastic transformation of human keratinocytes by human papillomavirus type 16 and an activated *ras* oncogene. Virology 1989;173:767–71.

15. Klaes R, Woerner SM, Ridder R, et al. Detection of high-risk cervical intraepithelial neoplasia and cervical cancer by amplification of transcripts derived from integrated papillomavirus oncogenes. Cancer Res 1999;59:6132–6.

16. Denny LA, Wright TC Jr. Human papillomavirus testing and screening. Best Pract Res Clin Obstet Gynaecol 2005;19:501–15.

17. Peyton CL, Schiffman M, Lorincz AT, et al. Comparison of PCR- and hybrid capture-based human papillomavirus detection systems using multiple cervical specimen collection strategies. J Clin Microbiol 1998;36:3248–54.

18. Davies P, Kornegay J, Iftner T. Current methods of testing for human papillomavirus. Best Pract Res Clin Obstet Gynaecol 2001;15:677–700.

19. Gravitt PE, Peyton CL, Alessi TQ, et al. Improved amplification of genital human papillomaviruses. J Clin Microbiol 2000;38:357–61.

20. de Roda Husman AM, Walboomers JM, van den Brule AJ, Meijer CJ, Snijders PJ. The use of general primers GP5 and GP6 elongated at their 3′ ends with adjacent highly conserved sequences improves human papillomavirus detection by PCR. J Gen Virol 1995;76:1057–62.

21. Denny L, Kuhn L, De Souza M, et al. Screen-and-treat approaches for cervical cancer prevention in low-resource settings: a randomized controlled trial. JAMA 2005;294:2173–81.

22. Franco EL. Chapter 13: Primary screening of cervical cancer with human papillomavirus tests. J Natl Cancer Inst Monogr 2003:89–96.

23. Cuzick J, Szarewski A, Cubie H, et al. Management of women who test positive for high-risk types of human papillomavirus: the HART study. Lancet 2003;362:1871–6.

24. Schiffman M, Herrero R, Hildesheim A, et al. HPV DNA testing in cervical cancer screening: results from women in a high-risk province of Costa Rica. JAMA 2000;283:87–93.

25. Ho GY, Bierman R, Beardsley L, Chang CJ, Burk RD. Natural history of cervicovaginal papillomavirus infection in young women. N Engl J Med 1998;338:423–8.

26. Burk RD, Kelly P, Feldman J, et al. Declining prevalence of cervicovaginal human

papillomavirus infection with age is independent of other risk factors. Sex Transm Dis 1996;23:333–41.

27. Saslow D, Runowicz CD, Solomon D, et al. American Cancer Society guideline for the early detection of cervical neoplasia and cancer. CA Cancer J Clin 2002;52:342–62.

28. American College of Obstetricians and Gynecologists. ACOG Practice Bulletin 45: Cervical Cytology Screening. Obstet Gynecol 2003;102:417–27.

29. Wright TC Jr, Cox JT, Massad LS, Twiggs LB, Wilkinson EJ. 2001 Consensus Guidelines for the management of women with cervical cytological abnormalities. JAMA 2002;287: 2120–9.

30. Wright TC Jr, Schiffman M, Solomon D, et al. Interim guidance for the use of human papillomavirus DNA testing as an adjunct to cervical cytology for screening. Obstet Gynecol 2004;103:304–9.

31. Sherman ME, Lorincz AT, Scott DR, et al. Baseline cytology, human papillomavirus testing, and risk for cervical neoplasia: a 10-year cohort analysis. J Natl Cancer Inst 2003;95: 46–52.

32. Castle PE, Wacholder S, Sherman ME, et al. Absolute risk of a subsequent abnormal pap among oncogenic human papillomavirus DNA-positive, cytologically negative women. Cancer 2002;95:2145–51.

33. Denny L, Kuhn L, Risi L, et al. Two-stage cervical cancer screening: an alternative for resource-poor settings. Am J Obstet Gynecol 2000;183:383–8.

34. Solomon D, Schiffman M, Tarone R. Comparison of three management strategies for patients with atypical squamous cells of undetermined significance: baseline results from a randomized trial. J Natl Cancer Inst 2001;93:293–9.

35. Arbyn M, Buntinx F, Van Ranst M, et al. Virologic versus cytologic triage of women with equivocal Pap smears: a meta-analysis of the accuracy to detect high-grade intraepithelial neoplasia. J Natl Cancer Inst 2004;96: 280–93.

36. Kim JJ, Wright TC, Goldie SJ. Cost–effectiveness of alternative triage strategies for atypical squamous cells of undetermined significance. JAMA 2002;287:2382–90.

37. Cox JT. Evaluating the role of HPV testing for women with equivocal Papanicolaou test findings. JAMA 1999;281:1645–7.

38. A randomized trial on the management of low-grade squamous intraepithelial lesion cytology interpretations. Am J Obstet Gynecol 2003;188:1393–400.

39. Paraskevaidis E, Arbyn M, Sotiriadis A, et al. The role of HPV DNA testing in the follow-up period after treatment for CIN: a systematic review of the literature. Cancer Treat Rev 2004;30:205–11.

40. Nobbenhuis MA, Meijer CJ, van den Brule AJ, et al. Addition of high-risk HPV testing improves the current guidelines on follow-up after treatment for cervical intraepithelial neoplasia. Br J Cancer 2001;84:796–801.

41. Brockmeyer AD, Wright JD, Gao F, Powell MA. Persistent and recurrent cervical dysplasia after loop electrosurgical excision procedure. Am J Obstet Gynecol 2005;192:1379–81.

42. Nobbenhuis MA, Walboomers JM, Helmerhorst TJ, et al. Relation of human papillomavirus status to cervical lesions and consequences for cervical-cancer screening: a prospective study. Lancet 1999;354:20–5.

43. Sherman ME, Wang SS, Wheeler CM, et al. Determinants of human papillomavirus load among women with histological cervical intraepithelial neoplasia 3: dominant impact of surrounding low-grade lesions. Cancer Epidemiol Biomarkers Prev 2003;12:1038–44.

44. Ylitalo N, Sorensen P, Josefsson AM, et al. Consistent high viral load of human papillomavirus 16 and risk of cervical carcinoma in situ: a nested case–control study. Lancet 2000;355:2194–8.

45. Josefsson AM, Magnusson PK, Ylitalo N, et al. Viral load of human papilloma virus 16 as a determinant for development of cervical carcinoma in situ: a nested case–control study. Lancet 2000;355:2189–93.

46. Khan MJ, Castle PE, Lorincz AT, et al. The elevated 10-year risk of cervical precancer and cancer in women with human papillomavirus (HPV) type 16 or 18 and the possible utility of type-specific HPV testing in clinical practice. J Natl Cancer Inst 2005;97: 1072–9.

47. Castle PE, Solomon D, Schiffman M, Wheeler CM. Human papillomavirus type 16 infections and 2-year absolute risk of cervical precancer in women with equivocal or mild cytologic abnormalities. J Natl Cancer Inst 2005;97:1066–71.

48. Wright JD, Li J, Gerhard DS, et al. Human papillomavirus type and tobacco use as predictors of survival in early stage cervical carcinoma. Gynecol Oncol 2005;98:84–91.

49. Schwartz SM, Daling JR, Shera KA, et al. Human papillomavirus and prognosis of invasive cervical cancer: a population-based study. J Clin Oncol 2001;19:1906–15.

50. Im SS, Wilczynski SP, Burger RA, Monk BJ. Early stage cervical cancers containing human papillomavirus type 18 DNA have more nodal metastasis and deeper stromal invasion. Clin Cancer Res 2003;9:4145–50.

51. van Muyden RC, ter Harmsel BW, Smedts FM, et al. Detection and typing of human papillomavirus in cervical carcinomas in Russian women: a prognostic study. Cancer 1999;85: 2011–16.

52. Viladiu P, Bosch FX, Castellsague X, et al. Human papillomavirus DNA and antibodies to human papillomavirus 16 E2, L2, and E7 peptides as predictors of survival in patients with squamous cell cervical cancer. J Clin Oncol 1997;15:610–19.

53. Lombard I, Vincent-Salomon A, Validire P, et al. Human papillomavirus genotype as a major determinant of the course of cervical cancer. J Clin Oncol 1998;16:2613–19.

54. Rose BR, Thompson CH, Simpson JM, et al. Human papillomavirus deoxyribonucleic acid as a prognostic indicator in early-stage cervical cancer: a possible role for type 18. Am J Obstet Gynecol 1995;173:1461–8.

55. Winkelstein W Jr. Smoking and cancer of the uterine cervix: hypothesis. Am J Epidemiol 1977;106:257–9.

56. Zehbe I, Voglino G, Wilander E, Genta F, Tommasino M. Codon 72 polymorphism of p53 and its association with cervical cancer. Lancet 1999;354:218–19.

57. Rosenthal AN, Ryan A, Al-Jehani RM, Storey A, Harwood CA, Jacobs IJ. p53 codon 72 polymorphism and risk of cervical cancer in UK. Lancet 1998;352:871–2.

58. Wang JL, Zheng BY, Li XD, Angstrom T, Lindstrom MS, Wallin KL. Predictive significance of the alterations of p16^{INK4A}, p14^{ARF}, p53, and proliferating cell nuclear antigen expression in the progression of cervical cancer. Clin Cancer Res 2004;10:2407–14.

Molecular imaging of cervical cancer

20

Matthew A Powell and Perry W Grigsby

INTRODUCTION

For the past 50–60 years little changed in the initial evaluation of cervical cancer – until recently. Staging of cervical cancer has relied on clinical methods with a limited radiologic assessment based on the classification system of the International Federation of Gynecology and Obstetrics (FIGO). Multiple imaging modalities, including computed tomography (CT), magnetic resonance imaging (MRI), ultrasound, and lymphangiography, have been evaluated with intent to improve the staging, treatment planning, and prognostic accuracy of the initial tumor assessment, all with disappointing results. Over the past decade, molecular imaging has been rapidly changing the evaluation and management of cervical cancer. In this chapter, we will review the use of the only molecular imaging test currently approved by the US Center for Medicare and Medicaid Services: positron emission tomography (PET) with the glucose analog 2-[^{18}F]-fluoro-2-deoxy-D-glucose (FDG). Patient preparation with a focus on unique features of imaging cervical cancer by PET will be discussed. In the past few years, PET combined with CT (image fusion) appears to also be a further step forward, and currently represents the molecular/anatomic imaging modality of choice. A clinician-focused review of PET and PET/CT for staging, lymph node assessment, treatment planning, prognostication, response assessment, and disease surveillance will be presented. Other novel molecular imaging modalities (^{64}Cu-ATSM–PET, [^{18}F]fluoromisonidazole, [^{11}C]choline, and nanoparticle-enhanced MRI) are under development to evaluate other important tumor biologic properties that may impact survival, and these will be briefly reviewed.

BACKGROUND

Initial diagnosis, staging, and treatment planning of most cervical cancers are achieved by physical examination and with the use of basic imaging studies. Improving the accuracy of staging is important both for selecting appropriate therapies and for predicting prognosis. Cervical cancers initially spread locally and then via the lymphatic system before dissemination to distant organs. The status of pelvic and para-aortic lymph nodes is one of the most important determinants of prognosis, and is necessary for treatment planning in patients undergoing radiotherapy. Approximately 30–40% of patients with cervical cancer will have positive lymph nodes. Nodal positivity is associated with other factors, including tumor stage, size of primary lesion, and tumor histology.[1] Given the inaccuracies of previous imaging modalities and the importance of determining nodal status, this has resulted in many oncologists recommending surgical assessment of pelvic and para-aortic lymph nodes even when chemoradiotherapy is the treatment of choice for the locally advanced primary tumor.[2] CT is currently the most widely used imaging method for assessment of nodal involvement and detection of distant metastatic disease. Despite high resolution and excellent depiction of anatomy, CT is limited by its inability to detect small-volume metastatic involvement in normal-size lymph nodes (<1 cm) or to determine whether enlarged nodes represent metastasis or reactive changes. Cervical cancers are often necrotic, which leads to a significant inflammatory response that can cause significant noncancerous lymphadenopathy.

Over the last decade, FDG–PET has become an established oncologic imaging tool for many forms of cancer. The functional information about regional glucose metabolism provided by FDG–PET provides for greater sensitivity and specificity in most cancer imaging applications in comparison with CT and other anatomic imaging methods. FDG is molecularly similar to glucose and is transported into the cell and phosphorylated, but then cannot proceed through glycolysis past hexose-6-phosphate, and thus remains trapped within the cell and when radiolabeled allows for localizing of metabolically active cells. Cervical cancers overexpress glucose transporter 1 (Glut-1) and glycolytic enzymes (hexokinase I and II), and therefore readily accumulate the FDG radiotracer. FDG uptake is usually expressed in standardized uptake value (SUV), which represents the ratio of FDG concentration in a region compared with the total body dose. PET scan resolution has reported detection of lesions as small as 2–4 mm.[3,4]

PATIENT PREPARATION AND IMAGING

Patient preparation for imaging of cervical tumors is similar to that for other cancers. However, because of the potential for artifacts related to FDG activity in urinary tract structures (e.g. streak artifacts and confusion of ureteral activity with lymph nodes), various interventions to minimize the amount of FDG in the urinary tract have been employed. In some centers, urinary tract preparation is performed. Most often, this involves placement of a urinary catheter, intravenous administration of fluids (1000–1500 ml of saline solution to be infused during the course of the study), and intravenous administration of 20 mg furosemide near the time of injection of FDG. The urinary catheter should be placed before injection of FDG to minimize radiation exposure to technical or nursing staff. For PET/CT, oral contrast administration is useful for delineating bowel. Several investigators have suggested that delayed PET imaging (>2–3 hours after injection of FDG) may improve the sensitivity for detection of nodal and peritoneal metastasis.[5]

CERVICAL CANCER STAGING

Cervical cancer typically progresses in a predictable fashion, with initial spread locally to the cervix and to immediately surrounding structures. Regional lymphatics then become involved in an orderly fashion (pelvic nodes, followed by common iliac, then para-aortic, and finally supraclavicular). Spread to distant organs tends to occur later, likely via hematogenous spread. Cervical cancer is staged clinically based on the FIGO staging system. Figure 20.1 shows the progression-free survival of 500 patients treated at our institution with

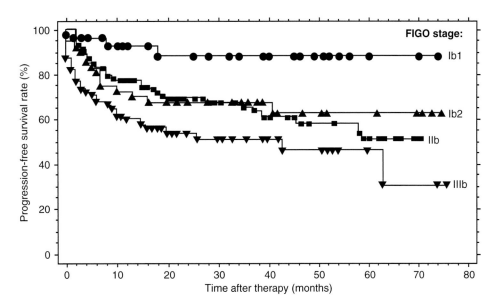

Figure 20.1 Progression-free survival by FIGO clinical stage (*n* = 500).

radiotherapy or combined-modality therapy based on their clinical stage. Involvement of pelvic or para-aortic lymph nodes does not alter the FIGO clinical stage of disease, but is associated with a worse prognosis and may have an important impact on therapy.

T staging

In general, most primary cervical cancers avidly accumulate FDG, and the accumulation does not seem to be dependent on histologic subtype but is limited by tumor size. Thus, this limits its use in evaluation of stage IA and early IB tumors. PET is not very accurate in determining the true extent of stage IA–IIB lesions, given that local spread to the parametrium and upper vagina is often microscopic and below the level of resolution of PET. Clinical examination remains the standard, with MRI being used when complementary information is required.

N and M staging

Multiple studies have demonstrated PET to be superior to conventional imaging methods for detecting metastatic disease, particularly lymph node metastasis.[6,7] A recent systematic review of the literature of PET in patients with newly diagnosed cervical cancer reported that the pooled sensitivity of PET was 79% (95% confidence interval (CI) 65–90%), with a pooled specificity of 99% (95% CI 96–99%) for detection of pelvic lymph node metastasis.[3,6–8] Two studies comparing PET with MRI and CT[6,7] found that MRI had a pooled sensitivity of 72% (95% CI 53–87%) and a pooled specificity of 96% (95% CI 92–98%), whereas CT had a pooled sensitivity of 47% (95% CI 21–73%). In four prospective studies using histology after para-aortic lymphadenectomy as the reference standard, the pooled sensitivity of PET for the detection of para-aortic nodal metastasis was 84% (95% CI 68–94%) and the pooled specificity was 95% (95% CI 89–98%).[7,9–11] In three of these studies, the inclusion criteria for study entry included a negative CT or MRI of the abdomen.[9,11,12] Thus, a direct comparison of accuracy of conventional imaging CT/MRI to PET could not be made.

False-negative results for detection of nodal metastasis appear to be related to the size resolution of PET, and thus its inability to detect microscopic disease and small macroscopic tumor deposits. In a study evaluating the sensitivity of FDG–PET in patients with early-stage cervical cancer undergoing radical hysterectomy, we found that the mean size of tumor deposits was larger in PET-positive pelvic nodes (15.2 mm; range 2–35 mm) than in PET-negative nodes (7.3 mm; range 0.3–20 mm).[4] False-positive results are most likely related to uptake of FDG in inflammatory/hyperplastic nodes or misinterpretation of physiologic activity in bowel or the urinary tract as nodal metastasis.

Studies from Washington University have shown that FDG–PET is superior to CT and lymphangiography in revealing unsuspected sites of metastasis in pelvic lymph nodes, extrapelvic lymph nodes, and distant metastasis in patients with newly diagnosed locally advanced cervical cancer.[13] FDG–PET showed abnormalities consistent with metastasis more often than did CT in pelvic lymph nodes (67% vs 20%) and in para-aortic lymph nodes (21% vs 7%). PET also demonstrated disease in clinically occult supraclavicular lymph nodes in 8%.[11] These results have been sustained in subsequent evaluations of data from our prospective registry, which now includes over 500 patients. Figure 20.2 shows our updated data on over 500 patients who have received pretreatment PET or PET/CT scans. Eighty percent of PET-positive lymph nodes identified have been found to be <1 cm.

The precise role of combined (fusion) PET/CT in the staging of cervical cancer needs to be further evaluated. The literature currently contains limited data on the use of fusion PET/CT in cervical cancer.[14] Choi et al[15]

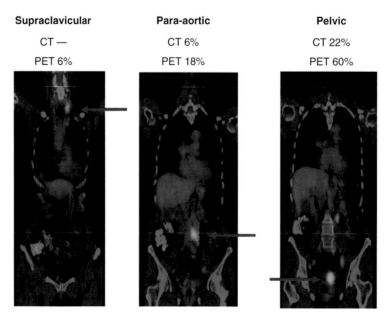

Figure 20.2 Nodal metastasis: FDG–PET/CT versus CT (*n* = 500). Nodes are marked with red arrows.

recently published a comparison of PET/CT versus MRI compared with histology in 22 stage IB–IVA patients, and found improved sensitivity with PET/CT (57.6% vs 30.3%; $p = 0.026$). There was also a trend toward improved accuracy with PET/CT (85.1% vs 72.7%; $p = 0.18$).

DIRECTING THERAPY

The use of FDG–PET in pretreatment evaluation appears to have a significant impact on the treatment planning in patients with cervical carcinoma. In our series of over 500 patients, approximately 40% have had modification of their treatment based on their pretreatment PET results. For nearly all stage IA, most IB1, and rarely IB2–IIA lesions, surgery with simple extrafascial (IA1) or radical (IA2–IIA) hysterectomy is often utilized. If these patients are found to have positive lymph nodes or other poor prognostic factors, they will typically be treated adjuvantly with radio- and/or chemoradiotherapy (trimodality therapy). Identifying patients with positive lymph nodes or other metastatic disease prior to subjecting them to radical surgery may allow for less toxic bimodality (chemoradiotherapy) rather than trimodality therapy (surgery plus chemoradiotherapy), without a demonstrated decreased survival rate. The use of PET in early-stage cancers continues to be evaluated. We have reported our experience with 59 stage IA–IIA patients undergoing pretreatment PET and PET/CT.[4] Thirty-two percent of patients had positive pelvic lymph nodes and PET/CT was 75% sensitive in detection. As one would predict, the lymph node metastases are smaller with the smaller primary tumors; thus, the sensitivity of PET was less. Nonetheless, when there is evidence of PET-positive lymph nodes in a patient with apparent early-stage disease,

one should carefully consider treatment options to minimize morbidity and consider extraperitoneal lymph node assessment or proceeding with chemoradiotherapy without radical surgery.

The current standard treatment of locally advanced cervical carcinoma (stage IB–IVA) is radiotherapy with concurrent chemotherapy.[16–18] Radiotherapy is directed at the pelvis to encompass primary disease as well as pelvic lymph nodes. Using the tumor volume as assessed by PET as the target volume for the radiotherapy should allow maximal efficacy balanced with minimizing the normal tissues treated. Figure 20.3 is an example of how PET scan results can be used to drive treatment planning. The radiotherapy port is expanded to include the para-aortic lymph node region only in patients who have evidence of para-aortic nodal disease. Patients who have evidence of disease beyond the para-aortic lymph nodes at the time of initial diagnosis have little chance of a cure, and should receive therapy with palliation as the goal. We now routinely administer curative-intent para-aortic irradiation to patients with CT-negative, FDG-positive para-aortic nodal disease, whereas irradiation to this region would have been administered to such patients in the past before the use of PET.[19]

In an effort to further minimize morbidity and maximize efficacy, we are investigating the use of PET/CT-guided intensity-modulated radiotherapy (IMRT) to deliver higher doses to the PET-positive para-aortic nodal basin.[20] Fused PET/CT images can be used to differentiate tumor from adjacent normal structures more reliably and thus to deliver higher doses of radiation to the tumor while decreasing radiation dose to normal structures (Figure 20.3).

FDG–PET may also be useful in determining whether concurrent chemotherapy should

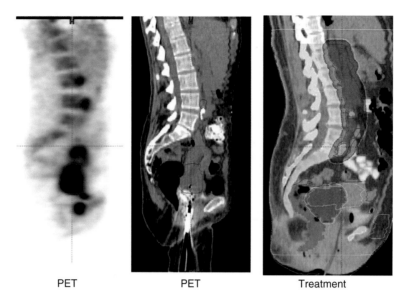

PET   PET   Treatment

Figure 20.3 Treatment planning based on PET scan results.

be administered to patients undergoing radio-therapy. We reviewed our experience in patients with locally advanced cervix cancer with no evidence of metastatic lymph node involvement as evaluated by FDG–PET treated with primary irradiation alone ($n = 15$) versus chemoradiotherapy ($n = 50$). There were no differences in survival (5-year survival rate 85% vs 81%) or sites of recurrence. Thus, if further study supports this preliminary data, one could use PET to tailor the use of sensitizing chemotherapy to those who stand to benefit most.

PROGNOSIS

Several prognostic factors have been identified for patients with carcinoma of the cervix. These include patient age, tumor histology, tumor stage, tumor size, lymph node metastasis, and tumor hypoxia.[21,22] Grigsby et al[19] demonstrated that the pelvic and para-aortic lymph node status determined by pretreatment FDG–PET is predictive of progression-free and overall

survival in patients with cervical cancer treated with radio- or chemoradiotherapy ($n = 111$). Based on the imaging findings in the pelvic lymph nodes, the 2-year disease-free survival rate was 84% for CT-negative/PET-nagative patients, 64% for CT-negative/PET-positive patients, and 48% for CT-positive PET-positive patients ($p = 0.05$). For the para-aortic nodes, the 2-year disease-free survival rate was 78% in CT-negative/PET-negative patients, 31% for CT-negative/PET-positive patients, and 14% for CT-positive/PET-positive patients ($p \leq 0.0001$). No patients with PET-positive supraclavicular lymph nodes survived 2 years. Survival based on PET status in 500 patients treated is shown in Figure 20.4. The status of the para-aortic nodes as determined by PET was the strongest predictor of survival in a multivariate logistic regression analysis. In a review of 56 patients in our prospective registry, we also found that the extent of lymph node involvement was inversely correlated with survival.[23] We have also found that FDG–PET demonstrated metastatic involvement in the left supraclavicular lymph

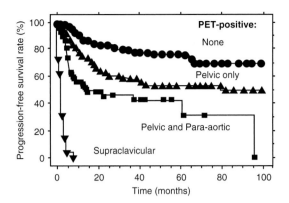

Figure 20.4 Progression-free survival based on FDG–PET lymph node status (all stages: *n* = 500).

nodes in 8% of our patient population;[24] this finding had a 100% concordance with histologic assessment and indicates a dismal prognosis, despite therapy. Similarly, the cause-specific survival for patients with FIGO stage IIIB carcinoma is highly dependent upon the extent of lymph node metastasis demonstrated by whole-body FDG–PET at initial diagnosis.[25] The 3-year cause-specific survival rates were 73% for those with no lymph node metastasis on PET, 58% for those with only pelvic lymph node metastasis, 29% for those with pelvic and para-aortic lymph node metastasis, and 0%

for those with pelvic, para-aortic, and supraclavicular lymph node metastasis ($p = 0.0005$). Survival for patients with stage IB cancers treated with radical surgery, radiotherapy, and/or chemoradiotherapy is highly variable and a pretreatment PET seems to accurately predict survival (Figure 20.5). The SUV of the primary tumor has been evaluated as a predictor of survival, and appears to be independent of tumor size (Figure 20.6). Table 20.1 summarizes the association of PET assessment of lymph nodes on ultimate distant failure of disease. Both PET tumor volume and PET SUV of the primary lesion also appear to accurately predict local failure (Tables 20.2 and 20.3). A post-treatment PET or PET/CT scan appears to have the best predictive ability of survival; this will be summarized in the following section.

SURVEILLANCE

Post-treatment surveillance PET or PET/CT studies performed approximately 3 months following the completion of therapy are very predictive of patient survival (Figure 20.7).[26] Clinical and radiologic techniques have been

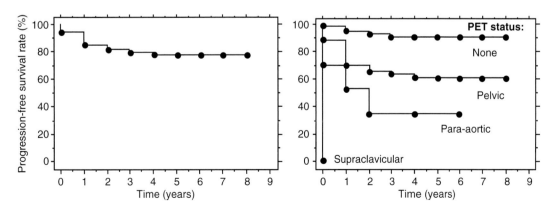

Figure 20.5 Progression-free survival of stage IB patients with pretreatment PET scan: (a) all patients; (b) according to PET nodal status.

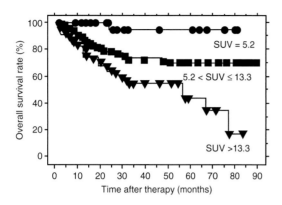

Figure 20.6 Overall survival: standardized uptake value (SUV) of primary tumor.

Table 20.2 PET volume of primary tumor related to local failure of radiotherapy or chemoradiotherapy

PET volume (cm³): all stages	Cervix failure rate (%)
<50 (4.5 cm diameter)	15
50–100 (5.7 cm diameter)	12
100–150 (6.5 cm diameter)	13
>150	40

used for early detection of recurrent disease without much success. Most patients with recurrent cervix cancer are found secondary to symptoms and not Pap smear or clinical examination findings.[27] FDG–PET has also been shown to have a role in the post-treatment monitoring of patients with cervical cancer. In a large retrospective study from Korea by Ryu et al,[28] 249 women with previously treated cervical cancer without overt evidence of recurrence underwent FDG–PET as part of their follow-up. Eighty patients (32%) had abnormal FDG uptake and ultimately 28 (11%) had clinically or histologically confirmed

recurrent disease within 6–18 months of diagnosis. Havrilesky et al[29] reported on 22 patients being evaluated for recurrent disease, and found the sensitivity and specificity of PET to detect recurrence to be 85.7% and 86.7%, respectively. Grigsby et al[26] reported on 152 patients previously treated with radiotherapy with or without concurrent chemotherapy who were free of FDG-avid sites on PET obtained an average of 3 months post-therapy. These patients had 5-year cause-specific and overall survival rate of 80% and 92%, respectively. Persistent abnormal uptake in the cervix or lymph nodes was found in 20 patients, and their cause-specific survival rate was 32%. New areas of increased FDG uptake in previously unirradiated regions were found in 18 patients, none of whom was alive at 5 years. Post-treatment PET abnormalities were found to be

Table 20.1 PET lymph node status on pretreatment PET or PET/CT scan and association with outcome (distant failure)

PET-positive lymph nodes: all stages	Distant failure rate (%)
None	12
Pelvic	25
Pelvic and para-aortic	41
Pelvic, para-aortic, and supraclavicular	100

Table 20.3 Standardized uptake value (SUV) on PET of the primary cervical tumor related to local failure of radiotherapy or chemoradiotherapy

PET SUV: all stages	Cervix failure rate (%)
<5	3
5–10	13
10–15	13
>15	24

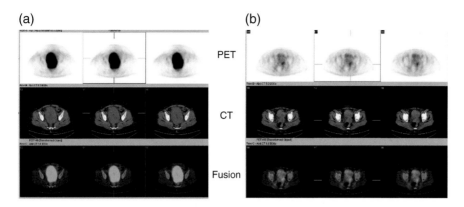

Figure 20.7 PET/CT with fusion (a) pre- and (b) post-treatment.

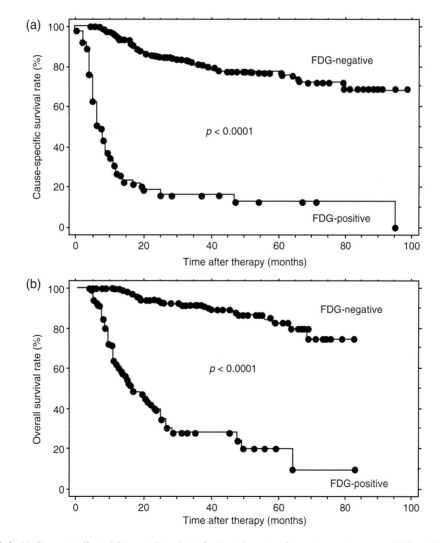

Figure 20.8 (a) Cause-specific and (b) overall survival of patients based on 3-months post-treatment PET or PET/CT (*n* = 293).

the most significant predictor of death from cervical cancer in this study. Together, these results point to a significant impact of FDG–PET findings on treatment strategy after primary therapy. Figure 20.8 shows cause-specific and overall survival of our updated post-treatment scans involving 293 patients who underwent PET or PET/CT approximately 3 months after the completion of therapy.

Additionally, Yen et al[30] have reported on two prospective studies from Taiwan examining the role of FDG–PET in patients with biopsy-confirmed relapse of disease or unexplained elevation of tumor marker serum levels with documented relapse after PET. Fifty-five women were enrolled: 36 (65.5%) had treatment modifications due to PET findings; the remaining 19 were treated according to the initial plan. Of those patients whose plans were modified, 25% received curative-intent salvage therapy but with the modality or field of irradiation changed, and 75% received palliative treatment. Together, these results demonstrate the usefulness of FDG–PET imaging for recurrent cervical cancer in determining the optimal salvage or palliative therapy.

OTHER NOVEL MOLECULAR IMAGING MODALITIES

In patients with cervical cancer, tumor hypoxia is an important prognostic factor indicating decreased overall and disease-free survival and this correlates with levels of hypoxia-inducible factor-1α (HIF-1α).[31] We have shown that a new tracer, ^{60}Cu-labeled diacetyl-bis-(N^4-methylthiosemicarbazone) (^{60}Cu-ATSM), accumulates avidly in hypoxic tissues but washes out rapidly from normoxic tissues. Twenty-seven patients with advanced cervical cancer were evaluated. There was an inverse relationship between tumor uptake of ^{60}Cu-ATSM and response to therapy (Figure 20.9).[32] Progression-free and overall survival were significantly worse in patients with increased uptake of ^{60}Cu-ATSM in the primary tumor prior to initiation of therapy. In these same patients, we found no significant difference in tumor FDG uptake in subjects with hypoxic (ATSM-avid) tumors versus those with normoxic tumors. Thus, ^{60}Cu-ATSM–PET imaging appears to provide additional prognostic information and has the potential to be used to identify patients requiring more

^{60}Cu-ATSM–PET

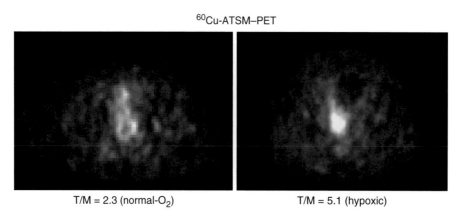

T/M = 2.3 (normal-O$_2$)　　　　　T/M = 5.1 (hypoxic)

Figure 20.9 ^{60}Cu-ATSM–PET scan with T = tumor: M = muscle ratio. The example on the left depicts a tumor with normal oxygen conditions, while the tumor on the right depicts hypoxic conditions.

aggressive/alternate therapies due to their predicted poor outcome.

Torizuka et al[33] evaluated [^{11}C]choline as a useful radiotracer in gynecologic malignancies, the main advantage being that it is not concentrated in the urinary system like FDG, allowing perhaps for better pelvic imaging. However, increased uptake in the intestine and limited availability of the radiotracer limit this application.

A lymph node-specific contrast agent has been developed for MRI that allows the identification of malignant nodal infiltration independent of nodal size.[34] The contrast agent is composed of an iron oxide core coated with low-molecular-weight dextran. This class of molecules are called ultrasmall particles of iron oxide (USPIO). Administered intravenously, the particles are taken up by macrophages within lymph nodes. Rockall et al[34] evaluated 29 cervical and 44 endometrial cancer patients with MRI before and after administration of USPIO. Scan results were compared with final pathologic specimen results. Rockall et al[34] concluded that USPIO significantly increased the sensitivity of MRI in the prediction of lymph node metastases, with no loss of specificity.

SUMMARY

Molecular imaging with FDG–PET shows great promise in aiding the clinician in the management of cervical cancer patients.[35] Current uses that appear beneficial to the patient include: (i) as an initial adjunct to clinical staging to more accurately define the extent of disease; (ii) to identify patients with metastatic disease not detected by other modalities to help define and plan treatment options (surgery vs radiations vs extent of radio- and/or chemotherapy); (iii) to provide better prognostic information at the completion of therapy; and (iv) to possibly identify recurrence earlier when cure may still be possible. Experimental uses include the use of PET/CT to define the most appropriate treatment fields for intensity-modulated radiotherapy in an effort to maximize efficacy and minimize morbidity. Other molecular imaging modalities may also prove useful. ^{60}Cu-ATSM–PET imaging appears to provide additional prognostic information, and may identify patients at very high risk of failure who should be targeted for more aggressive/novel therapies.

REFERENCES

1. Buchsbaum HJ. Extrapelvix lymph node metastasis in cervical carcinoma. Am J Obstet Gynecol 1979;133:814–24.

2. Goff BA, Muntz HG, Paley PJ, et al. Impact of surgical staging in women with locally advanced cervical cancer. Gynecol Oncol 1999;74:436–42.

3. Adam LE, Karp JS, Daube-Witherspoon ME, Smith RJ. Performance of a wholebody PET scanner using curve-plate NaI(T1) dectectors. J Nucl Med 2001;42:1821–30.

4. Wright JD, Dehdashti F, Herzog TJ, et al. Preoperative lymph node staging of early-stage cervical carcinoma by [^{18}F]-fluoro-2-deoxy-D-glucose–positron emission tomography. Cancer 2005;104:248–91.

5. Ma SY, See LC, Lai CH, et al. Delayed 18-F-FDG PET for detection of paraaortic lymph node metastases in cervical cancer patients. J Nucl Med 2003;44:1775–83.

6. Belhocine T, Thille A, Fridman V, et al. Contribution of whole-body ^{18}FDG PET

imaging in the management of cervical cancer. Gynecol Oncol 2002;87:90–7.

7. Reinhardt MJ, Ehritt-Braun C, Vogelgesang D, et al. Metastatic lymph nodes in patients with cervical cancer: detection with MR imaging and FDG PET. Radiology 2001;218: 776–82.

8. Havrilesky LJ, Kulasingam SL, Matchar DB, Myers ER. FDG–PET for management of cervical and ovarian cancer. Gynecol Oncol 2005;97:183–91.

9. Rose PG, Adler LP, Rodriguez M, et al. Positron emission tomography for evaluating para-aortic nodal metastasis in locally advanced cervical cancer before surgical staging: a surgicopathologic study. J Clin Oncol 1999; 17:41–5.

10. Yeh LS, Hung YC, Shen YY, et al. Detecting para-aortic lymph nodal metastasis by positron emission tomography of ^{18}F-fluorodeoxyglucose in advanced cervical cancer with negative magnetic resonance imaging findings. Oncol Rep 2002;9:1289–92.

11. Lin WC, Hung YC, Yeh LS, et al. Usefulness of ^{18}F-fluorodeoxyglucose positron emission tomography to detect para-aortic lymph nodal metastasis in advanced cervical cancer with negative computed tomography findings. Gynecol Oncol 2003;89:73–6.

12. Sugawara Y, Eisbruch A, Kosuda S, et al Evaluation of FDG PET in patients with cervical cancer. J Nucl Med 1999;40:1125–31.

13. Grigsby PW, Dehdashti F, Siegel BA. FDG–PET evaluation of carcinoma of the cervix. Clin Pos Imag 1999;2:105–9.

14. Subhas N, Patel PV, Pannu HK, Jacene HA, Fishman EK, Wahl RL. Imaging of pelvic malignancies with in-line FDG PET–CT: case examples and common pitfalls of FDG PET. RadioGraphics 2005;25:1031–43.

15. Choi HJ, Roh JW, Seo SS, et al. Comparison of the accuracy of magnetic resonance imaging and positron emission tomography/computed tomography in the presurgical detection of lymph node metastases in patients with uterine cervical carcinoma: a prospective study. Cancer 2006;106:914–22.

16. Rose PG, Bundy BN, Watkins EB, et al. Concurrent cisplatin-based radiotherapy and chemotherapy for locally advanced cervical cancer. N Engl J Med 1999;340:1144–53.

17. Morris M, Eifel PJ, Lu J, et al. Pelvic radiation with concurrent chemotherapy compared with pelvic and para-aortic radiation for high-risk cervical cancer. N Engl J Med 1999;340: 1137–43.

18. Keys HM, Bundy BN, Stehman FB, et al. Cisplatin, radiation, and adjuvant hysterectomy compared with radiation and adjuvant hysterectomy for bulky stage IB cervical carcinoma. N Engl J Med 1999;340:1154–61.

19. Grigsby PW, Siegel BA, Dehdashti F. Lymph node staging by positron emission tomography in patients with carcinoma of the cervix. J Clin Oncol 2001;19:3745–9.

20. Esthappan J, Mutic S, Malyapa RS, et al. Treatment planning guidelines regarding the use of CT/PET-guided IMRT for cervical carcinoma with positive para-aortic lymph nodes. Int J Radiat Oncol Biol Phys 2004; 58:1289–97.

21. Dehdashti F, Grigsby PW, Mintun MA, et al. Assessing tumor hypoxia in cervical cancer by positron emission tomography with ^{60}Cu-ATSM: relationship to therapeutic response – a preliminary report. Int J Radiat Oncol Biol Phys 2003;55:1233–8.

22. Grigsby PW. 4th International Cervical Cancer Conference: Update on PET and cervical cancer. Gynecol Oncol 2005;99 (3 Suppl 1):S173–5.

23. Stehman F, Bundy B, DiSaia P, et al. Carcinoma of the cervix treated with irradiation therapy. I. A multivariate analysis of prognostic variables in the Gynecologic Oncology Group. Cancer 1991;67:2776–85.

24. Tran BN, Grigsby PW, Dehdashti F, Siegel BA. Frequency and prognostic significance of

clinically occult supraclavicular lymph node metastases in cervical cancer patients identified by FDG–PET. Int J Radiat Oncol Biol Phys 2002;54(2 Suppl 1):69.

25. Singh AK, Grigsby PW, Dehdashti F, Herzog TJ, Siegel BA. FDG–PET lymph node staging and survival of patients with FIGO stage IIIB cervical carcinoma. Int J Radiat Oncol Biol Phys 2003;56:489–93.

26. Grigsby PW, Siegel BA, Dehdashti F, Rader J, Zoberi I. Posttherapy [18F]-fluorodeoxyglucose positron emission tomography in carcinoma of the cervix: response and outcome. J Clin Oncol 2004;22:67–71.

27. DiSaia PJ, Creasman WT. Clinical Gynecologic Oncology, 6th edn. St Louis, MO: Mosby, 2001.

28. Ryu SY, Kim MH, Choi SC, Choi CW, Lee KH. Detection of early recurrence with 18F-FDG PET in patients with cervical cancer. J Nucl Med 2003;44:347–52.

29. Havrilesky LJ, Wong TZ, Secord AA, et al. The role of PET scanning in the detection of recurrent cervical cancer. Gynecol Oncol 2003;95:546–51.

30. Yen T-C, See L-C, Lai C-H, et al. 18F-FDG uptake in squamous cell carcinoma of the cervix is correlated with glucose transporter 1 expression. J Nucl Med 2004;45:22–9.

31. Burri P, Djonov V, Aebersold DM, et al. Significant correlation of hypoxia-inducible factor-1α with treatment outcome in cervical cancer treated with radical rediotherapy. Int J Radiat Oncol Biol Phys 2003;56:494–501.

32. Grigsby PW, Mutch DG, Rader J, et al. Lack of benefit of concurrent chemotherapy in patients with cervical cancer and negative lymph nodes by FDG–PET. Int J Radiat Oncol Biol Phys 2005;61:444–9.

33. Torizuka T, Kanno T, Futatsubshi M, et al. Imaging of gynecologic tumors: comparison of 11C-choline PET with 18F-FDG PET. J Nucl Med 2003;44:1051–6.

34. Rockall AG, Sohaib SA, Harisinghani MG, et al. Diagnostic performance of nanoparticle-enhanced magnetic resonance imaging in the diagnosis of lymph node metastases in patients with endometrial and cervical cancer. J Clin Oncol 2005;23:2813–1.

35. Grigsby PW. Cervical cancer: combined modality therapy. Cancer J 2001;7(Suppl1) S47–50.

Neuroendocrine cancer of the cervix: prognostic and predictive factors

21

John K Chan and Daniel S Kapp

INTRODUCTION

Neuroendocrine tumors of the cervix are relatively uncommon. The variety of terms used to describe this cancer have resulted in confusion as to its true incidence, clinical features, prognostic factors, clinical behavior, and optimum treatment. A workshop sponsored by the College of American Pathologists and the US National Cancer Institute (NCI) recommended four general categories for endocrine tumors of the uterine cervix: typical (classical) carcinoid tumor, atypical carcinoid tumor, large cell neuroendocrine carcinoma, and small (oat) cell carcinoma.[1] This chapter will concentrate on the small (oat) cell tumors of the cervix. Their incidence, morphologic and molecular markers, prognostic factors, and treatment will be reviewed. Histologically, small (oat) cell carcinomas are composed of small round or fusiform cells with scant cytoplasm and hyperchromatic nuclei that grow in a diffuse manner or in nests, trabeculae, or cords (Figure 21.1). Although immunohistochemical stains are not required to make the diagnosis, the majority of these tumors stain positive for at least one of the common neuroendocrine markers (neuron-specific enolase (NSE), chromogranin, and synaptophysin) and this is often used to aid in the classification.[2]

INCIDENCE

The reported incidence of small (oat) cell carcinoma of the uterine cervix has ranged widely in the literature from 0.17% to 10.4% (Table 21.1). The variation in incidence is based, at least in part, on the selection criteria employed to identify patients with neuroendocrine cancers of the cervix and, to a lesser extent, the denominator used (e.g. all cervical cancers seen during the same time period, invasive cancers only, or only those with a given stage of disease). The incidence in most recent reports is approximately 1% of all invasive cervical cancers, probably a more realistic estimate than the higher figures noted in earlier series.

MORPHOLOGIC AND MOLECULAR MARKERS

Early studies identifying small cell carcinoma of the cervix based the diagnosis on histologic findings of tumors resembling small (oat) cell carcinomas of the lung, supplemented with Grimelius stains showing argyrophilic granules and electron microscopy studies demonstrating neurosecretory-type granules.[3,4] More recent series have utilized immunohistochemical (IHC) staining for neuroendocrine markers (including NSE, synaptophysin and chromogranin),

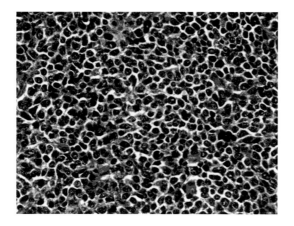

Figure 21.1 Small cell neuroendocrine carcinoma, showing small round or fusiform cells with scant cytoplasm, hyperchromatic nuclei with stippled granular chromatin, nuclear molding, high mitotic rate, and extensive necrosis. Courtesy of Dr Teri Longacre, Stanford University, Stanford, CA.

cytokeratin markers, and carcinoembryonic antigen (CEA), and staining for the presence of specific polypeptides, (including calcitonin and somatostatin) and serotonin (Figure 21.2). Since varying groups of IHC stains were employed in different series, the exact incidence of positive markers can only be estimated. The incidences of the more commonly employed markers are summarized in Tables 21.2 and 21.3. It should be noted, however, that several studies used the presence of one or more positive markers as inclusion criteria, thereby biasing the results.

The high percentage of tumors staining positive for NSE (80%) suggests that serum levels of NSE could be used to identify patients with otherwise occult residual disease, monitor response to therapy, and aid in early detection

Table 21.1 Incidence of small cell carcinoma of the uterine cervix

Ref	No. of small cell carcinomas	No. of cervical cancers	% small cell carcinomas	Selection criteria
54	25	3 511	0.7	Only small cell carcinomas; other neuroendocrine tumors were excluded
55	11	1 370	0.8	—
28	10	998	1.0	Only stage IB
56	10	449	2.2	Only invasive cancers
27	239	18 697	1.3	Compared with incidence of squamous cell + small cell cancers
32	20	1 362	1.5	—
40	11	2 899	0.38	—
57	7	>5 000	<0.14	Invasive cancers
2	12	370	3.24	Stage I, IIA patients treated with radical hysterectomy
39	26	NA	<1.0	Denominator not reported
15	14	1 412	1.0	—
20	12	1 154	1.0	Invasive cancers > stage I
58	9	546	1.6	Invasive cancers
59	10	365	2.7	Only small cell carcinomas
30	25	2 201	1.1	Invasive cancers
60	33	2 932	1.1	Of all stages of squamous cell cancer
61	20	193*	10.4	*Wide range of neuroendocrine types
62	6	3 507	0.17	Poorly differentiated carcinoid tumors
3	2	97	2.1	Small cell carcinomas only

NA, not available.

Included poorly-differentiated adenocarcinoma and adenosquamous carcinomas as well as undifferentiated carcinoma.

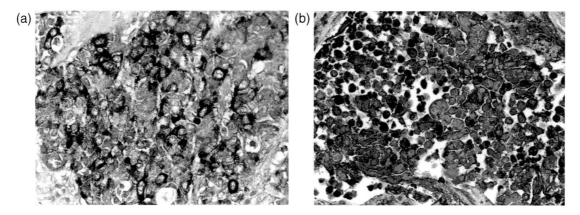

Figure 21.2 Immunohistochemical staining for the neuroendocrine markers – chromogranin (a) and synaptophysin (b). Courtesy of Dr Teri Longacre, Stanford University, Stanford, CA.

of recurrence. This approach has been successfully reported in small cell cancers of the lung.[5,6] Nakata et al[7] monitored the response to radiotherapy in a patient treated for stage III small cell carcinoma of the cervix, demonstrating a fall in serum NSE during treatment. Normal levels were maintained during follow-up. Chen et al[8] reported elevated serum NSE in 4 of 6 patients with small cell carcinomas of the cervix (versus none of 13 patients with squamous cell carcinomas). They noted an

extremely high level in one patient at the time of recurrence, suggesting that it correlated with disease extension. Other molecular markers have been studied in small series of patients with small cell cervical carcinomas, including mutations or loss of *TP53*,[9–13] with rates of loss varying from 10% to 50%. Loss of heterozygosity (LOH) at chromosome 3p has been reported in two series.[9,11] Aneuploidy has been noted in 27–100% of the cases studied,[14–16] and may be related to human papillomavirus 18

Table 21.2 Morphologic and molecular markers in small cell carcinomas of the cervix: neurosecretory granules

	No. positive/No. tested	
Ref	*Grimelius (argyrophilic granules)*	*Electron microscopy (neurosecretory granules)*
56	4/5	ND
37	ND	7/8
63	7/10	ND
58	ND	2/4
64	3/10	7/10
65	ND	3/5
66	10/15	ND
67	9/9	3/9
62	4/6	4/4
3	5/5	3/3
Total	42/60 (70%)	29/43 (67%)

ND, not done.

Table 21.3 Morphologic and molecular markers in small cell carcinomas of the cervix: neuroendocrine markers on immunohistochemical staining[a]

Ref	No. positive/No. tested			Marker inclusion criteria[b]
	NSE	Synaptophysin	Chromogranin	
55	9/11	8/11	7/11	None
10	ND	7/10	9/10	≥2 positive
28	ND	19/21	16/21	≥1 positive
31	6/6	ND	6/9	None
56	5/7	4/6	7/8	None
12	12/16	8/16	8/16	None
32	15/18	8/18	9/18	None
47	10/10	5/10	7/10	None
40	9/9	6/9	6/9	None
39	19/24	7/24	5/24	None
37	18/20	5/20	13/20	None
58	8/9	ND	ND	None
30	5/15	ND	3/15	None
Total	116/145 (80%)	77/145 (53%)	96/171 (56%)	

NSE, neuron-specific enolase; ND, not done.

[a]Included series with ≥9 patients with small cell carcinoma of the cervix.

[b]For patient to be included in study.

(HPV-18) infection[17] and associated with a worse prognosis.[16]

One of the most significant advances in understanding the pathobiology of cervix cancer has been the demonstration that infection with HPV is necessary for the development of nearly all cervical cancers.[18] HPV-16 is the most frequently detected HPV type (50–60%) in cervical cancer in North America, while HPV-18 is the next most common type found (10–14%).[18,19] The incidence of the common types of HPV in small cell carcinomas is summarized in Table 21.4. As noted, the incidence of HPV-18 is, in most series, much higher than the approximately 3:1 ratio of HPV-16-positive to HPV-18-positive cancers seen in nonsmall cell cancers of the cervix. The reason for the absence of HPV-18-positive tumors in the study from Pao et al[20] is not clear. HPV-18 has also been reported to be more commonly associated

with adenocarcinomas of the cervix, and may contribute, controlling for other prognostic parameters, to a worse prognosis. Thus, the poor clinical results seen for small cell carcinomas of the cervix may, in part, be related to fundamental changes in tumor biology related to HPV-18 interaction, which warrants further investigation.

Two recent investigations have looked for the expression of Kit in small cell carcinomas of the cervix. One study, using a polyclonal antibody against Kit protein, demonstrated cytoplastic staining in 6 of 22 (27%) of cases. However, the immunoreactivity was only focal and/or weak in 5 of these cases.[21] A second study identified overexpression of Kit (>25% of tumor cells stained) in 9 of 21 patients (43%).[22] These investigations suggest the potential use of imatinib (Gleevec/Glivec) or other tyrosine kinase inhibitors in the treatment of a select

Table 21.4 Human papillomavirus (HPV) types in small cell carcinomas of the cervix

| Ref | No. patients positive/total patients | | Comments |
	HPV-16	HPV-18	
54	1/26	17/26	No HPV: 8/26 patients
10	0/10	9/10	HPV-18-positive in 5/5 pure, 4/5 mixed small cell carcinomas
56	1/10	9/10	—
68	13/25	11/25	HPV-45: 1/25 patients
9	1/6	3/8	No HPV: 4/8 patients
39	7/25	10/25	No HPV: 8/25 patients
37	1/20	14/20	All cases HPV-positive
20	0/12	0/12	—
14	1/5	3/5	Only small cell carcinomas
Total	25/139 (18%)	76/141 (54%)	—

group of patients with small cell carcinomas of the cervix.

PARANEOPLASTIC SYNDROMES

A variety of paraneoplastic syndromes have been reported associated with the secretion of bioactive peptides in patients with small cell carcinomas of the cervix. Most cases satisfy some, but not all, of the vigorous criteria to establish that the tumor is producing the aberrant peptide with hormonal activity.[23] Table 21.5 summarizes the reported cases, and includes two reports[24,25] of patients with cervical cancer that were possibly small cell cancers (but were reported prior to the establishment of the current criteria for classification). The majority of cases had Cushing syndrome (8 patients), either at initial presentation or at relapse; and elevated levels of adrenocorticotropic hormone (ACTH) were found in the tumor, in the serum, or both. Other clinical syndromes included the syndrome of inappropriate antidiuretic hormone secretion (SIADH) (3 patients), severe hypoglycemia secondary to

secretion of insulin or insulin-like peptides (2 patients), carcinoid syndrome (1 or 2 patients), Lambert–Eaton Myasthenic Syndrome (LEMS), and peripheral leukocytosis (due to secretion of granulocyte colony-stimulating factor, G-CSF). Prompt identification of these syndromes in patients could lead to earlier detection of small cell carcinoma of the cervix. In addition, monitoring the serum levels of these inappropriately secreted peptides could be used to follow response to treatment and tumor recurrence. For example, serum insulin levels initially fell in response to radiotherapy and chemotherapy, paralleling clinical improvement in a patient with an insulin-secreting small cell carcinoma of the cervix.[26]

PROGNOSTIC FACTORS

Patients with small cell carcinomas of the cervix have a very poor prognosis, with a high frequency of initial lymph node involvement, presentation at late stage of disease, and rapid widespread dissemination.[27] For stage IB1 patients with small cell carcinoma of the cervix,

Table 21.5 Small cell carcinoma of the cervix: paraneoplastic syndrome

Ref	Patient age (years)/ Stage/Outcome[a] (months)	Hormonal activity[b]	Comments[b,c]
Cushing syndrome			
69	42/IB/DOD 9	ACTH	Plasma ACTH returned to normal after surgery, increased with liver metastasis
70	35/IB/DOD 4	ACTH	Elevated plasma ACTH; liver metastasis positive for ACTH on IHC
71	38/NA/DOD	ACTH	High levels of ACTH extracted from lung and pancreatic metastasis
72	28/IIA/DOD 12	ACTH	Elevated serum ACTH and tumor cells positive for ACTH on IHC
73	38/IB/DOD 31	ACTH	Elevated plasma ACTH; positive secretory granules in metastasis, staining for ACTH
74	40/IIA/DOD 4	ACTH	Greatly elevated ACTH; failure to suppress with dexamethasone; bilateral adrenal hyperplasia and normal pituitary at autopsy
25	—	ACTH	Severe hypokalemic acidosis: elevated urinary 17-hydroxycorticosteroids that did not suppress on dexamethasone; adrenal cortical hyperplasia at autopsy
SIADH			
47	45/IVB/DOD 8.5	ADH	ADH secretion and hypercalcemia
75	59/IVB/DOD 4	ADH	Tumor positive for ADH on IHC
76	69/IVB/DOD 6	ADH	Elevated serum ADH
Hypoglycemia			
26	29/IVB/DOD 1	Insulin	Elevated serum insulin, proinsulin, and C-peptide
24	25/IV/DOD 13	Insulin	Elevated serum and tumor insulin levels
Carcinoid syndrome			
77	38/IB/DOD 18	Cortisol, ADH	Elevated serum ACTH and cortisol, tumor cells stained for ACTH
78	34/IV/DOD 0.5		Elevated urinary 5-hydroxy indol
LEMS[d]			
79	37/IB/AWD 24	—	Symptoms responded to treatment of metastatic disease with chemotherapy
Peripheral leukocytosis			
80	70/IVB/DOD 11	G-CSF	Elevated serum G-CSF, leukocytes correlated with response of tumor to treatment

[a]DOD, dead of disease; AWD, alive with disease; NA, not available.

[b]ACTH, adrenocorticotropic hormone; ADH, antidiuretic hormone; G-CSF, granulocyte colony-stimulating factor.

[c]IHC, immunohistochemistry.

[d]SIADH, syndrome of inappropriate ADH secretion; LEMS, Lambert–Eaton myasthenic syndrome.

direct comparison with adenocarcinoma and squamous cell carcinoma of the cervix at the same stage has shown significantly poorer outcomes for the small cell cancer patients (10-year survival rates of approximately 55%, 76%, and 88%, respectively).[28] Age and International Federation of Gynecology and Obstetrics (FIGO) stage-adjusted hazards of death were 1.84 greater for endocrine tumors of the cervix compared with squamous cell carcinomas.[27] Similarly, using the Reagan and Wentz classification of cervical cancers,[29] controlling for stage, patients with small cell carcinomas had a significantly inferior 5-year

Table 21.6 Prognostic factors in small cell carcinoma of the cervix

Prognostic factor	Ref	Patients	Results[a]
Stage of disease	81	55	5-yr DSS: I–IIA (44%) vs IIB–IV (25%), ($p=0.045$)
	55	11	NED: IB (50%); >IB (0%)
	28	21	5-yr SR: IB1 (56%); >IB1 (0%)
	82	15	Only 1 NED survivor: stage IB1
	35	34	3-yr FFS: I, II (80%) vs IIB–IV (0%)
	31	34	5-yr OS: I, IIA (31.6%) vs IIB–IV (0%)
	56	10	OS: IB (2/6) vs IIA–IV (0/4)
	12	16	OS: stage of disease ($p=0.035$)
	32	20	5-yr OS: IA2–IB1 (85%) vs IB2–II (25%) vs IIIB–IVA (16%)
	47	10	Only survivor had IB
	83	26	5-yr SR: I (27%) vs II–IV (0%)
	16	38	OS: I, II (8/15) vs III–IV (0/23)
	84	15	DSS: IB (2/9) vs >IB (1/6) ANED
	59	14	DSS: I, II (1/9) vs III, IV (0/6) ANED
	30	29	FFF: I, II (53%) vs III, IV (0%)
Lymph node involvement	54	25	OS: negative (44%) vs positive (17%), $p=$NS
	85	12	OS: negative (32 months) vs positive (19 months)
	34	34	OS: negative (9/14) vs positive (3/15) ($p<0.001$)
	32	20	OS: negative (72%) vs positive (11%) ($p=0.01$)
	33	40	DSS: negative (70%) vs positive (35%) ($p=0.05$)
	2	12	DFI: negative (45.9 months) vs positive (27.9 months)
Tumor size	81	45	5-yr DSS: ≤2 cm (74.1%) vs >2 cm (39%) ($p=0.03$)
	35	34	FFS: ≤5 cm ($p=0.02$)
	31	34	Median OS: ≤2 cm (not reached) vs >2 cm (14.1 months) ($p=0.01$)
	32	20	OS: <4 cm (76%) vs >4 cm (18%) ($p=0.05$)
Smoking history	81	45	2-yr DSS: nonsmokers (55.6%) vs smokers (16.7%) ($p=0.01$)
	28	21	OS: all 6 survivors were nonsmokers; 7 smokers failed ($p>0.08$)
	31	34	MS: nonsmokers (19.3 months) vs smokers (11.6 months) ($p=0.04$)
			Multivariate analyses for early-stage patients: smoking, hazard ratio = 2.08

Continued

313

Table 21.6 *(cont)* Prognostic factors in small cell carcinoma of the cervix

Prognostic factor	Ref	Patients	Results[a]
Histology (pure small	31	34	MS: mixed (not reached) vs pure (14.1 months) (*p*=0.044)
cell carcinoma	32	20	OS: mixed (19%) vs pure (54%) (*p*<0.05) but all mixed tumors
or mixed)			were >4 cm
	16	38	OS: mixed (59%) vs pure (8%) DOD (in early-stage disease,
			mixed tumors were smaller)
	33	23	OS: mixed (60%) vs pure (50%) (*p*=0.97)
Adjuvant	34	34	OS: chemotherapy regimen: PE (10/17) vs VAC (4/9) vs other
chemotherapy			(1/10) (*p* <0.01)
	33	40	DSS: VAC or PE (68%) vs other (33%) (*p*=0.0078)
	54	25	OS: no significant benefit
	28	21	RFS: no significant benefit (*p*=0.4)
	31	34	MS: yes (15.8 months) vs no (15.1 months) (*p* = 0.56)
Resection margin status	31	34	MS: negative (37.7 months) vs positive (17.8 months) (*p*=0.016)
Chromogranin on	12	16	4-yr OS: negative (58%) vs positive (0%) (*p*=0.001)
immunohistochemistry			Multivariate analysis: relative risk = 21
DNA index	15	14	OS: index ≤1.9 (3/4 alive) vs >1.9 (0/6 alive)
Ploidy	16	38	OS: diploid (4/5 NED) vs hyperploid (0/11 NED)

[a]DSS, disease-specific survival; NED, no evidence of disease; SR, survival rate; FFS, failure-free survival; OS, overall survival; FFF, freedom from failure; DFI, disease-free interval; MS, median survival; DOD, dead of disease; PE, cisplatin and etoposide; VAC, vincristine, doxorubicin, and cyclophosphamide; RFS, relapse-free survival.

survival rate (55%) compared with those with large cell nonkeratinizing cancers (68%) and keratinizing squamous cell cancers (74%) (*p* <0.01).[30]

Table 21.6 summarizes the significant prognostic factors reported in patients with small cell carcinoma of the cervix from series with at least 10 patients. Pretreatment FIGO stage is the most frequently reported significant prognostic factor in univariate analyses (Figure 21.3a). Overall survival rates for advanced stages remain poor, with few long-term survivors with

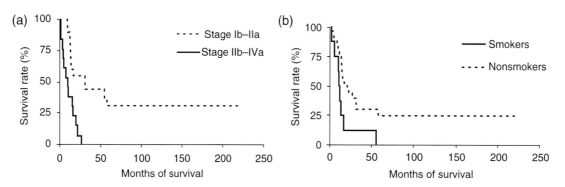

Figure 21.3 Kaplan–Meier survival analysis for FIGO stage (a) and smoking (b).

stage IIB or higher. Metastatic spread to regional lymph nodes found at the time of initial surgical treatment appears to be of significant prognostic importance. Survival in node-negative patients ranged from 44% to 72%, compared with 11–35% in patients with initial nodal involvement. In univariate analysis, larger tumor diameter (chosen as >2 cm, >4 cm or >5 cm in different studies) also correlated with worse outcome. Two reports noted a detrimental effect of smoking on outcome (Figure 21.3b). Conflicting results on the potential significance of pure versus mixed (with squamous cell carcinoma or adenocarcinoma) on outcome were noted. Two studies showed worse outcome for pure small cell carcinomas,[16,31] one showed worse outcome for patients with mixed tumors,[32] and one showed no significant effect of pure versus mixed tumors on outcome.[33] Confounding factors, such as correlation between tumor histology, size, and stage, may help explain these discordant results.[32] Single reports have also identified positive resection margins, immunohistochemical staining for chromogranin, high DNA index, and hyperploid tumors as adverse prognostic factors (Table 21.6). The influence of adjuvant chemotherapy on outcome, in particular the use of VAC (vincristine, doxorubicin, and cyclophosphamide) or PE (cisplatin and etoposide) has been shown in two studies to result in improved survival.[33,34] However, three other studies demonstrated no impact of chemotherapy on outcome.

Multivariate analyses, however, have consistently identified stage of disease as the only statistically significant prognostic factor.[28,31,35] One multivariate analysis identified both stage and IHC staining for chromogranin to be prognostically significant.[12] The small numbers of patients in each trial, the varying treatment approaches, and the retrospective nature of the analyses all limit the strength of these studies in attempting to determine clinically meaningful prognostic factors. Prospective trials, with standardized treatment regimens, stratified for stage, are needed to substantiate the important prognostic factors and to aid in the development of improved therapies.

TREATMENT

Small cell cervical carcinoma provides not only a diagnostic challenge for the pathologist but also a treatment dilemma for the gynecologic oncologist.[36,37] The Gynecologic Oncology Group (GOG) attempted to study small cell cervical carcinoma in GOG 66 from 1982 to 1986, but failed to accrue enough patients for this trial. Thus, most of the current therapeutic regimens have been derived from small single-institution series and advances made in the treatment of small cell lung cancer. Thus, the results from these small retrospective studies have made it difficult to assess the true impact of these multimodality approaches.

Surgery for early-stage disease

Primary surgery for early-stage disease has been the standard treatment for small cell neuroendocrine cervical carcinoma. van Nagell et al[30] reported on a series of patients who underwent surgery or radiotherapy without chemotherapy. Although the majority (70%) had stage I–II disease, 54% of the surgically treated patients had recurrence at any site. In another study of 14 patients with stage IB1 or IIA disease who underwent primary surgery with or without radiotherapy, Sheets et al[38] found nodal metastases in 57% of women, with only two survivors, both of whom had small (<2 cm) tumors without nodal disease. Sevin et al[2] also studied 12 patients who had undergone radical surgery, and found that although surgery is an important component in the multimodality treatment of early-stage cancer, the survival rate was only 36%. In a series of 34 patients, 23 women had early-stage disease and underwent primary surgery. Only those with small (<2 cm) lesions amenable to extirpation were cured.[31] All patients with tumors >2 cm or locally advanced tumors recurred or died of disease. Similarly, another series also showed that none of the patients who had disease more extensive than stage IB1 or clinical evidence of lymph node metastases survived, with an overall survival rate of only 29% at 5 years.[39] Thus, most studies have shown that large tumor size is correlated with survival in those with stage I disease.[2,31,38,39] Currently, there are no studies that have compared radical surgery alone with multimodality treatment in early-stage disease. Moreover, since women with more advanced disease were typically treated with radiation, it is difficult to compare these two treatment modalities. Although most patients with early-stage disease do not have metastatic disease at presentation, these tumors behave aggressively and have a proclivity to regional lymph node and distant metastasis. Thus, systemic chemotherapy should be considered as part of the standard treatment in all stages. Furthermore, given the high risk for metastatic and lymph node spread, surgical staging or more sensitive diagnostic imaging methods such as positron emission tomography (PET) may prove to be useful in detecting extrapelvic or para-aortic metastases requiring more extensive treatment.[28]

Neoadjuvant chemotherapy

Bermudez et al[32] have recommended neoadjuvant chemotherapy containing vincristine,

bleomycin, and cisplatin for patients with large lesions (>4 cm). Based on their series of 13 patients who received neoadjuvant chemotherapy, 9 patients had a >50% response to chemotherapy and 2 patients had complete response. The remaining 2 had a partial (<50%) response, 1 with stage IIB and the other with stage IIIB disease. Thus, Bermudez et al[32] suggested that preoperative chemotherapy may be a useful therapeutic tool to enhance the resectability of large tumors to improve outcome.

Adjuvant therapy

Given the aggressive nature of this disease, many authors have strongly recommended adjuvant chemotherapy after radical surgery or concurrent with radiation.[33–35] In a report assessing the patterns of recurrence, a significant number of patients have widespread dissemination of their disease involving bone, liver, lung, lymph nodes, and other soft tissues.[28] Other reports have also shown that distant metastasis is the major reason for failure.[30,38,40] Chang et al[33] treated 23 early-stage patients with postoperative chemotherapy, 14 received VAC (vincristine, doxorubicin, and cyclophosphamide) alternating with PE and 8 received PVB (cisplatin, vinblastine, and bleomycin). The 5-year survival rate was 68% for patients who received the VAC/PE regimen, compared with 33% for those treated with the PVB combination ($p = 0.0078$). In addition, Boruta et al[34] performed a multivariate analysis evaluating only patients with early-stage small cell cervical carcinoma treated with adjuvant chemotherapy with or without radiation. They found an improved survival for patients treated with chemotherapy containing VAC or PE compared with other regimens. In another series, 15 patients with poor prognostic factors on their hysterectomy specimen underwent postoperative radiotherapy with or without chemotherapy. Of these patients, 9 died of their disease secondary to distant and local recurrences, emphasizing the relative radioresistance and chemoresistance of this tumor. In this small subgroup of patients who underwent adjuvant treatment, there was no survival benefit in those who underwent radiotherapy with or without chemotherapy. However, it is notable that patients who received adjuvant therapy were those with large lesions and other poor pathologic risk factors.[31]

Hoskins et al[41] used four cycles of etoposide and cisplatin concurrent with radiotherapy similar to the regimens derived from small cell lung cancer.[42–44] In addition, prophylactic cranial radiotherapy was given in patients with no evidence of disease progression. Hoskins et al[35] subsequently developed another protocol that included carboplatin and paclitaxel with concurrent radiotherapy and did not find an improved efficacy but noted decreased toxicities associated with chemotherapy. Despite the use of these aggressive regimens, up to 35% of their patients experienced distant failure. Moreover, the 3-year overall survival rate was only 28%, with significant hematologic and gastrointestinal toxicity and two treatment-associated deaths.[35] Even though small series have shown some promising results associated with radical surgery followed by radiotherapy and chemotherapy, the true role of multimodality therapy is unclear and yields uniformly poor results, particularly in patients with advanced disease.[31,36,45–49]

Cranial irradiation

Similarly to small cell lung cancers, small cell carcinomas of the cervix have been found to have a high risk of brain metastasis in some series.[38,50,51]

A meta-analysis in small cell lung cancers showed that prophylactic cranial irradiation given to patients in complete remission can improve survival by decreasing the rate of brain metastasis.[52] Accordingly, some authors have included cranial irradiation as part of the multimodality treatment of small cell cervical carcinoma.[41] In a subsequent report, these authors no longer used cranial irradiation on a routine basis, because 23 (96%) of 24 nonirradiated patients did not recur in the central nervous system.[53] Likewise, others have not been able to demonstrate the high risk of brain metastasis. In one series of 21 patients who did not receive prophylactic cranial radiotherapy, only 2 had recurrences in the brain, and both of these were associated with concurrent lung metastases.[28]

SUMMARY

Radical hysterectomy and radiotherapy are effective therapeutic options in patients with early-stage disease; in fact, predominantly early-stage patients with small (<2 cm) tumors amenable to surgery were long-term disease-free survivors. Furthermore, smoking in early-stage and advanced-stage disease was an independent poor prognostic factors for survival. The role of primary or postoperative chemoradiotherapy is unclear and yields uniformly poor results, particularly with advanced lesions. Nevertheless, the typical approach is to treat advanced lesions with concurrent chemoradiotherapy followed by additional cycles of chemotherapy. An algorithm for the treatment of small cell cervical carcinoma based on review of the literature (Table 21.7) is provided in Figure 21.4. There has been an increased understanding of the biology of small cell lung cancer, leading to the subsequent development of innovative targeted therapeutics.

Table 21.7 Literature review of treatment and outcomes

Ref	Year	Patients	% Stage 1	Surgery	RT	Surgery + RT	CT	DFS (%)	Median OS (months)	Dead
30	1988	25	48	12	13	0	0	36	60	16
59	1988	14	29	2	11	0	3	8	12	13
84	1988	15	60	1	11	4	5	33	11	10
15	1991	14	43	≤3	6	4	≤7	—	9	8
36	1992	10	70	2	7	1	10	40	28	5
33	1998	23	100*	23	3	3	23	—	69	—
39	1994	26	58	12	5	9	Some	11	—	22
2	1996	12	83	5	0	7	0	36	20	—
40	1999	11	—	2	7	2	5	36	—	7
35	2003	31	52	0	27	4	31	54	>36	10
31	2003	34*	62	23	10	14	4	33	31	14

RT, radiotherapy; CT, chemotherapy; DFS, disease-free survival; OS, overall survival. *Stage I-II. Chart modified from Hoskins et al. J Clin Oncol 2003;21:3495-501[35] with permission from the American Society of Clinical Oncology.

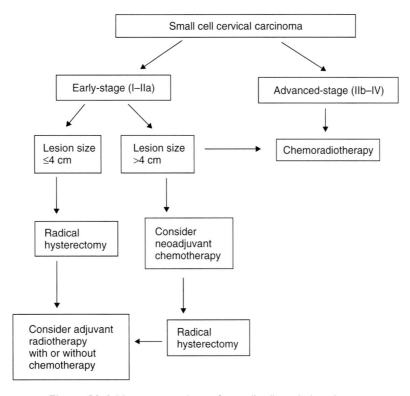

Figure 21.4 Management scheme for small cell cervical carcinoma.

Some of these promising approaches include matrix metalloproteinases, imatinib, and antisense oligonucleotides directed against *BCL2*.[53]

Clearly, advances in targeted therapies and multi-institutional clinical trials are needed for this aggressive subtype of cervical cancer.

REFERENCES

1. Albores-Saavedra J, Gersell D, Gilks CB, et al. Terminology of endocrine tumors of the uterine cervix: results of a workshop sponsored by the College of American Pathologists and the National Cancer Institute. Arch Pathol Lab Med 1997;121:34–9.

2. Sevin BU, Method MW, Nadji M, Lu Y, Averette HA. Efficacy of radical hysterectomy as treatment for patients with small cell carcinoma of the cervix. Cancer 1996;77:1489–93.

3. Tateishi R, Wada A, Hayakawa K, Hongo J, Ishii S. Argyrophil cell carcinomas (apudomas) of the uterine cervix. Light and electron microscopic observations of 5 cases. Virchows Arch A Pathol Anat Histol 1975;366:257–74.

4. Albores-Saavedra J, Larraza O, Poucell S, Rodriguez Martinez HA. Carcinoid of the uterine cervix: additional observations on a new tumor entity. Cancer 1976;38:2328–42.

5. Akoun GM, Scarna HM, Milleron BJ, Benichou MP, Herman DP. Serum neuron-specific enolase. A marker for disease extent and response to therapy for small-cell lung cancer. Chest 1985;87:39–43.

6. Burghuber OC, Worofka B, Schernthaner G, et al. Serum neuron-specific enolase is a useful

tumor marker for small cell lung cancer. Cancer 1990;65:1386–90.

7. Nakata SI, Yamamoto K, Kobayashi Y, et al. Excellent results of radiotherapy for neuroendocrine carcinoma of the uterine cervix. Oncol Rep 2001;8:777–9.

8. Chen CA, Wu CC, Juang GT, et al. Serum neuron-specific enolase levels in patients with small cell carcinoma of the uterine cervix. J Formos Med Assoc 1994;93:81–3.

9. Wistuba II, Thomas B, Behrens C, et al. Molecular abnormalities associated with endocrine tumors of the uterine cervix. Gynecol Oncol 1999;72:3–9.

10. Ishida GM, Kato N, Hayasaka T, et al. Small cell neuroendocrine carcinomas of the uterine cervix: a histological, immunohistochemical, and molecular genetic study. Int J Gynecol Pathol 2004;23:366–72.

11. Mannion C, Park WS, Man YG, et al. Endocrine tumors of the cervix: morphologic assessment, expression of human papillomavirus, and evaluation for loss of heterozygosity on 1p, 3p, 11q, and 17p. Cancer 1998; 83:1391–400.

12. Straughn JM Jr, Richter HE, Conner MG, Meleth S, Barnes MN. Predictors of outcome in small cell carcinoma of the cervix – a case series. Gynecol Oncol 2001;83:216–20.

13. Holm R, Abeler VM, Skomedal H, Nesland JM. Overexpression of p53 protein and c-erbB-2 protein in small cell carcinoma of the cervix uteri. Zentralbl Pathol 1993;139:153–6.

14. Ambros RA, Park JS, Shah KV, Kurman RJ. Evaluation of histologic, morphometric, and immunohistochemical criteria in the differential diagnosis of small cell carcinomas of the cervix with particular reference to human papillomavirus types 16 and 18. Mod Pathol 1991;4:586–93.

15. Miller B, Dockter M, el Torky M, Photopulos G. Small cell carcinoma of the cervix: a clinical and flow-cytometric study. Gynecol Oncol 1991;42:27–33.

16. Silva EG, Gershenson D, Sneige N, et al. Small cell carcinoma of the uterine cervix: pathology and prognostic factors. Surg Pathol 1989;2: 105–15.

17. Ambros RA, Park JS, Shah KV, Kurman RJ. Evaluation of histologic, morphometric, and immunohistochemical criteria in the differential diagnosis of small cell carcinomas of the cervix with particular reference to human papillomavirus types 16 and 18. Mod Pathol 1991;4:586–93.

18. Stanley MA. Human papillomavirus (HPV) vaccines: prospects for eradicating cervical cancer. J Fam Plann Reprod Health Care 2004;30:213–15.

19. Bosch FX, Manos MM, Munoz N, et al. Prevalence of human papillomavirus in cervical cancer: a worldwide perspective. International Biological Study on Cervical Cancer (IBSCC) Study Group. J Natl Cancer Inst 1995;87: 796–802.

20. Pao CC, Lin CY, Chang YL, Tseng CJ, Hsueh S. Human papillomaviruses and small cell carcinoma of the uterine cervix. Gynecol Oncol 1991;43:206–10.

21. Wang HL, Lu DW. Detection of human papillomavirus DNA and expression of p16, Rb, and p53 proteins in small cell carcinomas of the uterine cervix. Am J Surg Pathol 2004; 28:901–8.

22. Ohwada M, Wada T, Saga Y, et al. c-kit overexpression in neuroendocrine small cell carcinoma of the uterine cervix. Eur J Gynaecol Oncol 2006;27:53–5.

23. Shane JM, Naftolin F. Aberrant hormone activity by tumors of gynecologic importance. Am J Obstet Gynecol 1975;121:133–43.

24. Kiang DT, Bauer GE, Kennedy BJ. Immunoassayable insulin in carcinoma of the cervix associated with hypoglycemia. Cancer 1973;31:801–5.

25. Berthelot P, Benhamou JP, Fauvert R. [Hypercorticism and cancer of the uterus. Study of a case and review of the literature]. Presse Med 1961;69:1899–902.

26. Seckl MJ, Mulholland PJ, Bishop AE, et al. Hypoglycemia due to an insulin-secreting small-cell carcinoma of the cervix. N Engl J Med 1999;341:733–6.

27. McCusker ME, Cote TR, Clegg LX, Tavassoli FJ. Endocrine tumors of the uterine cervix: incidence, demographics, and survival with comparison to squamous cell carcinoma. Gynecol Oncol 2003;88:333–9.

28. Viswanathan AN, Deavers MT, Jhingran A, et al. Small cell neuroendocrine carcinoma of the cervix: outcome and patterns of recurrence. Gynecol Oncol 2004;93:27–33.

29. Reagan JW, Hamonic MJ, Wentz WB. Analytical study of the cells in cervical squamous-cell cancer. Lab Invest 1957;6:241–50.

30. van Nagell JR Jr, Powell DE, Gallion HH, et al. Small cell carcinoma of the uterine cervix. Cancer 1988;62:1586–93.

31. Chan JK, Loizzi V, Burger RA, Rutgers J, Monk BJ. Prognostic factors in neuroendocrine small cell cervical carcinoma: a multivariate analysis. Cancer 2003;97:568–74.

32. Bermudez A, Vighi S, Garcia A, Sardi J. Neuroendocrine cervical carcinoma: a diagnostic and therapeutic challenge. Gynecol Oncol 2001;82:32–9.

33. Chang TC, Lai CH, Tseng CJ, et al. Prognostic factors in surgically treated small cell cervical carcinoma followed by adjuvant chemotherapy. Cancer 1998;83:712–18.

34. Boruta DM 2nd, Schorge JO, Duska LA, et al. Multimodality therapy in early-stage neuroendocrine carcinoma of the uterine cervix. Gynecol Oncol 2001;81:82–7.

35. Hoskins PJ, Swenerton KD, Pike JA, et al. Small-cell carcinoma of the cervix: fourteen years of experience at a single institution using a combined-modality regimen of involved-field irradiation and platinum-based combination chemotherapy. J Clin Oncol 2003;21: 3495–501.

36. Morris M, Gershenson DM, Eifel P, et al. Treatment of small cell carcinoma of the cervix with cisplatin, doxorubicin, and etoposide. Gynecol Oncol 1992;47:62–5.

37. Stoler MH, Mills SE, Gersell DJ, Walker AN. Small-cell neuroendocrine carcinoma of the cervix. A human papillomavirus type 18-associated cancer. Am J Surg Pathol 1991;15:28–32.

38. Sheets EE, Berman ML, Hrountas CK, Liao SY, DiSaia PJ. Surgically treated, early-stage neuroendocrine small-cell cervical carcinoma. Obstet Gynecol 1988;71:10–14.

39. Abeler VM, Holm R, Nesland JM, Kjorstad KE. Small cell carcinoma of the cervix. A clinicopathologic study of 26 patients. Cancer 1994;73:672–7.

40. Sykes AJ, Shanks JH, Davidson SE. Small cell carcinoma of the uterine cervix: a clinicopathological review. Int J Oncol 1999;14: 381–6.

41. Hoskins PJ, Wong F, Swenerton KD, et al. Small cell carcinoma of the cervix treated with concurrent radiotherapy, cisplatin, and etoposide. Gynecol Oncol 1995;56:218–25.

42. Ueoka H, Kiura K, Tabata M, et al. A randomized trial of hybrid administration of cyclophosphamide, doxorubicin, and vincristine (CAV)/cisplatin and etoposide (PVP) versus sequential administration of CAV–PVP for the treatment of patients with small cell lung carcinoma: results of long term follow-up. Cancer 1998;83:283–90.

43. Fukuoka M, Furuse K, Saijo N, et al. Randomized trial of cyclophosphamide, doxorubicin, and vincristine versus cisplatin and etoposide versus alternation of these regimens in small-cell lung cancer. J Natl Cancer Inst 1991;83:855–61.

44. Roth BJ, Johnson DH, Einhorn LH, et al. Randomized study of cyclophosphamide, doxorubicin, and vincristine versus etoposide and cisplatin versus alternation of these two regimens in extensive small-cell lung cancer: a phase III trial of the Southeastern Cancer Study Group. J Clin Oncol 1992;10: 282–91.

45. Lim P, Aquino-Parsons CF, Wong F, et al. Low-risk endometrial carcinoma: assessment of a treatment policy based on tumor ploidy and identification of additional prognostic indicators. Gynecol Oncol 1999;73:191–5.

46. Kim YB, Barbuto D, Lagasse LD, Karlan BY. Successful treatment of neuroendocrine small cell carcinoma of the cervix metastatic to regional lymph nodes. Gynecol Oncol 1996;62:411–14.

47. Delaloge S, Pautier P, Kerbrat P, et al. Neuroendocrine small cell carcinoma of the uterine cervix: What disease? What treatment? Report of ten cases and a review of the literature. Clin Oncol (R Coll Radiol) 2000;12:357–62.

48. O'Hanlan KA, Goldberg GL, Jones JG, et al. Adjuvant therapy for neuroendocrine small cell carcinoma of the cervix: review of the literature. Gynecol Oncol 1991;43:167–72.

49. Lewandowski GS, Copeland LJ. A potential role for intensive chemotherapy in the treatment of small cell neuroendocrine tumors of the cervix. Gynecol Oncol 1993;48:127–31.

50. Weed JC, Shoup B, Tawfik O. Small cell carcinoma of the cervix: a clinical study of 15 patients and review of the literature. Prim Care Update Ob Gyns 1998;5:159.

51. Perrin L, Ward B. Small cell carcinoma of the cervix. Int J Gynecol Cancer 1995; 5:200–3.

52. Auperin A, Arriagada R, Pignon JP, et al. Prophylactic cranial irradiation for patients with small-cell lung cancer in complete remission. Prophylactic Cranial Irradiation Overview Collaborative Group. N Engl J Med 1999;341:476–84.

53. Wistuba II, Gazdar AF, Minna JD. Molecular genetics of small cell lung carcinoma. Semin Oncol 2001;28(2 Suppl 4):3–13.

54. Wang KL, Yang YC, Wang TY, et al. Neuroendocrine carcinoma of the uterine cervix: a clinicopathologic retrospective study of 31 cases with prognostic implications. J Chemother 2006;18:209–16.

55. Tsunoda S, Jobo T, Arai M, et al. Small-cell carcinoma of the uterine cervix: a clinicopathologic study of 11 cases. Int J Gynecol Cancer 2005;15:295–300.

56. Masumoto N, Fujii T, Ishikawa M, et al. p16 overexpression and human papillomavirus infection in small cell carcinoma of the uterine cervix. Hum Pathol 2003;34:778–83.

57. Wang SJ, Wang MB, Calcaterra TC. Radiotherapy followed by neck dissection for small head and neck cancers with advanced cervical metastases. Ann Otol Rhinol Laryngol 1999;108:128–31.

58. Huang SF, Shueh S, Chang TC. Small cell carcinoma of the uterine cervix: pathologic analysis of 9 cases. Taiwan Yi Xue Hui Za Zhi 1988;87:297–303.

59. Walker AN, Mills SE, Taylor PT. Cervical neuroendocrine carcinoma: a clinical and light microscopic study of 14 cases. Int J Gynecol Pathol 1988;7:64–74.

60. Saul PB. The clinical management of small cell carcinoma of the cervix. In: Rutledge RF, Gershenson D, eds. Gynecologic Cancer. Austin: University of Texas Press, 1987:245–250.

61. Barrett RJ 2nd, Davos I, Leuchter RS, Lagasse LD. Neuroendocrine features in poorly differentiated and undifferentiated carcinomas of the cervix. Cancer 1987;60: 2325–30.

62. Albores-Saavedra J, Larraza O, Poucell S, Rodriguez Martinez HA. Carcinoid of the uterine cervix: additional observations on a new tumor entity. Cancer 1976;38:2328–42.

63. Ueda G, Shimizu C, Shimizu H, et al. An immunohistochemical study of small-cell and poorly differentiated carcinomas of the cervix using neuroendocrine markers. Gynecol Oncol 1989;34:164–9.

64. Ulich TR, Liao SY, Layfield L, et al. Endocrine and tumor differentiation markers in poorly

differentiated small-cell carcinoids of the cervix and vagina. Arch Pathol Lab Med 1986;110:1054–7.

65. Groben P, Reddick R, Askin F. The pathologic spectrum of small cell carcinoma of the cervix. Int J Gynecol Pathol 1985;4:42–57.

66. Yamasaki M, Tateishi R, Hongo J, et al. Argyrophil small cell carcinomas of the uterine cervix. Int J Gynecol Pathol 1984;3:146–52.

67. Silva EC, Kott MM, Ordonez NG. Endocrine carcinoma intermediate cell type of the uterine cervix. Cancer 1984;54:1705–13.

68. Herrington CS, Graham D, Southern SA, Bramdev A, Chetty R. Loss of retinoblastoma protein expression is frequent in small cell neuroendocrine carcinoma of the cervix and is unrelated to HPV type. Hum Pathol 1999;30:906–10.

69. Hashi A, Yasumizu T, Yoda I, et al. A case of small cell carcinoma of the uterine cervix presenting Cushing's syndrome. Gynecol Oncol 1996;61:427–31.

70. Iemura K, Sonoda T, Hayakawa A, et al. Small cell carcinoma of the uterine cervix showing Cushing's syndrome caused by ectopic adrenocorticotropin hormone production. Jpn J Clin Oncol 1991;21:293–8.

71. Inoue T, Yamaguchi K, Suzuki H, Abe K, Chihara T. Production of immunoreactive-polypeptide hormones in cervical carcinoma. Cancer 1984;53:1509–14.

72. Lojek MA, Fer MF, Kasselberg AG, et al. Cushing's syndrome with small cell carcinoma of the uterine cervix. Am J Med 1980;69:140–4.

73. Matsuyama M, Inoue T, Ariyoshi Y, et al. Argyrophil cell carcinoma of the uterine cervix with ectopic production of ACTH, β-MSH, serotonin, histamine, and amylase. Cancer 1979;44:1813–23.

74. Jones HW, Plymate S, Gluck FB, Miles PA, Greene JF. Small cell nonkeratinizing carcinoma of the cervix associated with ACTH production. Cancer 1976;38:1629–35.

75. Ishibashi-Ueda H, Imakita M, Yutani C, et al. Small cell carcinoma of the uterine cervix with syndrome of inappropriate antidiuretic hormone secretion. Mod Pathol 1996;9: 397–400.

76. Kothe MJ, Prins JM, de Wit R, Velden KV, Schellekens PT. Small cell carcinoma of the cervix with inappropriate antidiuretic hormone secretion. Case report. Br J Obstet Gynaecol 1990;97:647–8.

77. Stockdale AD, Leader M, Phillips RH, Henry K. The carcinoid syndrome and multiple hormone secretion associated with a carcinoid tumour of the uterine cervix. Case report. Br J Obstet Gynaecol 1986;93:397–401.

78. Driessens J, Clay A, Adenis L, Demaille A. [Cervico-uterine tumor and biologic syndrome of carcinoidosis]. Arch Anat Pathol (Paris) 1964;12:200–3.

79. Sutton GP, Siemers E, Stehman FB, Ehrlich CE. Eaton-Lambert syndrome as a harbinger of recurrent small-cell carcinoma of the cervix with improvement after combination chemotherapy. Obstet Gynecol 1988;72: 516–18.

80. Watanabe A, Wachi T, Omi H, et al. Granulocyte colony-stimulating factor-producing small-cell carcinoma of the uterine cervix: report of a case. Diagn Cytopathol 2000;23:269–74.

81. Lee NK, Nguyen S, Cheung MK, et al. Neuroendocrine small cell cervical carcinoma – an analysis of prognostic factors. Proceedings of Western Association of Gynecologic Oncologists, 2006.

82. Weed JC Jr, Graff AT, Shoup B, Tawfik O. Small cell undifferentiated (neuroendocrine) carcinoma of the uterine cervix. J Am Coll Surg 2003;197:44–51.

83. Abeler VM, Holm R, Nesland JM, Kjorstad KE. Small cell carcinoma of the cervix.

A clinical study of 26 patients. Cancer 1994; 73:672–7.

84. Gersell DJ MG, Mutch DG, Rudloff MA. Small-cell undifferentiated carcinoma of the cervix. A clinicopathologic, ultrastructural, and immunocytochemical study of 15 cases. Am J Surg Pathol 1988;12:684–98.

85. Yu A, Zhang P, Lou H. Clinicopathologic characteristics and treatment of small cell carcinoma of uterine cervix. Zhonghua Zhong Liu Za Zhi 2002;24:400–3.

Predictive values of sentinel lymph nodes

22

Michael Frumovitz, Robert L Coleman, and Charles F Levenback

HISTORY OF SENTINEL NODES IN SURGICAL ONCOLOGY

Anatomists proposed in the 17th century that cancer spread from primary tumors to regional lymph nodes.[1] By the end of the 19th century, surgical and anesthetic techniques improved to allow major surgical procedures for patients with cancer. William Halsted pioneered radical mastectomy and axillary lymphadenectomy to treat patients with breast cancer. The operation was designed to remove the tumor, primary organ, regional lymph nodes, and intervening skin, fat, and lymphatic channels. Widespread application of this approach resulted in dramatically improved survival outcomes; however, short- and long-term morbidity was high. This was considered an acceptable alternative to a slow, agonizing death from a locally advanced tumor.

The Halsted model was replicated for most solid tumor sites. Stanley Way and others[2–4] pioneered radical vulvectomy and en bloc inguinal femoral and pelvic lymphadenectomy for patients with vulvar cancer. The first radical hysterectomy was performed in 1893 by John Goodrich Clark, and then replicated and popularized throughout the world. Surgical mortality rates at the start of the 20th century for radical hysterectomy series ranged up to 30%. At the time, this high mortality rate was considered tolerable, as these radical procedures cured patients with tumors previously believed incurable. Medical and social norms shifted leading to increasing detection and treatment of smaller tumors. This in turn led to the development of surgical techniques to reduce the mortality, morbidity, and mutilating effects of these operations. Nevertheless, certain complications, especially lymphedema, remain prominent.

Throughout the 20th century and into the 21st century, clinical experience has shown repeatedly that the single most important adverse prognostic factor in most patients with stage I solid tumors is the presence of metastatic disease in regional lymph nodes.[5] The importance of this observation has increased in the modern era as detection of smaller and smaller primary tumors has become possible with screening methods such as cervical cytology and mammography. Detection of small-volume metastatic disease associated with small primary tumors can only be reliably achieved with the removal of lymph nodes and with histologic analysis. There are no imaging techniques – cross-sectional, ultrasound, or molecular – that achieve the same sensitivity and specificity as histologic analysis.

For these reasons, regional lymphadenectomy has been a cornerstone in the surgical treatment of stage I solid tumors at multiple sites, including cancer of the female reproductive tract. Extensive clinical experience has repeatedly shown that the majority of stage I patients do not have lymph node metastases, while regional lymphadenectomy is associated with a significant risk of complications. Lymphedema is an especially troubling complication, with both cosmetic and functional sequelae, as treatment for this complication is limited and largely ineffective.

It is important to note that regional lymphadenectomy is generally considered diagnostic, not therapeutic. Patients with positive regional lymph nodes in any disease site almost always receive some form of adjuvant therapy – implicit acknowledgement that patients with positive regional lymph nodes are at increased risk for relapse.

The morbidity of regional lymphadenectomy led many investigators to develop techniques to enhance the detection of lymph node metastases while reducing morbidity. For years, clinical investigators have been injecting various compounds in vivo to study lymphatic anatomy and local sites of metastases. These efforts include injecting India ink into the cervix,[6] Indigo Carmine into the appendix,[7] Sky Blue into the stomach,[8] and Patent Blue into the female reproductive tract,[9–11] as well as utilizing ethiodized oil for penile lymphography.[12]

A group led by Donald Morton is credited with introducing lymphatic mapping and sentinel lymph node biopsy into modern surgical oncology with the systematic development of the techniques that are now in common use.[13–15] The sentinel lymph node is defined as the lymph node that is the first site of metastatic disease. Lymphatic mapping is the procedure used to identify the sentinel lymph node, and usually includes peritumoral injection of a weak radiocolloid and or a vital blue dye.

Numerous studies at multiple disease sites confirm that the sensitivity and negative predictive value of the sentinel lymph node are very high. These early results, as well as very

high surgeon and patient acceptance, led to wide adoption of the technique,[16] which in turn drove changes in the American Joint Commission on Cancer (AJCC) staging manual. In 2002, the melanoma TMN (tumor, lymph node, metastasis) classification underwent several major changes. Prior to 1997, the N1 category was any number of metastases <3 cm in size. In 2002, N1a became one lymph node with micrometastases and N1b one lymph node with macrometastases. The N1a category become possible due to the widespread use of sentinel lymph node biopsy.[17,18]

The impact of sentinel lymph node biopsy on breast cancer staging is even more dramatic. The 2002 AJCC modifications include specific reference to pathologic staging of sentinel lymph nodes. The pN category is subdivided into categories: no regional lymph node metastases histologically; lymph nodes with positive immunohistochemical findings <0.2 mm or positive by reverse transcriptase polymerase chain reaction (RT–PCR), lymph nodes histologically positive with metastases between 0.2 and 2 mm, and lymph nodes histologically positive with metastases >2 mm. These changes recognize that small clusters of malignant cells in the sentinel lymph node do not imply the same adverse prognosis as larger deposits of malignant cells. Lymph node status, at least in breast cancer patients, is no longer a simple binary function, either positive or negative.

Modern lymphatic mapping and sentinel lymph node biopsy requires a team approach. Nuclear medicine specialists assist surgeons in locating sentinel lymph nodes, especially in situations where there is complex lymphatic drainage to multiple regional lymphatic basins (e.g. truncal melanoma). Surgical specialists need the training and experience to accurately identify sentinel lymph nodes to minimize the risk of false-negative sentinel lymph nodes.

Detection of micrometastases in a sentinel lymph node depends on expert histopathology laboratories and pathologists. The full potential of this approach is only realized when all three specialties are performing at a high level of competence.

SENTINEL NODES IN GYNECOLOGIC MALIGNANCIES

As previously mentioned, the status of regional lymph nodes is the most important prognostic factor in patients with cancer of the uterus, cervix, and vulva. For that reason, regional lymph node dissections are routinely performed in the surgical treatment of these malignancies. Lymphatic mapping and sentinel lymph node biopsy are appealing possibilities for the identification of those lymph nodes most at risk for metastatic disease in women with vulvar, cervical, and uterine cancers, and have been studied extensively for these malignancies. Preoperative and intraoperative modalities can direct surgeons to the key lymph node basins draining the primary tumor (Figures 22.1 and 22.2). These techniques may discover multiple or aberrant lymph node basins. Once a sentinel lymph node has been identified, ultrastaging with immunohistochemistry may be performed to determine if micrometastatic disease is present in the sentinel lymph node.

SENTINEL LYMPH NODES IN VULVAR CANCER

Identification rate, sensitivity, false-negative rate, and negative predictive value (Table 22.1)

A meta-analysis of 279 patients who underwent lymphatic mapping as part of their treatment for vulvar cancer found the procedure to be highly feasible, with a sentinel node identification rate of 83.3%. The seemingly high rate of 16.7% with no sentinel node identified must be considered in light of the fact that the reported rate is per groin, not per patient. Therefore, patients with a lesion that approaches midline likely had bilateral groin dissections performed even though lymphatic drainage was probably only to the ipsilateral groin. Overall, the sensitivity of the sentinel node for detecting metastatic disease was 97.7% and the false-negative rate for the procedure, defined as positive lymph node metastasis in the lymphadenectomy specimen in the absence of metastatic tumor in the sentinel node identified, was 2.3%.[19] Of the 279 patients reviewed, only 2 false-negatives were reported – both at the same institution.[20] These investigators utilized blue dye only and found 14 groin metastases in 9 patients. In those patients, 9 groins had sentinel nodes positive for disease, 2 had false-negative sentinel nodes found, and 3 groins had no sentinel node found. The other study that used blue dye only had no false-negative sentinel nodes, but did have two groins with metastatic disease and no sentinel node found.[21] The remaining five studies utilized radiocolloid with or without blue dye, and had a sensitivity of 100% with no false-negative sentinel nodes.[22–26] The overall negative predictive value was 99.3%.

Location and identification of sentinel lymph node basins

One of the advantages of lymphatic mapping and sentinel lymph node identification is localization of those lymph node basins most at risk for metastatic disease. For example, primary lesions approaching, but not crossing, the midline typically have ipsilateral groin drainage. Preoperative lymphoscintigraphy could delineate

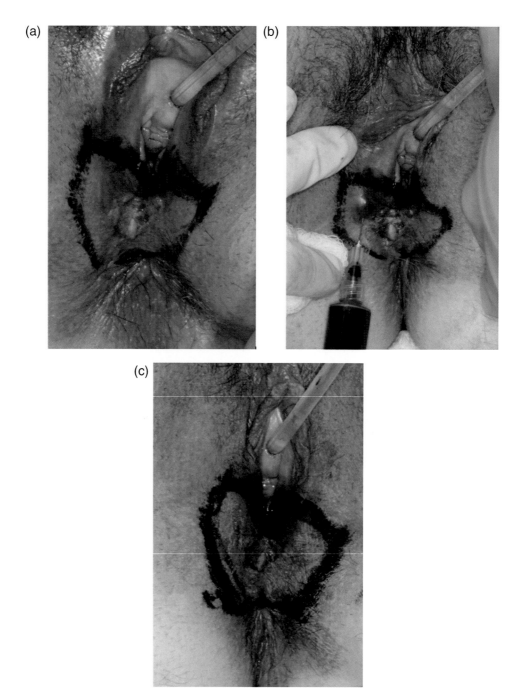

Figure 22.1 Lymphatic mapping of a midline perineal vulvar cancer. The lesion is (a) marked with a 2 cm margin and (b) then injected with Patent Blue dye intradermally in four quadrants around the tumor. (c) The dye is taken up by the lymphatics and transported to the draining nodal basins.

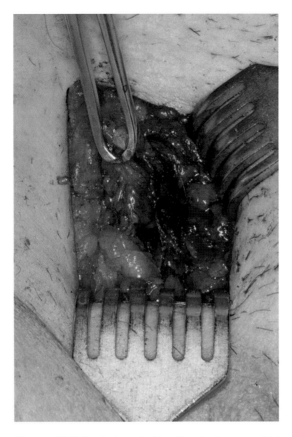

Figure 22.2 Sentinel node identified in the superficial inguinofemoral triangle.

an ipsilateral exploration would have been done otherwise. For lesions that cross the midline, we recommend bilateral groin exploration regardless of preoperative imaging.

Intraoperatively, sentinel nodes may be difficult to localize, depending on the anatomic location of the primary lesion. Although universally found below Camper's fascia, the position within the inguinal triangle may vary for lateral, midline, or clitoral lesions. Patients with clitoral lesions have been noted to have short afferent lymph channels, with sentinel nodes often located in a very medial location just lateral to the adductor longus muscle. This differs from the lateral lesions, whose draining nodes are often found just below the inguinal ligament.[21] The difficulty in locating the sentinel lymph node in patients with clitoral lesions may predict a higher risk of groin recurrence.[29] These 'recurrences' are likely due to residual disease left in situ at the time of primary groin dissection due to their medial location.

unilateral or bilateral lymphatic drainage of the primary tumor and potentially spare appropriate patients from bilateral groin dissections. Even lesions that are seemingly lateralized have been shown to have lymphatic drainage to the contralateral groin.[27,28] For these women, bilateral groin dissections can be performed when

Ultrastaging

The identification of micrometastasis in the sentinel lymph nodes of patients with vulvar cancer has been explored. Hematoxylin and eosin (H&E) staining after ultrastaging of sentinel nodes, described as the cutting of paraffin-embedded tissue in 400–500 μm intervals as opposed to 2–3 mm intervals, and immunohistochemical staining with cytokeratin has led to the identification of micrometastasis in sentinel lymph nodes thought to be negative on traditional pathologic processing.[25,30] Others have performed ultrastaging on all of the nodes in complete vulvar lymphadenectomy specimens and have found that as many as 42% of women with node-negative disease by H&E staining were actually positive for

Table 22.1 Overall identification (ID) rate, sensitivity, false-negative rate (FNR), and negative predictive value (NPV) for sentinel nodes in vulvar and cervical cancers

Site	ID rate (%)	Sensitivity (%)	FNR (%)	NPV (%)
Vulva	83.3	97.7	2.3	99.3
Cervix	89.0	91.3	8.7	97.0

micrometastatic disease.[31] Furthermore, the women with micrometastases were 20 times more likely to recur than those who were node-negative with immunohistochemistry. These numbers have not been replicated in other studies, and may not apply to sentinel nodes. Therefore, detection of micrometastases in sentinel nodes of patients with vulvar cancer is of unknown importance. However, at least one case report of a groin recurrence in a patient with a micrometastasis in a sentinel lymph node has been reported.[32] We believe that ultrastaging of sentinel nodes only and H&E staining of nonsentinel lymph nodes is acceptable for patients who undergo lymphatic mapping. Should sentinel node biopsy be accepted as standard of care, thereby excluding complete lymphadenectomy, we will likely continue to perform ultrastaging on the sentinel nodes removed.

SENTINEL LYMPH NODES IN CERVICAL CANCER

Identification rate, sensitivity, false-negative rate, and negative predictive value (Table 22.1)

In a review of 649 patients with cervical cancer who underwent lymphatic mapping and sentinel lymph node biopsy, the overall rate for detecting at least one sentinel lymph node in the patient was 89%. There did not appear to be much difference in sentinel node detection when comparing those studies that used blue dye only (88%) with those that used radiocolloid only (87%) with those that used the combined modalities (91%). Sentinel node identification may be decreased, however, in patients with large tumors (>4 cm)[33] or locally advanced disease.[34] Some investigators have reported a decreased identification rate in

patients with prior conization,[35] but others have not found this relationship valid.[36] The effect of benign gynecologic conditions such as endometriosis or past pelvic inflammatory disease, obstetric trauma, or prior cesarean section on successful identification of the sentinel node are not currently known.

In the combined studies, the overall sensitivity of the sentinel lymph node for detecting metastatic disease in patients with cervical cancer was 91.3%. The overall false-negative rate was 8.7% and the overall negative predictive value for the combined studies was 97%.

Location and identification of sentinel lymph node basins

Marnitz et al[37] reviewed the location of sentinel nodes in 151 patients with cervical cancer who underwent lymphatic mapping as part of their surgical staging. They found that 91% of all sentinel nodes were located in the pelvis, below the bifurcation of the internal and external iliac vessels. An additional 5% of sentinel nodes were located along the common iliac vessels and another 4% were para-aortic or precaval, above the bifurcation of the aorta. They used a variety of intraoperative methods to identify sentinel nodes, including Patent Blue dye, radiocolloid, and both. Preoperative lymphoscintigraphy was not part of their protocol, however.

We reviewed our experience, with the addition of preoperative lymphoscintigraphy to intraoperative mapping with blue dye and radiocolloid in women with cervical cancer, and found minimal usefulness in identifying additional at-risk nodes over intraoperative mapping techniques alone.[38] In contrast to a lateralized vulvar carcinoma, cervical cancer affects a midline structure, with all primary lymph node basins in the pelvis or on the abdominal portion of the aorta. The addition of lymphoscintigraphy therefore does not determine surgical approach or incision type, as it might in certain vulvar cancers. Also, the entire field of lymph nodes draining the primary lesion are in view of the surgeon intra-operatively, so blue dye and radiocolloid can be followed under direct visualization and with a hand-held gamma counter. We have therefore abandoned preoperative lymphoscintigraphy in women with cervical cancer, as it is expensive and time-consuming with unproven clinical benefit.

Ultrastaging

Controversy remains over the necessity of microsectioning and immunohistologic stain-ing of sentinel nodes in women with cervical cancer. Levenback et al[36] resubmitted sentinel nodes from 31 patients with no metastasis found on routine H&E sectioning. For these specimens, serial step sectioning was per-formed, with no additional metastasis being detected. Furthermore, 10 of these patients with no metastasis found on H&E staining or serial step sectioning had their sentinel nodes subjected to additional immunohistochemical analysis, with no additional metastasis being found. One patient with a documented metas-tasis on H&E in a pelvic sentinel node had a micrometastasis found in a contralateral sen-tinel node with microstaging. These conclu-sions are supported by Niikura et al,[39] who submitted all pathologically negative sentinel nodes on H&E staining for immunohisto-chemistry, with no additional metastasis being detected. Angioli et al[40] also reported no addi-tional metastasis found using immunohisto-chemistry on sentinel lymph nodes without tumor on H&E. In contrast, Barranger et al[41] found 12 sentinel nodes with metastatic disease

in eight patients. Of these 12 nodes, 4 (33%) had grossly positive, macroscopic disease, 5 (42%) were detected on H&E staining, and 3 (25%) were found on immunohistochemical staining. These results would argue for the importance of microstaging of sentinel lymph nodes. None of these studies has follow-up data that speak to the clinical significance of these micrometas-tases detected on immunohistochemistry.

SENTINEL LYMPH NODES IN UTERINE CANCER

Identification rate, sensitivity, false-negative rate, and negative predictive value

Comparatively, lymphatic mapping in corpus epithelial malignancy has been much less inves-tigated. Nonetheless, the value of identifying, with precision, metastatic lymphatic disease is just as important. Since the vast majority (approximately 85–90% of unselected cases) of clinical stage I and II patients will not have metastatic disease, the merit of systematic lymphatic dissection to determine spread is uncertain. However, in the absence of specific preoperative or intraoperative clues, such procedures are routinely performed to identify this important prognostic factor. In light of this situation, limited but directed evaluation as produced through a lymphatic mapping proce-dure would be of great value for patients with this disease, if validated.

Sentinel node mapping for endometrial cancer entered formal investigation in 1996, when Burke et al[42] reported on 15 patients undergoing intraoperative lymphatic mapping during laparotomy. They injected blue dye directly into the fundus at various points and at a depth felt to represent myometrial invasion. A sentinel node was identified in just 67%

of cases. The success of sentinel node identification has largely improved since this initial report, and has expanded to involve laparoscopic and hysteroscopic injection of both blue dye and radionuclide.

In a recent review of endometrial lymphatic mapping procedures,[43] we identified 12 publications in which the procedure was piloted. In all, 206 patients have been studied by various techniques, producing a global detection rate of approximately 85%. The lowest rate of success and highest false-negative rates were observed among the two trials where fundal injection of blue dye was performed at laparotomy (one with no sentinel nodes identified).[42,44] One other study of two cohorts utilized fundal or cervical and fundal injection with laparoscopic evaluation.[45] These investigators concluded that the number and detection rate of a sentinel node was improved by combining dye and nuclide and utilizing dual injection of the uterus. Unfortunately, hypothesis testing was not performed to define the sensitivity or false-negative rate in these two cohorts. Cervical injection, similar to the technique used in primary cervical cancer, appears to increase the detection rate of a sentinel node in several small series.[46–50] No false-negative cases were reported; however, the reliability and accuracy of the resulting nodal distribution following cervical injection in these series of uterine cancer patients is unknown. This has prompted investigators to perform direct peritumoral injection with hysteroscopic visualization. Arguably, this technique should produce the most accurate information on preferential node drainage. Limited recent investigation (four studies, with 82 patients) has identified a sentinel node in 93% of patients, with no false-negative lymphatic dissections.[51–54] Future studies are pursuing standardization of this approach.

Location and identification of sentinel lymph node basins

As beautifully illustrated in the monograph by Plentl and Friedman,[55] the lymphatic drainage of the corpus is diffuse and may preferentially utilize any of the dominant uterine trunks (femoral, interiliac, and aortic), depending on tumor residence in the corpus. The initial report of fundal injection by Burke et al,[42] while a crude estimation of an individual's tumor, highlighted the resulting ambiguity of lymphatic drainage basins and the spectrum of potential sentinel node locales. A unique finding in this study was the identification of sentinel nodes lying in the para-aortic chain above the root of the inferior mesenteric artery. Clinically, however, ordered cephalic flow and implantation of metastatic disease is more frequently apparent. Isolated para-aortic metastatic disease in the absence of pelvic metastases has been documented, but is uncommon. In a large clinicopathologic study from the Gynecologic Oncology Group (GOG), this event occurred in only 3% of patients.[56] Nonetheless, conditions such as deep invasion and fundal or cornual implantation of tumor may preferentially favor this mechanism. Since the tumor may be nonfocal and variably invasive, the spectrum of sentinel node locales is likely tumor-specific and determined by characteristics not easily defined preoperatively or intraoperatively.

As appears to be the case in primary cancer of the uterine cervix, nodal spread from endometrial malignancy accessing the paracervical/parametrial trunks has a distribution that favors the interiliac basins. In a recent study by Maccauro et al,[52] blue dye and radionuclide were injected hysteroscopically in 26 patients. A total of 65 sentinel nodes were identified, with approximately 63% being unilateral.

The sentinel node was in the pelvic basin in 79% of samples. The distribution of metastatic disease (five nodes in four patients) was reflective of the distribution of the identified sentinel nodes. However, a dominant laterality and predicted order (first-echelon) lymphatics based on tumor topography is not well defined. As such, both sides of the pelvic and para-aortic nodes must be evaluated. It is likely that successive secondary sites (second-echelon nodes) along these lymphatic chains will incorporate the lower and upper para-aortic locations. However, primary drainage to the upper para-aortic nodes can occur through lymphatics accompanying the ovarian vessels. While likely to be an uncommon primary mechanism, these minor trunks are important to evaluate in all mapping studies.

Ultrastaging

The previous discussion of sentinel node ultrastaging as it applies to vulvar and cervical cancer is relevant to uterine cancer. Since mapping investigation in this site is relatively new, adaptations of ultrastaging techniques are now routinely applied to discovered sentinel nodes, with similar concerns regarding implication and prognostic value of micrometastatic disease. Barranger et al[50] documented in five patients, 10 sentinel nodes with metastatic disease. None was positive by imprint cytology, and just three were positive by H&E staining. The rest were identified by cytokeratin immunohistochemistry. This group mapped all sentinel nodes to the pelvic drainage basins following cervical

injection of blue dye and radionuclide. Of interest, none of the patients with identified micrometastatic lymphatic disease was treated with adjuvant therapy. Clinical follow-up was not reported. In contrast, Niikura et al[54] reported on 28 patients undergoing hysteroscopic lymphatic mapping using a dual-tracer method. Out of 71 nodes, 70 were negative by H&E for metastatic disease. None was identified with cytokeratin staining. Currently, whether such micrometastatic disease is prognostic and warrants postoperative therapy (such as gross metastatic disease) or prognostic and warrants close surveillance (such as myometrial lymphovascular space invasion or high grade) or can be safely discounted is a matter of further study.

CONCLUSIONS

Most patients with gynecologic malignancy undergoing surgical staging will not have metastatic nodal disease. While identification of this factor is highly prognostic and defining for adjuvant therapy, the improvement of precision via lymphatic mapping stands to potentially benefit patients by limiting blinded evaluation and focusing sampling on the highest-risk areas. This latter result helps to identify those patients with aberrant lymphatic basins. Thus, sentinel node identification, if validated, provides a more accurate way to assess this important prognostic factor and, by identifying a limited number of 'at-risk' nodes, enables future biomarker discovery to further define clinical behavior and risk.

REFERENCES

1. Borgstein P, Meijer S. Historical perspective of lymphatic tumour spread and the emergence of the sentinel node concept. Eur J Surg Oncol 1998;24:85–9.

2. Way S. Carcinoma of the vulva. Am J Obstet Gynecol 1960;79:692.

3. Taussig FJ. Cancer of the vulva: an analysis of 155 cases. Am J Obstet Gynecol 1940; 40:764–73.

4. Twombly G. The technique of radical vulvectomy for carcinoma of the vulva. Cancer 1953;3:516–30.

5. Morton DL, Wanek L, Nizze JA, Elashoff RM, Wong JH. Improved long-term survival after lymphadenectomy of melanoma metastatic to regional nodes. Analysis of prognostic factors in 1134 patients from the John Wayne Cancer Clinic. Ann Surg 1991;214:499–501.

6. Zeit PR, Wilcoxon G. In vivo coloring of pelvic lymph nodes with India ink. Am J Obstet Gynecol 1950;59:1164–6.

7. Braithwaite L. Flow of lymph from iliocecal angle. Br J Surg 1923;11:7.

8. Weinberg J, Greaney E. Identification of Regional Lymph Nodes by Means of a Vital Staining Dye During Surgery of Gastric Cancer. Van Nuys, CA: University of California at Los Angeles, School of Medicine.

9. Eichner E, Bove ER. In vivo studies on the lymphatic drainage of the human ovary. Obstet Gynecol 1954;3:287–97.

10. Eichner E, Mallin LP, Angell ML. Further experience with direct sky blue in the in vivo studies of gynecologic lymphatics. Am J Obstet Gynecol 1955;69:1019–26.

11. Eichner E, Rubinstein L. Cervical stump lymphatics. Obstet Gynecol 1958;12:521–7.

12. Cabanas RM. An approach for the treatment of penile carcinoma. Cancer 1977;39:456–66.

13. Robinson DS, Sample WF, Fee HJ, Holmes C, Morton DL. Regional lymphatic drainage in primary malignant melanoma of the trunk determined by colloidal gold scanning. Surg Forum 1977;28:147–8.

14. Wong JH. Lymphatic drainage of skin in a sentinel lymph node in a feline model. Ann Surg 1991;214:637–41.

15. Morton DL, Wen DR, Wong JH, et al. Technical details of intraoperative lymphatic mapping for early stage melanoma. Arch Surg 1992;127:392–9.

16. Hampton T. Surgeons vote with their feet for sentinel node biopsy for breast cancer staging. JAMA 2003;290:3053–4.

17. Balch CM, Cascinelli N. Sentinel-node biopsy in melanoma. N Engl J Med 2006;355: 1370–1.

18. Morton DL, Hoon DS, Cochran AJ, et al. Lymphatic mapping and sentinel lymphadenectomy for early-stage melanoma. Ann Surg 2003;238:538–49.

19. Frumovitz M, Ramirez PT, Levenback C. Lymphatic mapping and sentinel node detection in gynecologic malignancies of the lower genital tract. Curr Oncol Rep 2005; 7:435–43.

20. Ansink AC, Sie-Go DM, van der Velden J, et al. Identification of sentinel lymph nodes in vulvar carcinoma patients with the aid of a patent blue V injection: a multicenter study. Cancer 1999;86:652–6.

21. Levenback C, Coleman RL, Burke TW, et al. Intraoperative lymphatic mapping and sentinel node identification with blue dye in patients with vulvar cancer. Gynecol Oncol 2001;83:276–81.

22. Sideri M, De Cicco C, Maggioni A, et al. Detection of sentinel nodes by lymphoscintigraphy and gamma probe guided surgery in vulvar neoplasia. Tumori 2000;86:359–63.

23. Sliutz G, Reinthaller A, Lantzsch T, et al. Lymphatic mapping of sentinel nodes in early vulvar cancer. Gynecol Oncol 2002;84: 449–52.

24. de Hullu JA, Hollema H, Piers DA, et al. Sentinel lymph node procedure is highly accurate in squamous cell carcinoma of the vulva. J Clin Oncol 2000;18:2811–16.

25. Puig-Tintore LM, Ordi J, Vidal-Sicart S, et al. Further data on the usefulness of sentinel lymph node identification and ultrastaging in

vulvar squamous cell carcinoma. Gynecol Oncol 2003;88:29–34.

26. Moore RG, Granai CO, Gajewski W, Gordinier M, Steinhoff MM. Pathologic evaluation of inguinal sentinel lymph nodes in vulvar cancer patients: a comparison of immunohistochemical staining versus ultrastaging with hematoxylin and eosin staining. Gynecol Oncol 2003;91:378–82.

27. Carlomagno G, Di Blasi A. Report of two cases of contralateral groin recurrence after ipsilateral groin node dissection for vulval cancer. Eur J Gynaecol Oncol 2005;26:665–6.

28. Jackson KS, Das N, Naik R, Lopes A, Monaghan JM. Contralateral groin node metastasis following ipsilateral groin node dissection in vulval cancer: a case report. Gynecol Oncol 2003;89:529–31.

29. Frumovitz M, Ramirez PT, Tortolero-Luna G, et al. Characteristics of recurrence in patients who underwent lymphatic mapping for vulvar cancer. Gynecol Oncol 2004;92:205–10.

30. Terada KY, Shimizu DM, Wong JH. Sentinel node dissection and ultrastaging in squamous cell cancer of the vulva. Gynecol Oncol 2000;76:40–4.

31. Narayansingh GV, Miller ID, Sharma M, et al. The prognostic significance of micrometastases in node-negative squamous cell carcinoma of the vulva. Br J Cancer 2005;92:222–4.

32. Tamussino KF, Bader AA, Lax SF, Aigner RM, Winter R. Groin recurrence after micrometastasis in a sentinel lymph node in a patient with vulvar cancer. Gynecol Oncol 2002;86:99–101.

33. O'Boyle JD, Coleman RL, Bernstein SG, et al. Intraoperative lymphatic mapping in cervix cancer patients undergoing radical hysterectomy: a pilot study. Gynecol Oncol 2000;79:238–43.

34. Barranger E, Coutant C, Cortez A, Uzan S, Darai E. Sentinel node biopsy is reliable in early-stage cervical cancer but not in locally advanced disease. Ann Oncol 2005;16:1237–42.

35. Dargent D, Enria R. Laparoscopic assessment of the sentinel lymph nodes in early cervical cancer. Technique–preliminary results and future developments. Crit Rev Oncol Hematol 2003;48:305–10.

36. Levenback C, Coleman RL, Burke TW, et al. Lymphatic mapping and sentinel node identification in patients with cervix cancer undergoing radical hysterectomy and pelvic lymphadenectomy. J Clin Oncol 2002;20:688–93.

37. Marnitz S, Kohler C, Bongardt S, et al. Topographic distribution of sentinel lymph nodes in patients with cervical cancer. Gynecol Oncol 2006; 103:35–44.

38. Frumovitz M, Coleman RL, Gayed IW, et al. Usefulness of preoperative lymphoscintigraphy in patients who undergo radical hysterectomy and pelvic lymphadenectomy for cervical cancer. Am J Obstet Gynecol 2006;194:1186–93; discussion 1193–5.

39. Niikura H, Okamura C, Akahira J, et al. Sentinel lymph node detection in early cervical cancer with combination ^{99m}Tc phytate and patent blue. Gynecol Oncol 2004;94: 528–32.

40. Angioli R, Palaia I, Cipriani C, et al. Role of sentinel lymph node biopsy procedure in cervical cancer: a critical point of view. Gynecol Oncol 2005;96:504–9.

41. Barranger E, Cortez A, Uzan S, Callard P, Darai E. Value of intraoperative imprint cytology of sentinel nodes in patients with cervical cancer. Gynecol Oncol 2004;94:175–80.

42. Burke TW, Levenback C, Tornos C, et al. Intraabdominal lymphatic mapping to direct selective pelvic and paraaortic lymphadenectomy in women with high-risk endometrial cancer: results of a pilot study. Gynecol Oncol 1996;62:169–73.

43. Coleman RL, Frumovitz M, Levenback CF. Current perspectives on lymphatic mapping in carcinomas of the uterine corpus and

cervix. J Natl Compr Canc Netw 2006; 4:471–8.

44. Echt ML, Finan MA, Hoffman MS, et al. Detection of sentinel lymph nodes with lymphazurin in cervical, uterine, and vulvar malignancies. South Med J 1999;92:204–8.

45. Holub Z, Jabor A, Kliment L. Comparison of two procedures for sentinel lymph node detection in patients with endometrial cancer: a pilot study. Eur J Gynaecol Oncol 2002;23:53–7.

46. Pelosi E, Arena V, Baudino B, et al Preliminary study of sentinel node identification with ^{99m}Tc colloid and blue dye in patients with endometrial cancer. Tumori 2002;88:S9–10.

47. Lelievre L, Camatte S, Le Frere-belda MA, et al. Sentinel lymph node biopsy in cervix and corpus uteri cancers. Int J Gynecol Cancer 2004;14:271–8.

48. Holub Z, Jabor A, Lukac J, Kliment L. Laparoscopic detection of sentinel lymph nodes using blue dye in women with cervical and endometrial cancer. Med Sci Monit 2004;10:CR587–91.

49. Gargiulo T, Giusti M, Bottero A, Leo L, Brokaj L, Armellino F, et al. Sentinel lymph node (SLN) laparoscopic assessment early stage in endometrial cancer. Minerva Ginecol 2003; 55:259–62.

50. Barranger E, Darai E. Relevance of the sentinel node procedure in endometrial cancer. Gynecol Oncol 2004;94:861–2; author reply 862–3.

51. Fersis N, Gruber I, Relakis K, et al. Sentinel node identification and intraoperative lymphatic mapping. First results of a pilot study in patients with endometrial cancer. Eur J Gynaecol Oncol 2004;25:339–42.

52. Maccauro M, Lucignani G, Aliberti G, et al. Sentinel lymph node detection following the hysteroscopic peritumoural injection of ^{99m}Tc-labelled albumin nanocolloid in endometrial cancer. Eur J Nucl Med Mol Imaging 2005;32:569–74.

53. Raspagliesi F, Ditto A, Kusamura S, et al. Hysteroscopic injection of tracers in sentinel node detection of endometrial cancer: a feasibility study. Am J Obstet Gynecol 2004;191:435–9.

54. Niikura H, Okamura C, Utsunomiya H, et al. Sentinel lymph node detection in patients with endometrial cancer. Gynecol Oncol 2004;92:669–74.

55. Plentl A, Friedman A. Lymphatic System of the Female Genitalia. Philadelphia: W.B. Saunders, 1971.

56. Creasman WT, Morrow CP, Bundy BN, et al. Surgical pathologic spread patterns of endometrial cancer. A Gynecologic Oncology Group study. Cancer 1987;60(8 Suppl):2035–41.

Index

Page references in *italics* refer to figures and Tables

Index

Printed and bound by CPI Group (UK) Ltd, Croydon, CR0 4YY

01/11/2024

01782641-0001